An atlas of nursing techniques

AN ATLAS OF
NURSING TECHNIQUES

Norma Greenler Dison, R.N., B.A.

Clinical Instructor, Medical-Surgical Nursing,
Department of Nursing, College of Saint Teresa,
Winona, Minnesota

SECOND EDITION

With 593 illustrations by Marita Bitans

5 4 6 7

The C. V. Mosby Company

SAINT LOUIS   1971

To cure sometimes, to relieve often, to comfort always.

—attributed to

EDWARD L. TRUDEAU

Preface

The basic purpose of this book, as in the first edition, is to provide an explanatory text and meaningful illustrations of techniques used in nursing. Many of the beliefs stated in the preface to the first edition have guided the thinking that has resulted in this revision.

The general format of the book is similar to that of the previous edition. Some content has been rearranged to enhance the meaningfulness of the presentation, and new material has been added. All text has been evaluated carefully and, when necessary, rewritten or expanded. All illustrations have been redrawn or developed by Marita Bitans, Medical Illustrator. The table of contents has been expanded to include a list of the major headings in each chapter. A glossary of terms including a pronunciation guide has been developed.

Content and illustrations new to this edition include surgical scrubs, closed method of gloving, the hand-E-vent II and Retec N-30 units used for assisted ventilation, the Teledyne oxygen detector, postural drainage, range of motion, use of intravenous and irrigation solutions packaged in plastic bags, the sump type of gastric tube, and the Laird colostomy irrigating tip.

Questions for discussion and exploration follow each chapter. Many of these are based on actual situations and are designed to stimulate thinking and further study and discussion. It is hoped that some of the questions will provoke additional questions. These questions can be answered by the application of knowledge, principles, and concepts, but they are intended to permit differences in approach. It is hoped that in discussion the climate will permit exploration of many factors that might influence each situation, not the least of which are the people involved and their reactions. This approach is time-consuming but results in creative learning. Students given independent responsibility for major parts of their learning should find these questions useful. No attempt has been made to include a listing of the many multimedia learning aids available from professional and allied sources. Selection of learning aids will be determined by the behavioral objectives established for a particular presentation or situation.

Throughout this revision I have been privileged to have the cooperation of many persons. With deep gratitude I acknowledge the assistance given me by Dr. H. Frederic Helmholz, Jr., Consultant in Physiology, The Mayo Clinic; Dr. A. D. Sessler, Consultant in Anesthesiology, The Mayo Clinic; Dr. Donald A. Wolochow, Department of Internal Medicine, Southern California Permanente Medical Group, San Diego, California; Mrs. Reneé Casperson, Registered Inhalation Therapist, The Mayo Clinic; Mrs. Mary Ann Sandersfeld, Radiologic Technologist, Department of Gastroenterology, The Mayo Clinic; Mrs. Eva Bennett, R.N., Department of Inservice Education, Saint Marys Hospital; the librarians at Saint Marys Hospital; and my good friend, Mrs. Jean Skar, Librarian, Rochester Methodist Hospital, who has been most helpful in locating sources of information and in providing encouragement. Others have also contributed to this book. Students, patients, colleagues in the Department of Nursing, College of Saint Teresa, Winona, Minnesota, members of the nursing staffs of Saint Marys Hospital and Rochester Methodist Hospital, Rochester, Minnesota, and physicians, therapists, and technicians of The Mayo Clinic, Rochester, Minnesota, have shared their knowledge and insight with me. Appreciation is extended to the manufacturers for their cooperation and for granting permission to illustrate their products. Special gratitude is given to Marita Bitans, Cleveland Metropolitan General Hospital, Cleveland, Ohio, who produced the illustrations for this edition. A special thank-you goes to those persons who commented on the previous edition after its publication.

Norma Greenler Dison

Contents

An atlas of nursing techniques

Chapter 1

Emergency action

The prevention, early recognition, and immediate treatment of emergencies are important nursing responsibilities. With adequate preparation, the nurse can do much to preserve function and save lives. Observation and assessment of the patient's condition are helpful in determining the nursing action indicated and in obtaining medical assistance before an acute emergency develops. The simple action of turning the patient's head to one side or otherwise positioning the lower jaw to remove the tongue from the airway may, if done when stertorous breathing or increased efforts to inhale are noted, prevent a respiratory emergency from developing. This is especially important when the patient is too exhausted or is unable to move.

Principles commonly used in nursing can be applied in emergency situations. For example, the principles of moving patients can be used to transfer victims of emergencies. Principles of providing support, understanding, and guidance to patients and relatives during the stress that accompanies illness can be applied in emergency situations also. However, the welfare of the patient is of primary importance during an acute emergency. When sufficient personnel are available or when the emergency is under control, relatives must be given explanations, guidance, and support. As the patient regains consciousness, he needs help to retain or regain his ability to function.

Cardiopulmonary resuscitation

Cardiopulmonary emergencies usually follow some form of accident or occur secondary to disease. A common example is myocardial infarction secondary to arteriosclerosis. Inadequate ventilation allowed to persist long enough to produce myocardial hypoxia may lead to cardiac arrest. This is seen in the early postoperative period or following generous doses of drugs, such as the opiates, that depress the central nervous system. In these instances, accidental death can be prevented simply by assisting the patient to maintain an adequate ventilatory exchange until he is able to do this spontaneously.

When resuscitation is successful and the victim survives, it is almost always due to the immediate action of the person discovering him. Therefore, hospitals should expend the necessary time and effort to train a so-called first line of defense. This means that all floor personnel, regardless of their position or education, should be trained to act promptly in such situations. This training should include lectures, demonstrations, and an opportunity to practice the techniques. Manikins designed for such practice are available. Artificial ventilation can be practiced on live persons; cardiac massage should be practiced only on a manikin.

All floor personnel should have a clear understanding of the sequential steps that must be carried out when confronted with a situation demanding either rescue breathing or cardiopulmonary resuscitation. The following steps are suggested as being helpful:

1. Appraise the victim's physical status and determine whether cardiopulmonary resuscitation is indicated or not.
2. If cardiopulmonary resuscitation is indicated, start ventilation and external cardiac massage promptly.
3. Call the resuscitation team or the attending physician or both for definitive treatment.

Determination of the physical status of the victim is concerned with observations of any spontaneous respiration, assessment of circulatory status, and assessment of possible central nervous system damage by observing the pupils of the eyes.

If the patient shows any attempt at spontaneous respiration, he should be assisted immediately with artificial ventilation. If the patient is still attempting to breathe, one should assume that some circulatory function still exists. Restoration of an adequate ventilatory volume may be the only measure necessary to overcome this situation.

The rescuer assesses circulatory status by palpating the carotid artery. When circulatory function is poor or nonexistent, it is important to place the palpating fingers directly on the artery. The rescuer approaches the common carotid artery from the front and slides three fingers between the side of the wall of the larynx and the sternocleidomastoid muscle, pulling this mus-

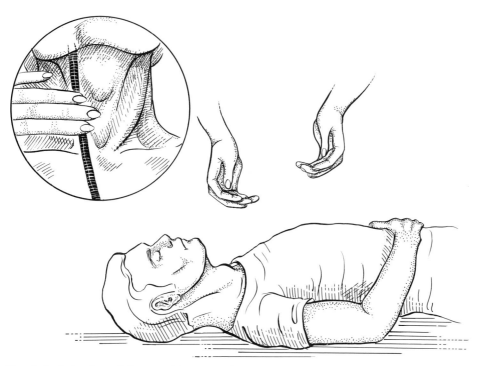

Fig. 1-1. Palpation of the carotid artery. The rescuer palpates the common carotid artery by approaching it from the front and sliding three fingers between the side of the wall of the larynx and the sternocleidomastoid muscle, pulling this muscle to the side.

cle to the side (Fig. 1-1). If no pulse is felt, it is assumed that cardiac arrest is present.

Hypoxic effects on the central nervous system can be assessed by examining the pupils of the eyes. When cerebral function ceases, the pupils begin dilating immediately and are dilated completely in about 45 seconds. After the pupils are maximally dilated, they will continue to contract when exposed to light for approximately 3 more minutes. After 4 minutes elapse, the pupils become centrally fixed, remain dilated, and fail to react when exposed to a bright light. An attempt to observe both pupils simultaneously should always be made. It is helpful for the physician to know if the pupils vary in size; this variance in size would indicate a cerebrovascular accident or central nervous system lesions. Deviation or movement of the pupils indicates very light stages of unconsciousness and means that resuscitation is quite likely to be successful.

It must be remembered that the aim of resuscitation is to **maintain life,** and it is indicated for the purpose of restoring the victim to a useful life when this is possible. Resuscitation is not indicated when cardiopulmonary arrest represents the termination of an irreversible disease process such as advanced malignancy. The decision not to follow resuscitation procedures should be made and communicated to appropriate personnel prior to the time when clinical death occurs.

Institution of resuscitation follows the ABC's of resuscitation, in that order. This means that one must restore first the air passages, *A*, second the breathing, *B*, and third the circulation, *C*.

Restoration of airway and rescue breathing

The obstruction of the upper airways is caused most commonly by the base of the tongue, which falls down and lies on the posterior wall of the pharynx (Fig. 1-2, *A*). In younger persons this type of obstruction can be relieved by hyperextending the neck (Fig. 1-2, *B*). In older persons or in those with neck injury, hyperextending the neck, as shown in Fig. 1-2, *B*, may not be

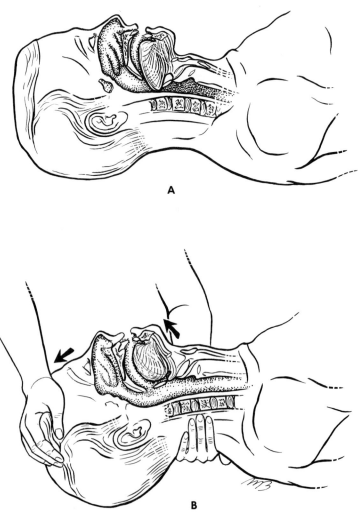

A

B

Fig. 1-2. Mouth-to-mouth breathing. **A,** Position of victim showing tongue pulled down by gravity and occluding the air passages. **B,** Hyperextension of the neck elevates the lower jaw, to which the tongue is attached, and opens the airway.

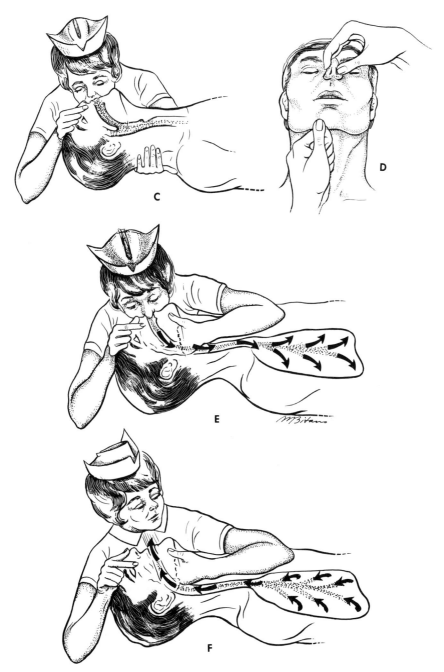

Fig. 1-2, cont'd. C, The nose is sealed with the thumb and index finger; then the rescuer seals his mouth over the mouth of the victim for inhalation. Note that the position of the victim's head is maintained in order to keep the airway open. **D,** An alternate method of maintaining the position of the victim's head. Pressure exerted on the forehead and the jaw is used to maintain hyperextension of the neck. The nostrils are occluded with the thumb and index finger of the hand that is exerting pressure on the forehead. **E,** The rescuer inflates the victim's lungs with her exhalation. **F,** The rescuer observes passive exhalation of the chest and listens for passive exhalation.

possible. Then the rescuer lifts the lower jaw forward into a jutting position until the lower teeth extend well in front of the upper teeth, positioning the head to remove the tongue from the airway.

The nasal pathways must be occluded with pressure by the thumb and index finger for effective mouth-to-mouth breathing, as shown in Fig. 1-2, *C* to *F*. The rescuer seals her mouth over

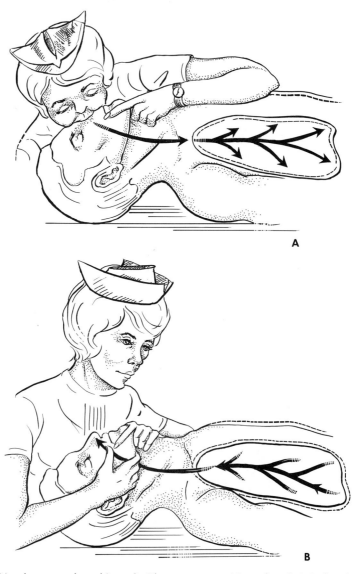

Fig. 1-3. Mouth-to-nose breathing. **A,** The rescuer positions the victim's head to remove the tongue from the airway, seals the victim's mouth with the index finger, and seals her mouth over the nose of the victim for the inhalation phase. **B,** The rescuer maintains the jaw in the jutting position while removing her mouth from the victim's nose and observing passive exhalation. The rescuer repeats these steps alternately until the victim is able to breathe spontaneously.

the mouth of the victim, and her exhalation is used to inflate the victim's lungs (Fig. 1-2, *E*). The rescuer seals the mouth with the index finger and seals her mouth over the victim's nose for the inhalation phase of mouth-to-nose breathing (Fig. 1-3, *A*) when this method is used. The jaw must be maintained in the jutting position while the rescuer removes her mouth from the victim's nose or mouth and observes passive exhalation (Fig. 1-3, *B*).

Before ventilation is started, the rescuer must remove loose dentures or foreign bodies that may cause obstruction. If stomach contents have been regurgitated into the pharynx, she must remove them also. Maintenance of open air passages may be difficult for the inexperienced. The insertion of an oropharyngeal airway (Fig. 1-4, *A*) may be helpful, but it must be remembered that this device alone is not designed to maintain open air passages. A nasopharyngeal airway inserted carefully through the widest part of the nose may be more helpful (Fig. 1-4, *B*).

Either mouth-to-mouth (Fig. 1-2) or mouth-to-nose rescue breathing (Fig. 1-3) may be employed for adequate ventilation. These techniques provide a form of intermittent positive pressure ventilation. Their effectiveness depends upon a leakproof system that does not allow air flow into spaces other than the lungs. The victim's exhalation is purely passive and is observed by watching deflation of the chest (Figs. 1-2, *F*, and 1-3, *B*). Tight clothing around the neck, which causes significant obstruction of the airway, or unnecessary weight on the thorax or abdomen may interfere with inflation of the lungs.

Although mouth-to-mouth and mouth-to-nose breathing are effective and have helped save lives, it must be understood that the exhaled air of the rescuer used to ventilate the victim is relatively poor in oxygen content and relatively rich in carbon dioxide. These factors are not in the best interest of the victim, and it is preferable to employ fresh air for each breath with a simple nonrebreathing technique. A self-inflating portable resuscitator is used for this purpose (Fig. 1-4).

Use of a portable resuscitator

When a portable resuscitator is used, the position of the patient is the same as that described for mouth-to-mouth and mouth-to-nose breathing (Fig. 1-4, *C* to *E*). This position may be improved somewhat by elevating the shoulders with a blanket folded to a thickness of about 2 inches.

If an oropharyngeal airway is used, the rescuer must position it properly (Fig. 1-4, *A*). It may stimulate gagging and can be occluded by the patient biting on it. These reflexes return as the patient regains consciousness. If a nasopharyngeal airway is available, it can be introduced by bending the tip of the nose upward and pushing the tube downward through the widest part

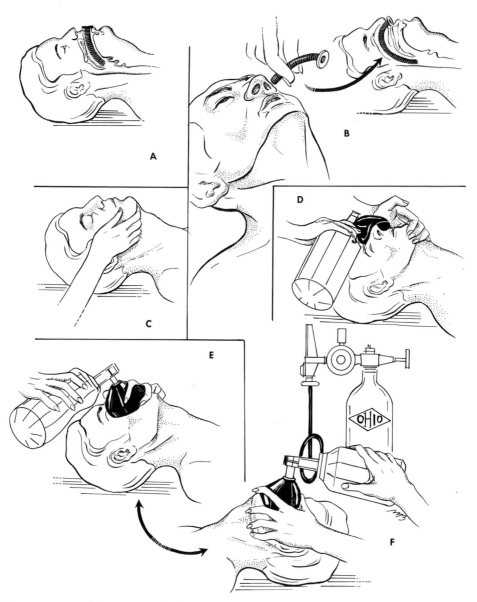

Fig. 1-4. Use of the Hope self-inflating portable resuscitator. **A,** An oropharyngeal airway in place. This helps to keep the tongue forward but does not guarantee an open airway. As the patient regains consciousness, this airway may stimulate gagging, vomiting, or biting. **B,** Placement of a nasopharyngeal airway. The nurse inserts the tube downward through the widest part of the nose. If any resistance is encountered, she should use the other nostril. This must be done gently in order to avoid damage to the vessels in the nose, resulting in hemorrhage as circulation is restored. **C,** The nurse places her fingertips on the angles of the jaw and pulls the lower jaw forward until the lower teeth extend over the upper teeth. **D,** The nurse maintains the position of the jaw with one hand while using the other hand to fit the narrowest part of the mask into the deepest depression at the bridge of the nose. **E,** The nurse brings the mask forward over the mouth, using care not to exert pressure on the eyes. She wraps her thumb and index finger around the mask to hold it firmly in place. **F,** The nurse uses the remaining fingers of the same hand to maintain the position of the jaw. With the other hand she compresses the bag to augment spontaneous inspiration and then releases it until exhalation is complete. All portable resuscitators should be connected to oxygen if it is available. (Courtesy Ohio Medical Products, Division of Air Reduction Co., Inc., Madison, Wis.)

of the nose (Fig. 1-4, *B*). If any resistance is encountered, the other nostril should be used. Forcible advancement of the airway is likely to damage blood vessels, resulting in nasal hemorrhage as the circulation is restored. As a guide, a soft latex tube, size 32 French, is used for the adult female, and size 34 French is used for the adult male.

The experienced person will probably find it convenient to position the head in the following manner. Place the tips of the index and middle fingers on the angle of the lower jaw and pull it forward until the lower teeth extend well over the upper teeth (Fig. 1-4, *C*). Move the fingers around the edge of the lower jaw. Be careful not to press on the soft tissues but yet maintain the position of the jaw. Fit the narrowest part of the mask into the deepest depression at the bridge of the nose (Fig. 1-4, *D*) and bring the mask forward over the mouth (Fig. 1-4, *E*). Wrap the thumb and index finger around the mask to hold it firmly in place, maintaining the position of the jaw with the remaining fingers of the same hand (Fig. 1-4, *F*). Use the other hand to compress the bag for inhalation. Then release the bag until passive exhalation occurs (Fig. 1-4, *F*). Squeezing the bag should coincide with any spontaneous efforts to inhale. If the bag is compressed rapidly and vigorously, air turbulence rather than entry of air into the lungs will occur.

If the chest does not rise and the bag does not empty when squeezed, an obstruction is present. Correction of the obstruction by removal of secretions, loosening the gown, and repositioning has been discussed previously. If the bag empties but the chest does not rise, air may be leaking between the mask and the face. This must be corrected by refitting the mask. Leakage that forces gases to flow over the eyes must not be allowed to persist because it may cause irreversible damage to vision. Continuous care must be exercised when a portable resuscitator is used so that the eyes are not damaged by exertion of pressure on them. It should always be assumed that the victim may be wearing contact lenses. These need not be removed if the mask is positioned properly.

Rescue breathing for infants and children

Rescue breathing is done for infants and children in a manner similar to that for adults. However, the volume of air used to inflate the lungs of infants will be less than that for an adult, the pressure needed to inflate the lungs of an infant will be greater than that for an adult. The volume of air needed for children can be determined best by observing the inflation of the chest.

If the stomach rises during inflation, the nurse should press the abdomen with her hand to remove the air. Regurgitation may result, and therefore the head should be turned to the side prior to putting pressure on the abdomen. If regurgitation occurs, the nurse must remove secretions before the patient is repositioned and rescue breathing is continued. There is usually no need for an oropharyngeal or nasopharyngeal airway.

Rescue breathing through a stoma

If the patient is to be ventilated through a stoma, the nurse should elevate his shoulders slightly and align his head with his body. She should not turn his head to either side, for doing so may change the shape of the stoma and occlude the airway. The airway is suctioned through the stoma (Chapter 4, pages 113 to 116). It is not necessary to remove obstructions above the stoma or to occlude the mouth and nose prior to administering ventilation through a stoma.

If the tracheostomy tube is fitted with an inflatable balloon, inflation of the balloon will seal the space between the tube and the wall of the trachea, increasing the effectiveness of ventilation. (See Chapter 4, pages 116 and 117 for the technique of inflating a cuffed tracheostomy tube.)

The patient with a permanent stoma may not be wearing a tube in it. If a tube is in place, the inner cannula should be removed. If a breathing machine fitted with adaptors for the tube is readily available, it should be connected to the outer cannula. As soon as air exchange is occurring freely, secretions must be aspirated from the airway. If a breathing machine is not available immediately, the nurse positions the mask of a portable resuscitator to adjust to the contour of the neck. A seal between the mask and the neck is obtained by removing the plug from the mask, if it is of an inflatable type, or by packing a damp cloth around the mask. If equipment is not available, mouth-to-stoma breathing is used. The rescuer takes a deep breath, seals her mouth around the stoma, and inflates the patient's lungs by exhalation.

If it is known that the patient has a permanent stoma that has healed, there should be no hesitation about removing the cannula from the trachea. This is done by breaking the chain or cutting the cloth tapes that hold the cannula in place. **Removal of the outer cannula from the trachea of a patient with a fresh, temporary stoma will result in occlusion of the stoma within a matter of minutes.**

Restoring cardiac function
External cardiac massage

External cardiac massage must begin soon after cardiac arrest occurs, because irreversible brain damage begins within 3 to 5 minutes. The patient with cardiac arrest loses consciousness suddenly, becomes cyanotic rapidly, ceases to breathe, and has no pulse. Cardiac massage is sometimes indicated when the heart is beating so faintly and rapidly that adequate circulation is not maintained.

The nurse should position the patient on a firm surface as described for mouth-to-mouth resuscitation. A board ½ inch thick and 2½ feet square, placed directly under his thorax, is ideal. If such a board is not readily available, a closet shelf or a serving tray turned upside down will provide a firm surface, or the patient may be placed on the floor.

If she is alone, the nurse should use mouth-to-mouth resuscitation to blow 3 or 4 deep breaths into the patient's lungs in order to oxygenate the blood before she begins external cardiac massage. Until a trained person is available to apply continuous rescue breathing, the nurse must interrupt cardiac massage every 30 seconds to blow 4 deep breaths into the lungs. This interruption reduces the effectiveness of cardiopulmonary resuscitation significantly. Another trained person should be called as quickly as possible.

The nurse positions herself at a right angle to the patient's chest, with the major portion of her body above the level of his chest. If the bed cannot be lowered or if a footstool is not available, she can reach this position by kneeling on the bed. The sternum is located by palpation (Fig. 1-5, A).

The right-handed nurse places the heel of her right hand on **the lower third of the body of the sternum.** She places the heel of her left hand on top of her right hand and at a right angle to it. The fingers of both hands should be straight or slightly hyperextended to prevent trauma to adjacent tissues (Fig. 1-5, B). Finger rings may produce trauma also.

The nurse applies enough pressure to depress the sternum 1½ to 2 inches and releases pressure (Fig. 1-5, C). Placement of her hands on the sternum should be maintained during the recoil period, simultaneously allowing the heart to fill with blood. The rhythm of alternately applying and then releasing pressure should occur at a regular rate of approximately 60 times per minute. If the technique is effective, the carotid or femoral pulse will become palpable. A blood pressure cuff placed on the upper arm should register 100 mm. of mercury with each compression. The nurse continues resuscitation until the physician relieves her of this responsibility.

If the physician is resuscitating the patient, he may ask the nurse to check his timing and the effectiveness of cardiac massage or to relieve him while he performs other tasks. The nurse should direct others to bring needed equipment and supplies to the bedside. A special cart equipped with supplies, solutions, and needed equipment should be maintained in a convenient location within the hospital area. Supplies needed immediately frequently include an electrocardiogram machine, an external defibrillator, and 1 ml. of aqueous epinephrine (Adrenalin) in a syringe that is fitted with an intracardiac needle, usually a No. 22 needle

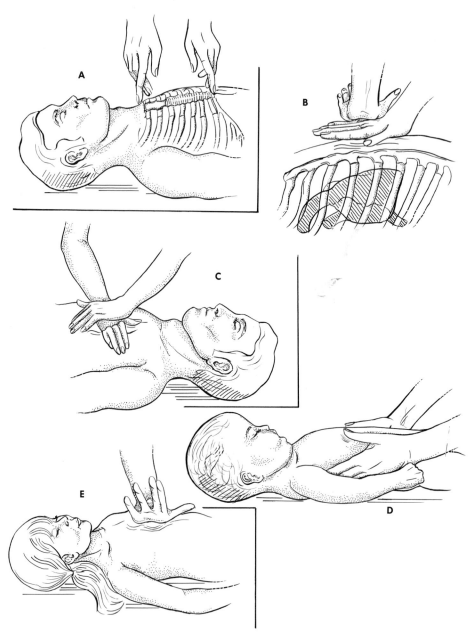

Fig. 1-5. External cardiac massage. **A,** The nurse locates the sternum by palpation. **B,** Back view of the nurse's hands. The right-handed nurse places the heel of her right hand on the lower third of the body of the sternum. She places the heel of her left hand on top of her right hand and at a right angle to it. The fingers are straight or slightly hyperextended to prevent trauma to the adjacent tissues. **C,** The nurse's hands are in position on the lower one third of the body of the sternum. She applies pressure alternately and releases it without removing the hands from the sternum. This conserves the resuscitator's energy and avoids any need to reposition the hands. **D,** The nurse may reach around the chest of a small infant and use her thumbs to depress the sternum. If preferred, she may use the index and middle fingers. **E,** The nurse can depress the sternum of an older child with the heel of one hand alone.

3½ inches long. Epinephrine stimulates the myocardium and the conduction tissue, electrocardiography monitors the heart, and defibrillation converts fibrillation to effective contraction of the heart. Injectable solutions of 10% calcium gluconate and sodium bicarbonate (approximately 1 mEq. of drug per milliliter of solution) should be readily available to combat electrolyte imbalance. Other drugs, solutions, and equipment needed are discussed by Jude and Elam.

Prior to using the defibrillator, the nurse applies sufficient electrode jelly to prevent skin damage and disconnects any electrical equipment attached to the patient. Contact with the patient must be avoided when the defibrillator is in use. If she is asked to hold the electrodes, the nurse must remember to touch **only the handles** of the electrodes.

External cardiac massage applied to children. Modification of the amount of pressure exerted on the sternum of the infant is achieved by using the index and middle fingers, or the thumbs only (Fig. 1-5, *D*). For the child 1 year old or older, pressure may be applied with the heel of one hand (Fig. 1-5, *E*).

Control of hemorrhage

The flow of blood to an area is limited by restricting activity, elevating the part, and applying direct pressure. If signs and symptoms of shock are present, the nurse should place the patient in a supine position with his legs elevated at approximately a 45° angle to the pelvis. The knees should be straight and the pelvis slightly higher than the chest. This is believed to be more useful than the traditional Trendelenburg position in aiding the supply of blood to the brain.

In addition, the nurse should supply the patient with increased concentrations of oxygen. Efforts to supply external warmth are no longer commonly practiced. Additional warmth increases metabolism and the need for oxygen.

The physician must be notified whenever evidence of shock is detected so that measures to correct the cause can be instituted. The action planned by the physician will depend upon the cause of the shock. The nurse should anticipate the need for replacement fluids, intravenous therapy, vasopressor drugs, ventilatory assistance, and equipment for monitoring central venous pressure, blood pressure, and urinary output.

Direct pressure

Applying a thick, sterile compress with manual pressure is a simple method of controlling most bleeding (Fig. 1-6, *A* and *B*). Pressure is exerted in such a way that the edges of the wound are brought together rather than forced apart. Sustained pressure can be achieved with a pressure dressing secured with bandage, tape, or elastic tape. An inflatable plastic splint or bandage can be used to apply uniform pressure to an extremity.

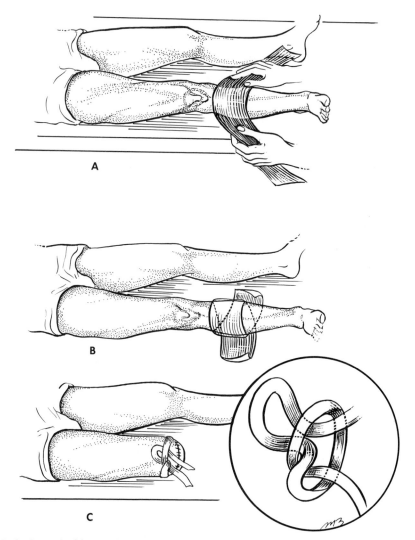

Fig. 1-6. Control of hemorrhage. **A,** The nurse applies pressure to the wound with bandage over a dressing on the wound. **B,** Preparation for securing the bandage with pressure. **C,** Application of a tourniquet proximal to the site of hemorrhage. A tourniquet is used with knowledge that the limb may have to be sacrificed. The surgeon may leave instructions for its use if hemorrhage occurs following amputation. The inset shows a method of applying a tourniquet that provides for easy removal.

Frequent inspection for signs of continued bleeding is necessary. A hematoma that forms beneath an elastic bandage may not be visible, but it will feel spongy when palpated.

Tourniquet   If a physician is available, a tourniquet should not be used without his order. In the absence of a physician, the nurse applies a tourniquet to save a life, recognizing that the limb may be sacrificed as a result. A tourniquet should always be attached to the

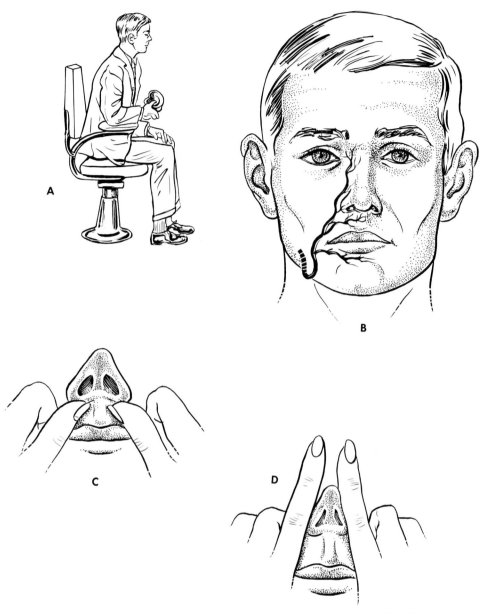

Fig. 1-7. Control of nosebleed. **A,** Sitting position reduces the flow of blood to the head and nose. The forward position of the head prevents swallowing of blood. **B,** Anatomic location of blood vessels supplying the nose. **C,** A common method of occluding the main artery supplying the nose. **D,** Alternate method of occluding the artery and its branches.

head of the bed so that it is readily available immediately following an amputation. It should be applied as closely as possible to the source of the bleeding (Fig. 1-6, *C*).

Tourniquets applied to occlude arterial circulation should be at least 2 inches wide to avoid damage to the underlying tissues, blood vessels, and nerves. After a tourniquet has been applied, it should be released only when medical assistance is available to control the hemorrhage and to restore blood volume. If a tourniquet is applied, the nurse should obtain medical assistance without delay. A tourniquet is rarely needed because bleeding can usually be controlled by other means.

Pressure points   Firm manual pressure on the main artery supplying the wound is used when direct pressure fails to control bleeding. This

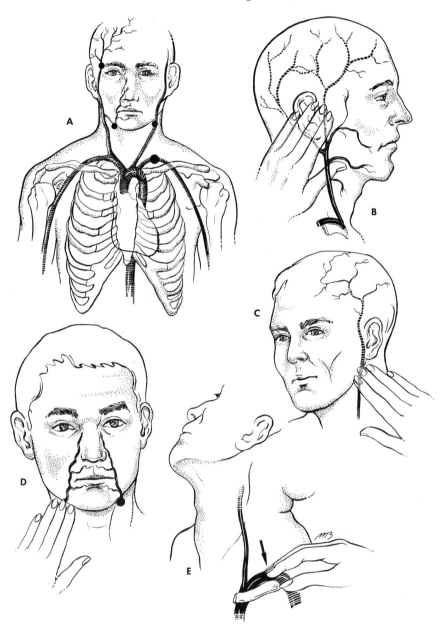

Fig. 1-8. Use of pressure points to control bleeding. **A,** Anatomic location of major blood vessels and pressure points. **B,** Pressure to stop scalp bleeding. **C,** Head and neck. **D,** Face. **E,** Chest wall and armpit.

method is particularly useful in the control of nosebleed (Fig. 1-7). Certain points commonly referred to as pressure points are used to control bleeding (Fig. 1-8). These same points can be used to obtain pulses.

Wound disruption   If a patient complains of a sensation of something giving way or leaking in the area of the wound, the nurse should inspect the wound for bleeding, dehiscence, or evisceration. If dehiscence is apparent, she should alleviate the tension on the wound by positioning the patient. The patient with an abdominal wound

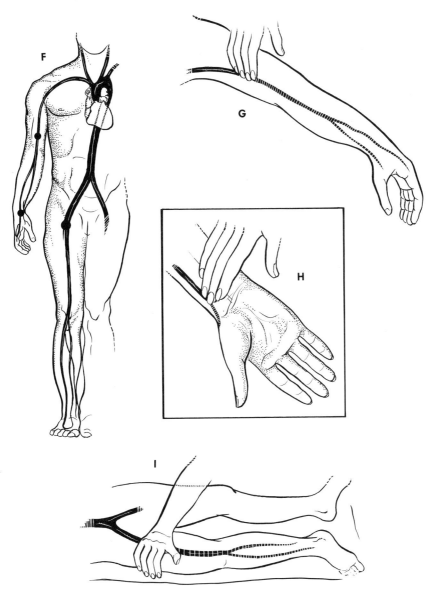

Fig. 1-8, cont'd. F, Anatomic location of blood vessels and pressure points. **G,** Pressure to stop bleeding of the upper arm. **H,** Wrist. **I,** Leg.

should lie supine with his knees flexed. The nurse should place a sterile dressing over the wound and apply pressure in an effort to prevent evisceration. A binder applied snugly is thought to be helpful. Evisceration is treated immediately by placing the patient in the supine position with the knees flexed and covering the protruding viscera with a sterile dressing moistened with sterile normal saline. The physician should be notified at once.

Eye injury   Immediate treatment is indicated whenever foreign material contacts the eye accidentally. Following contact with acid or alkali the eyes should be flushed with copious amounts of clean water. In an emergency, a person can flush the eye by holding his head over a drinking fountain, with the injured eye nearest the flow of water and the eyelids separated. Gently flowing water from a faucet or a clean container will suffice. The direction of flow should be from the inner angle of the eye to the outer angle (Chapter 11, pages 252 and 253).

To remove a foreign body from the eye, the nurse may need to evert the eyelid (Fig. 1-9), removing the foreign object with a cotton-tipped applicator that has been moistened with boric acid, normal saline, or sterile water. An applicator not much larger than the foreign object is preferred. Gentle swabbing or rotation of the applicator is used to remove the object. If the object is on the cornea or appears to be embedded, the nurse should bandage the eye and obtain medical treatment at once. Any evidence of hemorrhage or loss of vision should be evaluated by a physician.

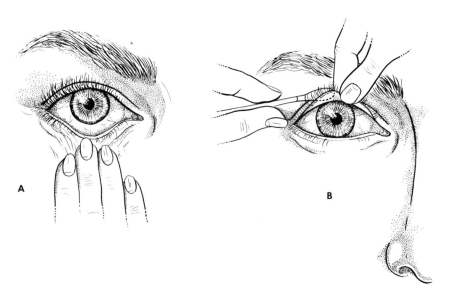

Fig. 1-9. Preserving sight. **A,** Traction on the tissues distal to the eye exposes the inner aspect of the lower eyelid. **B,** The upper eyelid being everted. The index finger may be used instead of a swab.

1. As you walk by a room you notice that a patient is snoring loudly and exerting effort to inhale. What may this indicate? What action should you take?
2. You are on your way to obtain some sterile supplies for a doctor who is waiting in his patient's room. Suddenly Mrs. X. runs into the hallway screaming, "He's dead!" List the actions you would take, the order in which you would carry them out, and the reasons for each action.
3. You see the relatives of Mr. X., who is being resuscitated, standing in the hallway near the door of his room, wringing their hands and crying. You are free to initiate supportive action. What can you say or do to help them and the other patients in the nursing unit?
4. When you are helping a postoperative patient to cough productively, he eviscerates. What must you do? In what order? Why?
5. A neighbor's child comes to you after being hit in the eye with a mud ball. What first aid can you initiate? On what basis will you decide whether he should be seen by a doctor?
6. You come upon an accident on your way home from vacation. One person has blood spurting from the popliteal area, another appears not to be breathing, and a third has blood on his forehead and an obvious fracture of the left arm. What will your actions be?
7. When you take a specimen to the laboratory, you learn that a technician has just gotten a chemical in her eye. She is holding her eye and saying, "I can't see!" What is the first thing you can do to help her? What is the rationale for your thinking?
8. List and discuss methods of preventing accidents in your hospital. In your home.
9. Mrs. Y. exhibits evidence of shock shortly after you have given her an injection of meperidine. What are the signs and symptoms of shock? What action must you take immediately?
10. If irreversible death occurs, what is your role in relation to the patient? The relatives? What are your feelings about death?

Selected references

Abramson, H., editor: Resuscitation of the newborn infant and related emergency procedures, ed. 2, St. Louis, 1966, The C. V. Mosby Co.

American Cancer Society: First aid for laryngectomees, New York, 1962, International Association of Laryngectomees.

American Heart Association: Instructor's manual in cardiopulmonary resuscitation, New York, 1965, American Heart Association.

American Nurses' Association: Emergency intervention by the nurse, Monograph 1, New York, 1962, American Nurses' Association.

American Red Cross: First aid, ed. 4, New York, 1957, Doubleday & Co., Inc.

Bergersen, B. S., and Krug, E. E.: Pharmacology in nursing, ed. 11, St. Louis, 1969, The C. V. Mosby Co.

Bordick, K. J.: Patterns of shock, New York, 1965, The Macmillan Co.

Cahill, D.: The nurse's role in closed-chest cardiac resuscitation, Amer. J. Nurs. 65:84-88, 1965.

Feldman, S., and Ellis, H.: Principles of resuscitation, Philadelphia, 1967, F. A. Davis Co.

Henderson, J.: Emergency medical guide, ed. 2, New York, 1969, McGraw-Hill Book Co.

Horgan, P.: The nurse's guide to rescue breathing, R.N. 60:35-45, 1960.

Jude, J. R., and Elam, J. O.: Fundamentals of cardiopulmonary resuscitation, Philadelphia, 1965, F. A. Davis Co.

Modell, W., editor: Drugs of choice, 1970-1971, St. Louis, 1970, The C. V. Mosby Co.

Nett, L., and Petty, T.: Acute respiratory failure, Amer. J. Nurs. 67:1847-1853, 1967.

Schneewind, J. H.: Medical and surgical emergencies, ed. 2, Chicago, 1968, Year Book Medical Publishers, Inc.

Simeone, F. A.: The nature of shock, Parts I and II, Amer. J. Nurs. **66:** 1287-1294, 1966.

Stephenson, H. E.: Cardiac arrest and resuscitation, ed. 3, St. Louis, 1969, The C. V. Mosby Co.

Vallari, R. M.: Mobile unit for cardiac arrest, Nurs. Outlook **64:**39, 1964.

von Morpurgo, D., and Gauder, P. J.: Coordinated action in cardiac arrest, Amer. J. Nurs. **62:**91-93, 1962.

White, J.: Closed chest cardiac massage, Amer. J. Nurs. **61:**57-59, 1961.

Zoll, P. M. and others: Use of external electric cardiac pacemaker in cardiac arrest, J.A.M.A. **159:**1428-1431, 1955.

Chapter 2

Safety

Principles that ensure patient safety are incorporated into all nursing procedures and many nursing activities. The simple act of placing the patient's bed in its lowest position and keeping the side rails raised prevents accidents and permits the patient to assist himself in changing his position or in getting out of bed. Any items that he may wish to use should be within easy reaching distance of the patient who is confined to bed. A means of summoning the nurse must be available at all times. The effectiveness of the system used to call for help is dependent upon the personnel, who should respond promptly. This provides needed assistance, prevents accidents, and increases the patient's feeling of security.

Certain techniques are designed to increase the patient's safety by lessening the risk of infection. A number of means are used to reduce the transmission of organisms. Others reduce contact with allergens, and some reduce the possibility of self-inflicted injury. Still other safety measures are discussed throughout the text.

Hand washing   The nurse washes her hands to remove bacteria and other contaminants that her hands are exposed to before and after caring for the patient, feeding him, handling food, preparing and administering medications, using bathroom facilities, and touching any part of the body or objects that may possibly be contaminated. This includes used linen and objects that have been in the patient's room or in contact with a contaminated area such as the floor.

An effective method of cleansing the hands is to wash them thoroughly with an approved cleansing agent. This may be soap

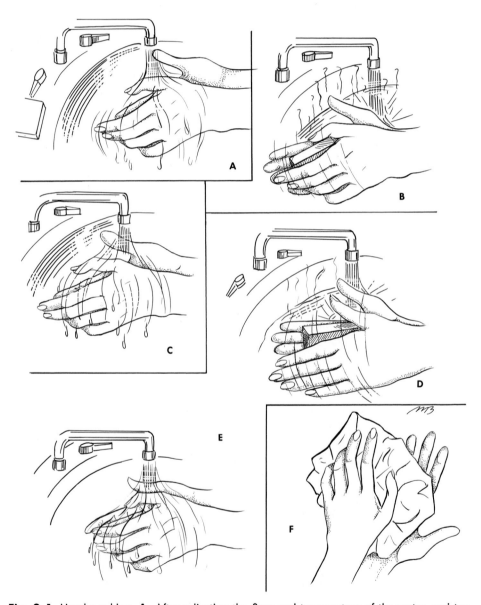

Fig. 2-1. Hand washing. **A,** After adjusting the flow and temperature of the water, moisten hands. **B,** Apply soap until a heavy lather covers the area to be cleansed, rubbing the hands against each other to produce friction. **C,** Rinse thoroughly. **D,** Apply more soap and repeat step B. **E,** Rinse well. **F,** Dry hands thoroughly. Use a paper towel to shut off flow of water, thus avoiding contamination from faucets.

or a germicidal compound in either liquid or solid form. The length of time required for effective hand washing depends upon the amount and kind of contamination, the amount of friction used, and the cleansing agent. Removal of bacteria appears to be directly related to the amount of friction used. Grossly contaminated hands should be washed thoroughly at least twice.

Prior to beginning hand washing, the nurse should remove her wristwatch, or move it well above her wrist, and should remove her rings. Initially, she should adjust the temperature and flow of the water to comfort, letting the water run throughout the technique. She should direct her hands downward throughout the washing and rinsing processes in order to prevent water from running back onto the hands after it has contacted the unwashed arms.

The nurse should wet the hand and wrist areas thoroughly and apply the cleansing agent in the amount needed to produce lather. If a solid soap is used, the nails may be pressed into it, forcing soap beneath them. Efforts to clean the areas beneath the nails and the spaces around the cuticle are important because these areas are known to harbor bacteria. The nurse should rub the hands together, interlacing the fingers to cleanse the spaces between them, then rub the back of each hand with the palm of the other. Each surface should be rubbed a minimum of ten times to ensure cleansing. Then the nurse should rinse the hands, still directed downward, thoroughly, and dry them with paper towels or a forced air blower. She should use a towel to turn off hand-operated faucets. This maintains the clean state of the hands (Fig. 2-1).

Skin preparation　　Preparation of the skin precedes surgical incision. The procedure is done in the patient's room, in a special area, or in the operating room. Little seems to be known of advantages to the patient of one method of preparation over another. Some procedure policies include surgical cleansing of the surface area prior to the patient's entrance into the operating suite. The method of hair removal may utilize depilatory agents or a razor. If a wet shave is given, the nurse should use liquid soap solution or another wetting agent to soften the hair and reduce friction. Powder reduces friction if a dry shave is given with a safety razor. It is thought that fewer epithelial cells are removed with the dry method. Avoiding irritation and abrasion of the skin is important because irritation and abrasion cause discomfort, alarm the patient, and injure the skin, a natural barrier to infection. To determine that a clean shave has been obtained, the nurse should view the dry surface against an adequate source of light.

The nature of the surgical procedure and the location and extent of the incision determine the area of the skin to be pre-

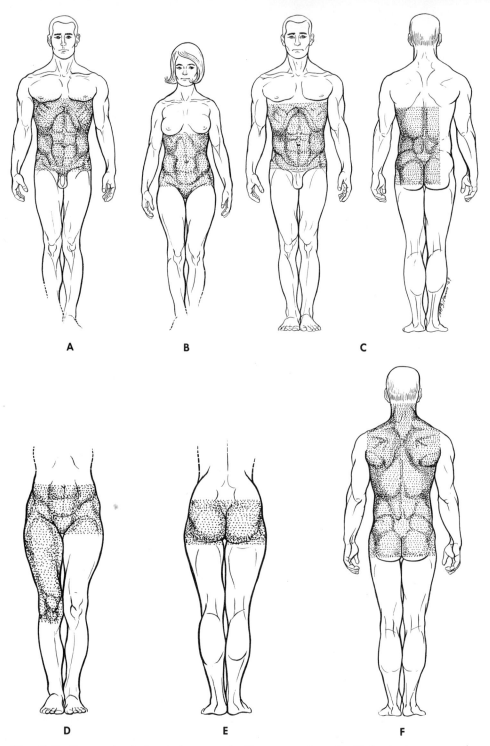

Fig. 2-2. Commonly designated areas of skin preparation. **A,** Abdominal surgery: the nipple line, symphysis pubis, and lateral aspects of the body serve as demarcation lines. **B,** Complete abdominal preparation (abdominoperineal preparation): abdomen and pelvic and perineal areas are prepared. **C,** Nephrectomy: abdominal area and three fourths of the back on the designated side are prepared. **D,** Inguinal hernia: lower abdomen plus anterior and lateral aspects of thigh are prepared. Preparation extends below the knee when fascial repair is planned. **E,** Rectal surgery: buttocks, anal area, and perineum are prepared. **F,** Neurosurgery and orthopedic surgery of the back: the entire back is prepared. Outermost borders of the area extend to top of scapula, lateral aspects of trunk, and distal portion of buttocks. If a bone graft is planned, the entire leg will be prepared to the ankle.

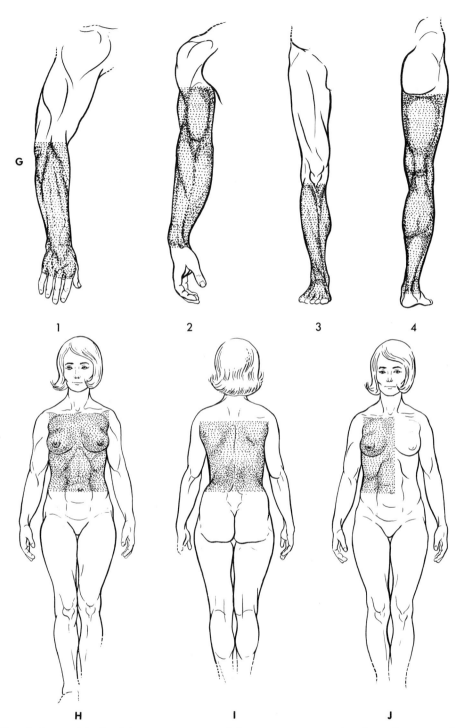

Fig. 2-2, cont'd. G, Other areas prepared for neurosurgery and orthopedic surgery include: **1,** lower arm and hand; **2,** arm; **3,** lower leg and foot; and **4,** entire leg. **H** and **I,** Chest surgery: the anterior area is demarcated by clavicle and umbilicus; the posterior area extends to upper border of scapula; the axilla is usually included. **J,** Unilateral mastectomy: clavicle, umbilicus, and opposite breast serve as demarcation lines; the axilla and the inner aspect of the upper arm are included.

Continued.

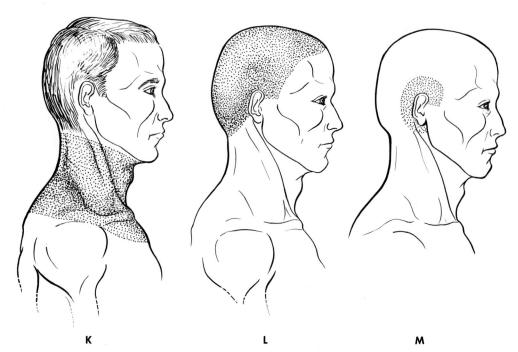

K   L   M

Fig. 2-2, cont'd. K, Neck: male patient may be permitted to shave the designated area; a female patient is not usually shaved. **L,** Head: written permission should be obtained from the patient prior to this preparation. **M,** Ear: the area extends 1 to 1½ inches behind, above, and below the external ear; male patients are asked to shave the beard in front of the ear.

pared. This area will be considerably larger than the predicted incision. Commonly designated areas of skin preparation should never supersede the order of the physician, who may specify a somewhat different area (Fig. 2-2).

It is wise to obtain a specific order from the physician as well as the written permission of the patient if certain areas are to be freed of hair: the face or neck of the female patient, the eyebrows, the head. If the head must be shaved, removed hair should be saved until the patient has recovered and indicates that it may be destroyed. Sometimes, women wish to fashion this hair into a hairpiece. In the event of the patient's death, it may be possible for a mortician to simulate a natural appearance if he is furnished with the hair that has been removed.

The nurse who prepares the skin for surgery should provide privacy for the patient, should use this opportunity to explain what she plans to do and why such preparation is necessary, and should reassure and encourage the patient.

Surgical scrub   The surgical scrub renders the hands and arms as free of contaminants as is possible with mechanical and chemical means (Fig. 2-3). The effectiveness of scrubbing is dependent upon mechanical action, which helps remove organisms from the ducts of the sebaceous glands in which they grow. As yet no means of rendering the skin sterile is available. The effectiveness of scrubbing also depends upon the chemical agent used. The system used should be chosen to fit the surgical procedure planned. An agent that acts slowly but over a long period of time is preferred when long procedures are planned. A rapid-acting agent is preferred for shorter procedures.

The scrub system used varies with institutional policy and individual preferences. Some prefer a scrub timed by the clock; others use a counted-stroke method. The time of the scrub or the number of strokes used varies also. This is affected by the cleansing agent used, the length of time between scrubs, the amount of contamination present, and the use of a preliminary wash or scrub or both. Differences of opinion exist concerning whether the scrub should extend to or above the elbow, whether a chemical rinse should follow the scrub, and what solution or solutions should be used for terminal rinsing. New systems of scrubbing are being investigated. If the system used is uniform, microbial studies can be obtained and used to determine when changes are indicated.

Preparation for scrubbing

The nurse begins the surgical scrub after she is dressed appropriately for the operating room. This means that she is wearing a clean surgical dress, conductive footwear, a cap that covers her hair completely, and a mask that covers her mouth and nose. If, during the scrub technique, any part of the hands or forearms touches the sink, faucet, or an unsterile object or surface, the nurse must begin the scrub again. For all the described scrubs, the nurse holds her hands and arms upward so that these parts are above the level of the elbow. With the hands and arms held upward, water used in scrubbing will drip from the elbow. Washing, scrubbing, and rinsing activities proceed from the fingertips toward the elbow. Prior to beginning to scrub, the temperature and rate of flow of the water are adjusted to the comfort of the practitioner. Water is left running throughout the scrub. Several methods of scrubbing are described. Variations from these will occur, depending upon where the nurse is employed.

Methods of scrubbing

Routine scrub (long scrub). Using the *timed method,* the nurse wets the hands and arms thoroughly and applies the cleansing agent. To remove surface contamination, she washes from the fingertips to the elbow, taking about 1 minute. Then she rinses the hands and arms, again proceeding from the fingertips to the elbow, and applies more cleansing agent. A sterile brush or sponge adds gentle friction. Scrubbing proceeds in short

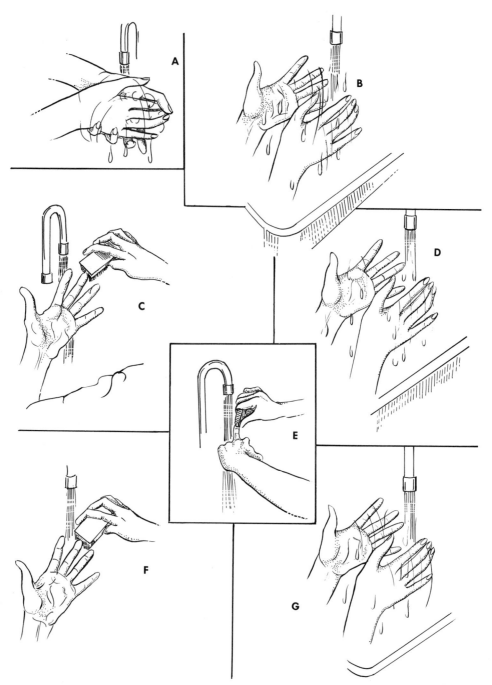

Fig. 2-3. The surgical scrub. **A,** Wet the hands and arms thoroughly, apply the cleansing agent, and wash the arms and hands. **B,** Rinse the hands and arms. **C,** Use a sterile brush or sponge to add gentle friction. **D,** Use additional water as needed to increase the lather. **E,** Clean the nails with a sterile file or orangewood stick. **F,** Apply more cleansing agent and use another sterile brush to scrub all surfaces of the hands and forearms. **G,** Rinse the hands and arms thoroughly.

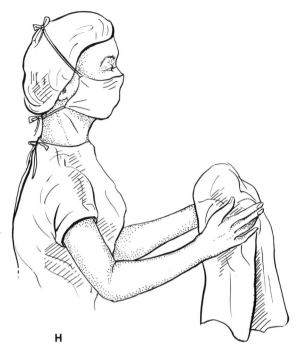

H

Fig. 2-3, cont'd. H, Blot the hands and arms dry with a sterile towel after the scrub is completed.

or circular strokes until the entire area is covered, about 4 minutes. The nurse adds water as needed to increase the lather. If soap is used, she may add additional soap for the same purpose. Next, she discards the brush and cleans the nails with a sterile file or orangewood stick. When this is discarded, she rinses the hands and arms thoroughly. She applies more cleansing agent and uses another sterile brush to scrub all surfaces of the hands and forearms for 4 more minutes. She rinses again and uses a sterile towel to blot the hands and arms until they are dry.

The *counted stroke method* differs from the timed method in that the parts of the hands and arms are scrubbed with a specified number of strokes. The nurse begins the scrub with initial washing and rinsing. A suggestion for the first scrubbing is as follows: 20 strokes to the nails, 10 strokes to the surfaces of the fingers and nails, and 6 strokes to all surfaces of the arms. The nurse does a second scrubbing with another sterile brush after she rinses and cleans the nails. She applies counted strokes during the second scrub as follows: 10 strokes to the nails, 6 strokes to the surfaces of the fingers and hands, and 3 strokes to each surface of the arms.

Short surgical scrub. The nurse uses the short surgical scrub between cases when contamination has not occurred, and she keeps the gown and gloves on until this scrub is begun.

Following the *timed method,* after the nurse removes the gown and gloves, she wets her hands and forearms thoroughly, applies the cleansing agent, and scrubs the areas with a sterile brush for 3 minutes. She discards the brush, rinses the hands and arms thoroughly, and dries them with a sterile towel.

Using the *counted stroke method,* after wetting the hands and arms, the nurse applies the cleansing agent, cleans the nails, and uses a sterile brush to stroke the nails 20 times, the surfaces of the fingers including the nails 10 times, and the surfaces of the arms 6 times. After rinsing, she dries the hands and arms with a sterile towel. The primary difference between the *long counted stroke method* and the *short counted stroke method* is that for the latter the scrub is considered complete after the initial scrubbing.

pHisoHex wash, surgical wash, and surgical scrub. The pHisoHex wash, surgical wash, and surgical scrub are used widely. pHisoHex is said to leave a minimal number of bacteria on the skin with a shorter scrub than when ordinary soap is used. In addition, it leaves a film on the skin that helps keep resident bacteria to a minimum. The surgical wash is useful for those whose skin is irritated by the trauma of scrubbing with a brush. When pHisoHex is used, small amounts of water are added as needed to produce more suds. Adding more pHisoHex is neither necessary nor recommended.

Drying hands and arms with a sterile towel. The nurse uses a sterile towel to dry her hands and forearms following the surgical scrub. She grasps the towel by one corner and raises it up to unfold it. The towel must not come in contact with anything that is unsterile. This means that the nurse will step into a space away from any objects and will hold the towel well away from her body while drying her hands and arms. She holds the towel in one hand and uses it to blot the surfaces of the fingers, hands, and arms until they are dry. She then moves the dry hand to the opposite end of the towel to hold it while drying the other hand. During this process, she manipulates the towel in order to ensure a dry surface. After drying the hands and arms, the nurse is ready to put on a sterile gown (Fig. 2-3, *H*).

Putting on a sterile gown   The method for putting on a sterile gown differs from the method illustrated for putting on an isolation gown. The sterile gown is folded in a manner that permits the hands to touch only the inside of the gown. The nurse grasps the gown from the inside, holds it up and away from unsterile areas to be unfolded, and slips her hands into the sleeves. The circulating nurse may touch the inside of the outer edges of the back of the gown to adjust it and also to tie it.

pHisoHex wash, surgical wash, and surgical scrub°

Preliminary wash (precedes surgical wash and surgical scrub)

1. Wet hands and forearms.
2. Apply about 2 ml. of pHisoHex.
3. Wash (without brush) for 30 seconds, adding small amounts of water. Avoid washing off lather.
4. Clean under nails (keep nails short and clean).
5. Rinse.

Surgical wash

1. Apply 2 to 4 ml. of pHisoHex.
2. Wash (without brush), as follows, while frequently adding small amounts of water.

Frequency of pHisoHex wash	Wash for	Benzalkonium (Zephiran) rinse
Routinely (twice daily or more often)	2 minutes	Unnecessary
Once daily	4 minutes	Optional
Infrequently	6 to 8 minutes	Recommended

3. Rinse.
4. Terminal rinse with benzalkonium solution 1:750. Do not rinse with alcohol alone.

Surgical scrub

1. Apply 2 to 4 ml. of pHisoHex.
2. Scrub (with brush), as follows, while frequently adding small amounts of water.

Frequency of pHisoHex scrub	Timed scrub	Counted stroke "anatomic" scrub (number of strokes lengthwise of brush for every area)		Benzalkonium (Zephiran) rinse
		Skin	Nails	
Routinely (twice daily or more often)	2 minutes	9	15	Unnecessary
Once daily	4 minutes	15	25	Optional
Infrequently	6 to 8 minutes	30	50	Recommended

3. Rinse.
4. Terminal rinse with benzalkonium solution 1:750.

°*Courtesy Winthrop Laboratories, New York, N. Y.*

Methods of gloving

Two methods of gloving may be used. The open method is also used when gloving is required for a technique not requiring the use of a gown, such as for catheterization.

Open method

After the package is opened (Fig. 2-4), the nurse grasps the glove for the right hand by the turned-down cuff with the left hand (Fig. 2-5, *A*) and slips the right hand into the glove. She places the right hand, now gloved, beneath the cuff of the left glove (Fig. 2-5, *B*) so that she may place the left hand in the glove. She places the right hand beneath the cuff of the left glove to pull it over the cuff of the gown (Fig. 2-5, *C*). After she pulls the cuff of the right glove similarly over the cuff of the gown (Fig. 2-5, *D*), she can adjust the fingers of the gloves. It is important to observe the position of the thumbs when pulling the gloves over the gown if contamination is to be avoided.

Closed method

The nurse slips the hands only partially through the sleeves of the gown so that they will remain covered by the sterile gown (Fig. 2-6, *A*). She grasps the inside seam of the end of the left sleeve and uses it to pick up the left glove (Fig. 2-6, *B*). She

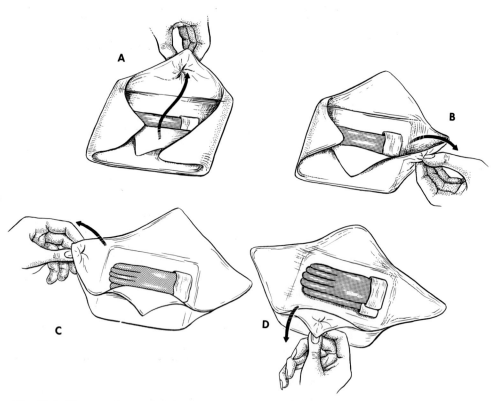

Fig. 2-4. Unwrapping sterile gloves. **A,** Unseal the package, fold the upper corner back, and open it away from the package. **B,** Reach the hand around the sterile field to unfold the next part of the wrapper by grasping the outside of the wrapper. **C,** Retract the next fold similarly. **D,** Expose the contents of the package.

places the left glove, palm down, on the right forearm of the gown (Fig. 2-6, *C*). Next, she pulls the glove, still held by the inside seam of the gown, on over the left hand (Fig. 2-6, *D*). She then uses the gloved hand to pick up the other glove, fitting it in a similar manner.

Isolation   If transmission of organisms to or from a patient constitutes a hazard to health, isolation is practiced. If this is done to prevent transmission of organisms from the patient to others, it is commonly said that isolation or isolation precautions are in effect. When transmission of organisms to the patient is to be avoided, a modified type of isolation is used. This may be referred to as reverse or protective isolation precautions, for the basic concept involved concerns transmission of organisms from other people to the patient. It should not be confused with reverse isolation in its more absolute form.*

*Seidler, F. M.: Adapting procedures for reverse isolation, Amer. J. Nurs. **65**:108-111, 1965.

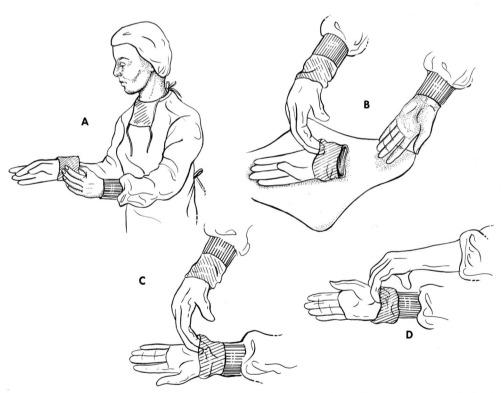

Fig. 2-5. Putting on sterile gloves by the open method. **A,** After washing and drying her hands, the nurse slips her right hand inside the right glove. She must take care to prevent contamination of the exterior part of the glove. **B,** She places her gloved hand beneath the cuff of the left glove to put it on. **C,** She places the gloved right hand beneath the cuff of the left glove to unfold it and pull it over the cuff of the gown. **D,** She pulls the cuff of the right glove similarly over the cuff of the gown.

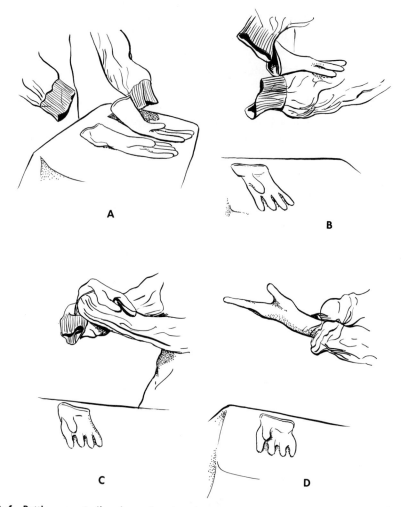

Fig. 2-6. Putting on sterile gloves by the closed method. **A,** The nurse does not slip her hands completely through the sleeves of the gown so they remain covered by the sterile gown. **B,** She grasps the inside seam of the end of the sleeve and uses it to pick up the left glove. **C,** She places the left glove, palm down, on the left forearm of the gown. **D,** She pulls the glove, still held by the inside seam of the gown, on over the left hand.

The exact procedure followed will vary with the physical facilities, the materials used, and the nature of the infection. The patient must be in an area or room equipped with facilities for hand washing and disposal of waste because the effective practice of isolation precautions depends upon correct application of principles derived from a knowledge of medical asepsis.

The purpose of isolation precautions must be understood if principles drawn from microbiology are to be applied correctly. Therefore, an understanding of what is to be considered clean or contaminated is essential. The source of contaminating organisms and mode of transfer will influence the techniques used.

For the purpose of reducing transmission of pathogens, sterilization of equipment with steam under pressure, in a gas sterilizer, or with chemicals is useful. Due to damage that ensues if these methods are applied to certain materials, a less than perfect method of frictional cleansing or airing, preferably in sunlight, may be necessary. Choice of method and cleansing agents differ with the established policies of institutions.

The use of disposable equipment, when practical, is recommended and is particularly important when organisms causing certain diseases such as infectious hepatitis are present. It is possible to obtain disposable items such as gowns, gloves, syringes, and dishes at relatively low cost. Many of these items are manufactured from plastic and have the added advantage of acting as a barrier to moisture. This quality helps reduce considerably the transmission of organisms. Lining waste containers with a bag made of such material or placing soiled linen in a similar bag should increase the safety with which waste and linen can be removed from the room. The bag can be sealed by folding the top and securing it with a rubber band or a cord. When the contaminated bag is removed from the room, it is placed within a clean bag held by an assistant who stands near the entrance to the isolation area. The receptacle for isolation linen should be plainly marked to warn laundry personnel that special precautions are in order.

Certain aspects of medical asepsis used when isolation is in effect are routinely incorporated into daily nursing practice. Hand washing (Fig. 2-1), for instance, is essential following known or possible contact with contaminants.

Use of gown   The nurse can protect her clothing by avoiding direct contact with contaminated areas or by wearing a gown. For example, if isolation is used to prevent transfer of organisms from a well-dressed wound, it may be permissible for the nurse to take an oral temperature without gowning if she is certain that she can avoid physical contact with the patient, furniture, or linen.

Gowns are available in various styles and materials, each with some advantages. They may be made of paper, plastic, or cloth. Design determines whether the gown has an open, semiclosed, or closed back. Fig. 2-7 illustrates the single use of a disposable gown. The gown shown is manufactured by the E. C. Ricter Company, Rochester, Minnesota, and features complete covering of the back, easy removal, and polyethylene construction. It is impervious to moisture and is considered disposable.

Some hospitals make repeated use of the same gown. This presumes that every person who uses the gown will have faultless technique. Cloth gowns are usually used. The technique of gowning in these circumstances is shown in Fig. 2-8.

*Use of mask and
hair covering*

If transmission of organisms to or from the nasopharynx and hair is to be avoided, a mask and a hair covering are worn. Both are applied prior to gowning. The mask should cover the mouth and nose, and all hair should be tucked under the cap. Method of removal depends upon their design.

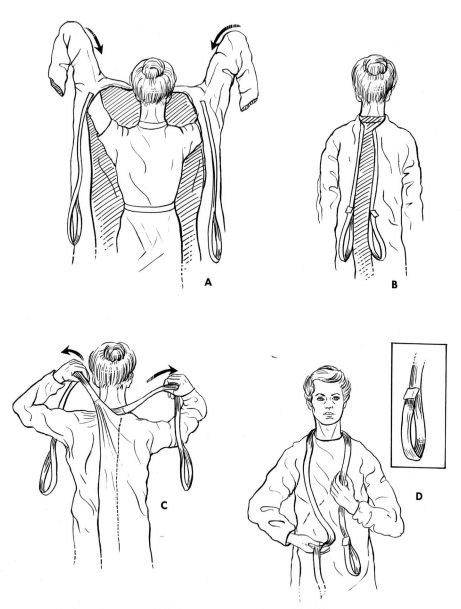

Fig. 2-7. Single use of a disposable protective gown. **A** to **F**, Gowning procedure. **A,** Open the gown and put it on with the opening in the back. **B,** View of gown before it is tied. **C,** Bring the tie from the right side over the left shoulder and the left tie over the right shoulder. **D,** Ends of the ties may be unfastened. Ends are taped onto the tie to prevent it from touching the floor prior to this step.

Dust-free environment Preparation and maintenance of a dust-free environment are essential to the control of certain allergenic responses. In addition, this environment serves to control transmission of organisms that dust transports.

Ideally, the room is emptied and scrubbed thoroughly to remove all traces of dust. All parts of the bed are scrubbed with soap and water, but the bed is not removed from the room.

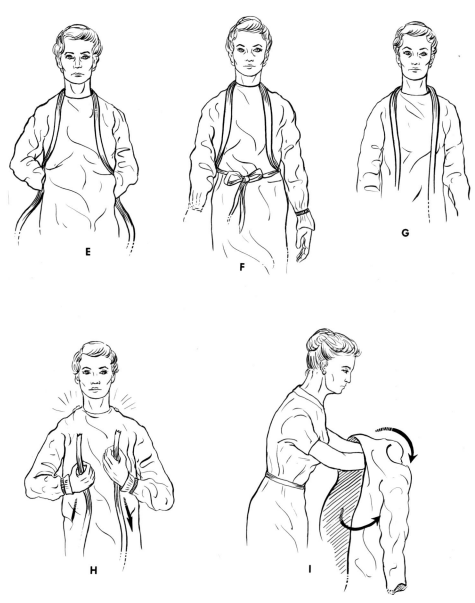

Fig. 2-7, cont'd. E, Ties are brought under the arms and cross in the back. **F,** Ties are adjusted in front until comfortable and are tied. **G to I,** Removing the gown. **G,** To remove the gown, untie the ties and bring them to the front. **H,** Break ties from the shoulders by exerting a firm pull on them. **I,** Remove gown by folding the inside over the outside. This avoids self-contamination. (Courtesy E. C. Ricter Co., Rochester, Minn.)

The allergies of the patient will determine the exact precautions used. Permissibility of oiling or waxing the floor must be evaluated in light of known allergy history and the ingredients of the product used. Flaxseed is one ingredient found in these products to which allergic reaction may occur. The pillows, mattress,

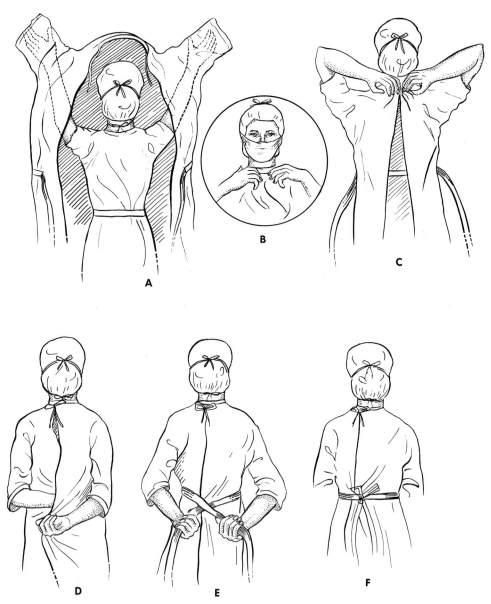

Fig. 2-8. Reuse of gowns. **A** to **F**, Technique of putting on the gown. **A,** Grasp the gown inside the back opening and slip hands into the sleeves. **B,** Adjust the neckband so that it fits comfortably and rather snugly. **C,** Secure the gown at the neck by tying it. **D,** Bring the left side of the gown across the back and the right side of the gown over the left. **E,** Bring ties to the back and cross them. **F,** Tie the gown in the back.

and box springs are enclosed in a dustproof cover, and the closures are sealed with adhesive tape. The need to do so when these items are said to be dustproof is determined by the allergist. His decision is based on experience and on knowledge of the porosity of such materials.

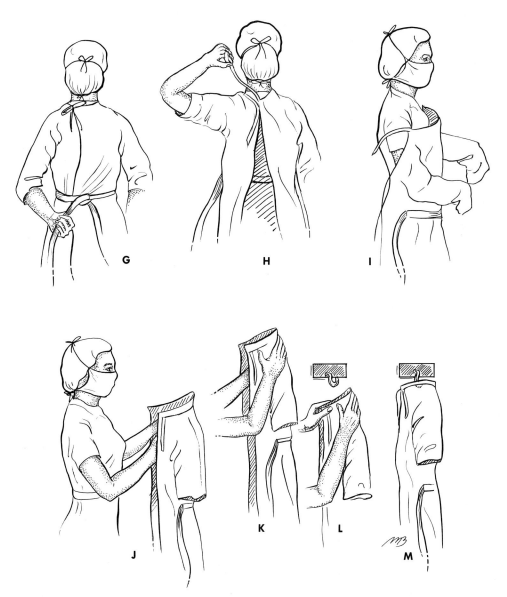

Fig. 2-8, cont'd. G to **M,** Technique of removing the gown preparatory to its reuse. **G,** Untie the gown at the waist. **H,** Untie the gown at the neck. Hands are washed prior to this step. **I,** Slip hands out of the gown, using care to prevent them from contamination by the outside surfaces of the gown. **J,** Grasp shoulder seams on the inside of the gown. **K,** Fold gown lengthwise with uncontaminated surfaces to the inside. Hands should not touch the gown below the neckline. **L,** Fold the gown at shoulder seams by grasping the neckline. **M,** Hang the gown by placing shoulder seams over the hook. The open back should be placed to facilitate putting the gown on when it is reused.

Linen for the bed must be freshly laundered and changed frequently. Choice of blankets necessarily eliminates those that have not been laundered, are fuzzy, or contain down. Wool blankets are preferred and are tolerated well.

Air conditioning and various types of filters that prevent entrance of dust or pollen are used appropriately. Hot air ducts are treated with a filter or are sealed. Filters should filter well and should be constructed in such a way that they may be cleansed thoroughly. Certain reusable filters retain particles of dust even after thorough washing, and some disposable filters are inadequate. Windows and doors should be kept closed.

Control of allergens, including dust, is further reinforced by storing clothing, stuffed articles such as toys, and fur materials outside the dust-free area. If curtains and drapes are used, they must be washed frequently.

Following initial preparation, this environment is maintained with a thorough cleaning each week and daily dusting of the furniture and the floor with a damp cloth or mop. If possible, the patient should move to another area during the cleaning, and the room should be sealed for an hour after it has been cleaned. If the patient must remain in the room during the cleaning, he should be furnished with a mask. Cloth masks should be of double thickness and should be moistened to increase filtering power. Disposable surgical masks that filter efficiently when worn dry are available. Moistening these masks increases discomfort, for the material becomes flimsy and is drawn into the nostril or mouth with inhalation, obstructing respiration.

Prevention of injury In special circumstances a decreased level of consciousness, mental confusion, or physical disability may predispose a patient to self-inflicted injury. The method of choice for preventing such misfortune should be evaluated for each such situation. The nurse should not restrain a patient forcibly without a physician's order or unless it is absolutely necessary.

The nurse should explain the purpose of any restraining device to the patient and his family. Adequate help during application must be available if injury to a highly active patient is to be avoided. The device itself must be applied correctly, for a carelessly applied restraint can be more dangerous than no restraint. For example, the nurse should not restrain one side of the patient's body only or fasten his hands to the head of the bed. It is safer to restrain opposite extremities, thus preventing potentially tragic activity. If inflexible materials are incorporated into the restraining device, the nurse should protect the underlying tissues with sufficient padding. For instance, padding is used beneath a leather cuff to prevent skin damage. Methods of securing the selected device vary. Commonly, ties, buckles, or locks are self-contained in the device.

Periodic removal of these devices is essential to prevent tissue injury. The skin should be cleansed, powdered, and observed for signs of irritation, and extremities should be exercised. Normal range of motion exercises are discussed in Chapter 3.

Improvised restraints

Modified clove-hitch restraint. Often the patient simply needs to be helped or reminded to restrain himself. A convenient method of reminding the patient that he is not to touch a particular wound is to apply a modified clove-hitch type of restraint. Its use in preventing self-inflicted injury following eye surgery may be combined with local application of a metal or other type of protective eye shield. Two-inch wide roller bandage may be used to form the modified clove hitch (Fig. 2-9).

Clove-hitch restraint. The nurse can fold a triangular bandage diagonally and apply it as a clove-hitch restraint. She can secure it by tying the free ends to the bed frame in a manner that allots a range of permissible movement. A distance of 12 inches or less is often desirable (Fig. 2-10).

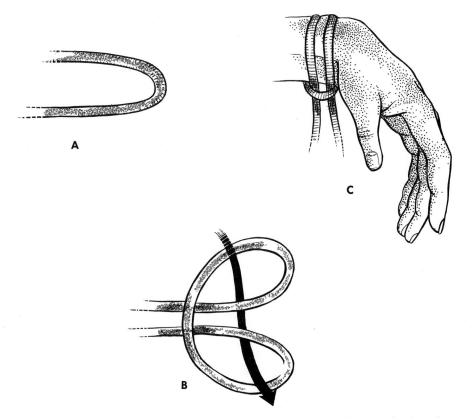

Fig. 2-9. Modified clove-hitch restraint. **A,** Form a loop. **B,** Fold the loop backward over itself. Enlarge as necessary to place the patient's arm through hitch as shown by arrow. **C,** Tighten the hitch to restrain the extremity.

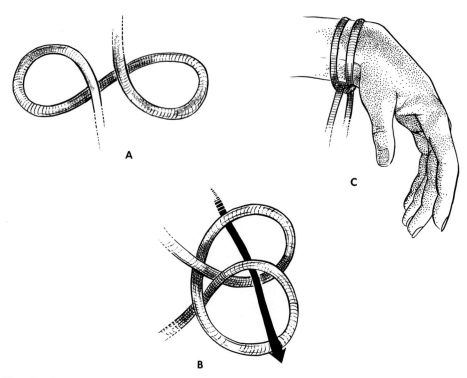

Fig. 2-10. Clove-hitch restraint. **A,** Make a double loop. **B,** Turn one loop in preparation for placing the extremity within the loops as shown by the arrow. **C,** Completed clove hitch.

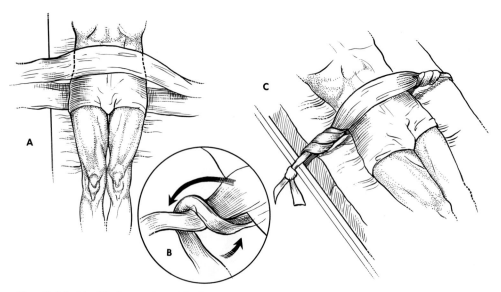

Fig. 2-11. Modified restraint with sheets. **A,** Fold two sheets diagonally. Place one under, the other over the abdominal area. **B,** Twist the ends of the sheets until they are snug. **C,** Tie the ends of the sheets to the bed frame.

If the patient is restless or confused, the restraint should be knotted securely. This prevents the restraint from tightening and impairing circulation. In this instance, adequate padding should be applied between the restraining device and the patient's skin.

Sheets. The nurse can fold two sheets diagonally and apply them around the lower trunk to remind the patient to stay in bed. She places one sheet beneath the abdomen, and the other on top of it. These must not extend over the rib cage, restricting respiration. The nurse twists the protruding ends of the sheets to form a snug cage around the body, draws them to the edge of the bed, and ties them securely to its frame (Fig. 2-11).

Questions for discussion and exploration

1. What are the differences between the ways the hands are held for hand washing and for surgical scrubbing? List situations in which hand washing is necessary.
2. What areas of the skin do the surgeons in your hospital commonly ask to be prepared for surgery?
3. If, during skin preparation, the patient tells you or indicates by his nonverbal communication that he is frightened about his forthcoming surgery, what can you do to help him?
4. A lady who has consented to have brain surgery objects to having her head shaved. For what reasons may she be concerned? How can you relieve her immediate anxiety? What alternatives can you offer until her own hair has grown back?
5. What are the basic differences between the short and long surgical scrubs used in your hospital? How do they differ from those described in the text?
6. What are the basic principles that should be followed when sterile technique is used?
7. Are the inside, outermost edges of a sterile package considered clean, sterile, or contaminated? Why?
8. What are the basic principles and concepts used in isolation technique? How can the nursing staff help the patient feel less lonely? What teaching must you do for the patient and his visitors?
9. What are the basic principles for opening a package of sterile gloves and putting them on?
10. If a person is being admitted to the hospital with severe asthma related to dust allergies, what preparations should be made to control his environment? What special attention should be given to his environment during his hospitalization? What teaching does he and his family need prior to dismissal? Of what value might follow-up visits at his home be?
11. What are the advantages and disadvantages of reusing the same gown for isolation technique? Of using paper, cloth, or plastic gowns?
12. If you are alone and a patient becomes very disturbed, how can you restrain him temporarily? What are your hospital policies regarding the application of restraints? Where are various types of restraints and materials for improvised restraints kept in your hospital? What care specific to the use of restraints must be given to the patient? What are some possible reasons that a patient may become confused?

Selected references

Alexander, E. L., Burley, W., Ellison, D., and Vallari, R.: Care of the patient in surgery, including techniques, ed. 4, St. Louis, 1967, The C. V. Mosby Co.

Berry, E. C., and Kohn, M. L.: Introduction to operating room technique, ed. 3, New York, 1966, McGraw-Hill Book Co.

Dumas, R. G.: Psychological preparation for surgery, Amer. J. Nurs. **63:** 52-55, 1963.

Feinberg, S. M.: Allergies and air conditioning, Amer. J. Nurs. **66:**1333-1336, 1966.

Foster, M.: A positive approach to medical asepsis, Amer. J. Nurs. **62:**76-77, 1962.

Fuerst, E. V., and Wolff, L.: Fundamentals of nursing, ed. 4, Philadelphia, 1969, J. B. Lippincott Co.

Gallivan, G. J., and Tovey, J. D.: Isolation for possible and proved Staph., Amer. J. Nurs. **67:**1048-1049, 1967.

Ginsberg, F., Brunner, L. S., and Cantlin, V. L.: A manual of operating room technology, ed. 2, Philadelphia, 1970, J. B. Lippincott Co.

Kline, P.: Isolating patients with staphylococcal infections, Amer. J. Nurs. **65:**102-104, 1965.

Kretzer, M. P., and Engley, F. B., Jr.: Effective use of antiseptics and disinfectants, R.N. **32:**48-53, 1969.

Laduke, M. M., Hrynus, G. W., Johnston, M. A., Alpert, S., and Levenson, S. M.: Germfree isolators, Amer. J. Nurs. **67:**72-79, 1967.

LeMaitre, G. D., and Finnegan, J. A.: The patient in surgery, ed. 2, Philadelphia, 1970, W. B. Saunders Co.

Louise, Sister M.: The operating room technician, ed. 2, St. Louis, 1968, The C. V. Mosby Co.

Matheney, R. V., Nolan, B. T., Ehrhart, A. M., and Griffin, G. J.: Fundamentals of patient-centered nursing, ed. 2, St. Louis, 1968, The C. V. Mosby Co.

Parrish, H. M., Weil, T. P., and Wolfson, B.: Accidents to patients can be prevented, Amer. J. Nurs. **58:**679-682, 1958.

Perkins, E. W., and Cibula, M. E.: Aseptic technique for operating room personnel, Philadelphia, 1964, W. B. Saunders Co.

Riley, R. L.: Air-borne infections, Amer. J. Nurs. **60:**1246-1248, 1960.

Rockwell, V. T.: Surgical hand scrubbing, Amer. J. Nurs. **63:**75-81, 1963.

Sather, M.: Environmental care of an asthmatic child, Amer. J. Nurs. **68:** 816-817, 1968.

Scheffler, G. L.: The nurse's role in hospital safety, Nurs. Outlook **10:**680-682, 1962.

Schneewind, J. H.: Medical and surgical emergencies, Chicago, 1968, Year Book Medical Publishers, Inc.

Seidler, F. M.: Adapting nursing procedures for reverse isolation, Amer. J. Nurs. **65:**108-111, 1965.

Smith, A. L.: Microbiology and pathology, ed. 9, St. Louis, 1968, The C. V. Mosby Co.

Tyler, V. R.: Gas sterilization, Amer. J. Nurs. **60:**1596-1599, 1960.

U. S. Department of Health, Education, and Welfare: Isolation techniques for use in hospitals, Public Health Service Publication No. 2054, U. S. Government Printing Office, Washington, D. C., 1970.

Werrin, M., and Kronick, D.: Salmonella control in hospitals, Amer. J. Nurs. **66:**528-531, 1966.

Yeager, M. E.: Operating room manual, ed. 2, New York, 1965, G. P. Putnam's Sons.

Chapter 3

Optimum activity

Maintenance and promotion of optimum activity are important nursing responsibilities. The nurse must individualize the degree of mobilization for each patient; for some patients, periods of immobility may be necessary, and this would represent optimum activity for them. The nurse's selection and implementation of an individualized program of positioning and exercise should be consistent with the needs of the patient and with the activity or restrictions prescribed by the attending physician. Utilization and involvement of physical therapists do not relieve the nurse from responsibility for the patient's musculoskeletal function.

Techniques that promote optimum activity are found in much of nursing, with their selection being guided by the amount and kind of assistance needed by the patient. Factors influencing the selection and frequency of using techniques involving positioning and exercise include the patient's level of consciousness, state of health, age, surgical trauma, and degree of mobility or paralysis. Unconscious and paralyzed patients require more assistance than those who respond to stimuli or voluntarily change position. The needs of patients for whom a period of immobilization is prescribed differ from those of ambulatory patients.

Pressure, friction, or moisture between the patient and linen, casts, braces, and other objects is damaging to the skin and underlying tissues. Knowledge of this should guide the modification of techniques used. For instance, pressure on bony prominences can be relieved by proper placement of pillows and other devices, friction from the rough edges of a cast can be reduced with petals of adhesive tape and positioning with pillows, and the perineal area of a body cast can be protected with waterproof material.

The nurse who utilizes the principles of body mechanics and obtains the assistance of other personnel when lifting or turning and when helping the patient to walk can avoid strain or trauma to the patient and herself. Mechanical devices to move the dependent patient may be indicated.

Whenever a positioning or exercise program is to be followed after discharge from the hospital, the nurse should teach the patient and at least one responsible family member the plan and techniques involved. Ideally, such teaching begins early, providing time for those involved to practice and gain confidence.

Positions Proper positioning is a part of preventative nursing. Pillows, lumbar pads, trochanter rolls, and other accessory aids help to maintain good body alignment and prevent prolonged pressure that results in complications. In addition, frequent rotation of selected positions that alternate flexion, extension, abduction, and adduction promotes range of motion and prevents contractures, muscle spasms, and other symptoms of disuse.

Keeping the foundation linen of the bed tight and free of wrinkles helps prevent irritation to the skin. Sheepskin or a substitute properly positioned reduces friction. Sponge rubber pads, silicone gel–filled pads, alternating air mattresses, and other commercial equipment may be used to redistribute pressure. Doughnut-shaped devices are likely to restrict circulation further, interfering with adequate oxygenation of the affected cells.

Prolonged pressure on certain points, such as a bony prominence or edges of the ribs, cheeks, nose, and ears, contributes to excoriation and formation of blisters and decubiti. Similarly, circulatory problems and nerve damage may result from incorrect positioning. For example, "gatching" the foot of the bed may produce pressure in the popliteal area that, along with the dependent position of the lower leg, contributes to the development of thrombophlebitis.

Elevation of the head of the bed produces gravitation of abdominal contents away from the chest, permitting the lungs to expand more fully. Conversely, flexion of the neck interferes with an adequate airway, and clothing tightened over the chest restricts respiration. Pressure from an arm lying across an injured chest further restricts respiration.

The nurse should maintain body alignment with each position. She may profit from assuming these positions herself to gain awareness of discomforts that result from improper positioning. For example, she can readily feel the tension on muscles of the leg if she assumes the side-lying position without elevating the uppermost leg.

The nurse must change the patient's position frequently to avoid complications that result from immobilization. Such complications may occur in a relatively short period of time. These changes are often planned for 2-hour to 3-hour intervals. However, the frequency should be dictated by the needs of the patient and his pathophysiologic condition.

Back-lying position   When the patient is in back-lying position, the nurse may use one or more pillows to align the head. These should extend to a level between the sixth cervical and first thoracic vertebrae, thereby preventing tension on the neck and shoulder muscles and flexion of the neck (Fig. 3-1, *A*). If she uses only one pillow, it should equal the thickness of the shoulders. She may place a second pillow on top of the first pillow, with its lower edge near the base of the neck to provide alignment or comfort.

The nurse may form a lumbar pad by folding a bath blanket or towels to an individualized size, placing the pad under the small of the back for added comfort. She may form a trochanter roll by folding a bath blanket into thirds lengthwise, then in half, tucking it under the thigh and rolling it firmly under itself to correct outward rotation of the thigh (Fig. 3-1, *B*). A folded towel under the area between the calf and the heel supports this area and relieves pressure on the heel (Fig. 3-1, *A* and *D*).

A substantial footboard supports the feet and also holds the top linen off the toes. It should be nearly the width of the mattress and should be constructed sturdily, for if the head of the bed is elevated at all, the patient tends to gravitate toward the footboard (Fig. 3-1, *A* and *D*).

Side-lying position   The back, in the side-lying position, should be as straight as if the patient were standing. The nurse flexes the lower arm to cradle the head in the hand and to maintain the position of the hand and extension of the fingers. She places a pillow between the head and the hand to align the head and reduce pressure on the hand.

Extension of the uppermost arm rests the hand on the hips, sustains extension of the fingers, and prevents pressure on the chest. Alternate positioning of this arm necessitates the use of pillows, hand rolls, and support of the wrist.

The uppermost leg is flexed and elevated with bolster pillows to prevent adduction and muscle tension. Padding may be needed to reduce pressure on the malleolus. Additional support of the foot maintains this position and prevents footdrop. The

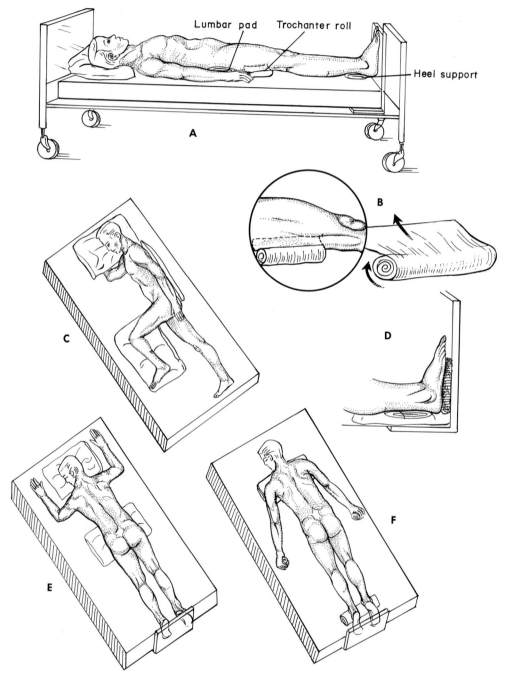

Fig. 3-1. Positions. **A,** Back-lying position showing the trochanter roll, heel support, and lumbar pad. **B,** The formation of a trochanter roll. **C,** Side-lying position. **D,** Support of the foot. **E** and **F,** Face-lying positions.

vertical bars of a side rail, previously attached to the bed, furnish a method of supporting the foot. A sandbag, folded towel, or other padding supports the instep area of the foot and prevents direct contact with the rail (Fig. 3-1, *C*).

The nurse may increase the stability and comfort of this position by placing pillows securely behind the back, tucking one edge under the patient while depressing the mattress, then pushing the free edge of the pillow under the anchored portion.

Face-lying position

The face-lying position is used unless contraindicated by conditions such as abdominal incisions and advanced pregnancy, which would cause unnecessary discomfort. The patient's feet project beyond the mattress to maintain their alignment and prevent pressure on the toes. When a footboard is in place, adequate toe space can be assured by placing 4-inch-square blocks at the outside edges of the footboard, between it and the mattress. A thin pillow under the abdomen aligns the spine and protects the breasts (Fig. 3-1, *E*). Usually it is unnecessary to support the area between the lower ribs and pelvis of a child.

The head may be turned to either side. The nurse positions prominences such as the ears, cheeks, and nose to prevent distortion and pressure. Abduction and external rotation of the arms promote full expansion of the chest. Shoulder rolls, made by rolling a towel, correct inward rotation of the shoulder when necessary. Two washcloths that have been formed into a roll limit flexion of the fingers if placement of the hands palms down with fingers extended is ineffective (Fig. 3-1, *F*).

Range of motion

Rotation of the previously described position produces range of motion unless effort is used to prevent it. However, additional exercises may also be used. These are conducted slowly, smoothly, without force, and within the existing range of motion. If pain occurs, discontinue exercises until further instructions are obtained from the physician, who also prescribes limitations to be observed, special devices such as skates, slings, and pulleys, and exercise programs to regain or increase range of motion.

Planning the bed bath, positioning, and other nursing care to include either active or passive range of motion may eliminate the need for designated exercise periods. Observation of alignment and correction of faulty movements, such as raising the shoulder during neck exercises, increase effectiveness.

Neck

To exercise his neck the patient bends his head forward until his chin rests on his chest. Then he bends the head back as far as possible, turning his head toward his left shoulder, then his right. Finally he tilts his head toward each shoulder in an attempt to touch his shoulder with his chin (Fig. 3-2, *A*).

Text continued on p. 54.

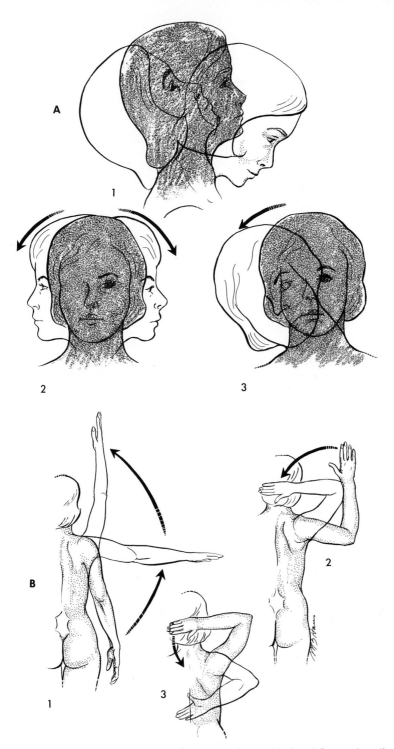

Fig. 3-2. Range of motion. **A,** Neck: **1,** the patient bends his head forward until the chin rests on the chest, then backward as far as possible; **2,** he turns his head toward the left shoulder, then toward the right shoulder; **3,** he tilts his head toward the right shoulder, attempting to touch the shoulder with the chin, then toward the left shoulder, attempting to touch the shoulder with the chin. **B,** Shoulder and elbow: **1,** the patient extends his arm at the side with the palm of his hand turned toward the hip and raises the extended arm up and backward until it is held directly above his head; **2,** he bends his elbow and moves the palm of his hand behind his head; **3,** finally, he moves his hand to the small of his back.

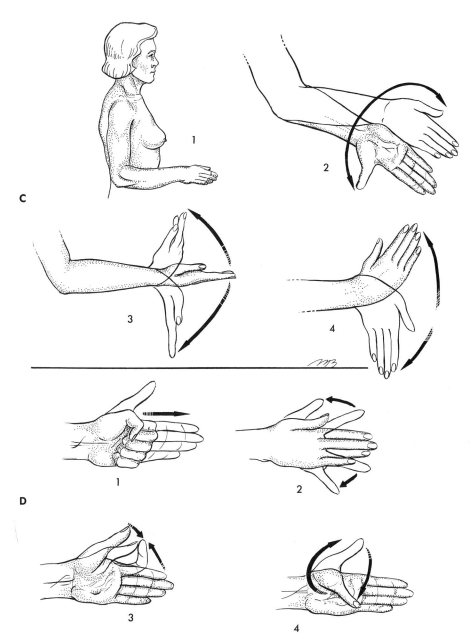

Fig. 3-2, cont'd. C, Wrist and lower arm: **1,** the patient holds the upper part of his arm in contact with the side of his body with the elbow at a right angle to it; **2,** he turns the palm up, then down; **3,** extending his fingers, he bends his hand down as far as possible, then up as far as possible; **4,** he aligns his hand with his lower arm, keeping the elbow bent, and moves the hand to either side as far as possible; then, he rotates the hand over and back as far as possible. **D,** Fingers and thumb: **1,** the patient makes a fist and then straightens the fingers and thumb; **2,** he spreads the fingers and thumb apart and then brings them together; **3,** he touches each finger with the thumb; **4,** then he rotates the thumb.

Continued.

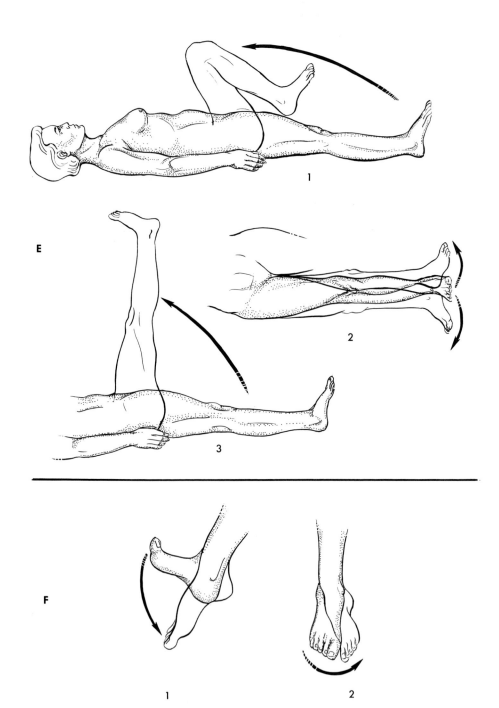

Fig. 3-2, cont'd. E, Hip and knee: **1,** after assuming a back-lying position, the patient bends his knee toward the body as far as possible; **2,** he straightens the leg, rolls it inward as far as possible, and then outward as far as possible; **3,** then he raises the leg straight up. **F,** Ankle and foot: **1,** after assuming a sitting position with the feet dangling, the patient bends his foot and toes downward, then upward; **2,** he rotates the entire foot inward, then outward and points the toes inward, finally circumducting the ankle.

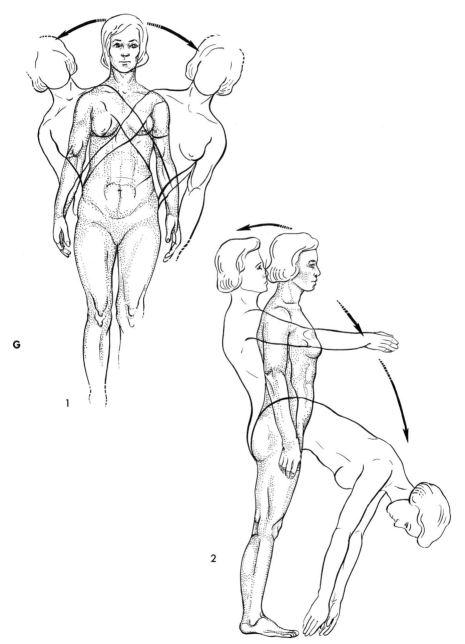

G

1

2

Fig. 3-2, cont'd. G, Trunk: **1,** the patient bends the upper trunk to the left, then to the right, and then he twists the upper trunk to the left, then to the right; **2,** with the knees straight, he touches the toes with the tips of the fingers and then bends his body backward.

Shoulder and elbow   Extending his arm at his side with the palm of his hand turned toward the hip and keeping the arm extended, the patient raises it up and backward through an arc until he holds it directly above his head, then bends his elbow and moves the palm of his hand behind his head, and finally to the small of his back (Fig. 3-2, *B*).

Wrist and lower arm   In exercising his wrist and lower arm, the patient holds the upper part of his arm in contact with the side of his body, with his elbow at a right angle to it. He turns the palm up, then down. Extending his fingers, he bends his hand down as far as possible, then up as far as possible. He aligns his hand with his lower arm, keeping the elbow bent, and moves his hand as far as possible to either side. He finishes by rotating his hand over and back as far as possible (Fig. 3-2, *C*).

Fingers and thumb   The patient, to exercise his fingers and thumb, makes a fist, straightens the fingers and thumb, spreads them apart, and brings them together. He touches each finger with the thumb, then rotates the thumb (Fig. 3-2, *D*).

Hip and knee   The hip and knee are exercised by having the patient, in a back-lying position, bend his knee as far toward the body as possible. Then, straightening the leg, he rolls it inward, then outward as far as possible. Finally he raises the leg straight up. He sits on the edge of the bed to dangle the lower leg and moves the foot inward, outward, forward, and back. He raises his knee toward his chest (Fig. 3-2, *E*).

Ankle and foot   The patient sits with his feet dangling. He bends the foot and toes downward, then upward, rotates the entire foot inward, then outward, and points the toes inward, finally circumducting the ankle (Fig. 3-2, *F*).

Trunk   Standing with the feet a few inches apart, the patient bends his upper trunk to the left, then to the right, and twists the upper trunk to the left, then to the right. With his knees straight, he touches his toes with the tips of his fingers and then bends backward (Fig. 3-2, *G*).

Transfers   The selection of transfer techniques is individualized. For example, horizontal transfer with a sheet moves patients with abdominal surgery from the stretcher to the bed, a three-man carry moves orthopedic patients through narrow doorways, mechanical devices such as lifts transfer patients with ease, and special frames or beds maintain body alignment during transfer. Precautions that prevent twisting or crepitation of the spine are employed in turning the patient with a spinal injury. If full range of motion is permitted, the patient may assist with the transfer or move himself independently.

Care to instruct the patient, to prevent trauma by positioning or supporting the extremities, to protect drainage tubes from tension, and to synchronize efforts of the persons involved contributes to safe, gentle transfer. The practice of transferring on the count of three serves the latter objective. Jolting or sudden movements are likely to cause physiologic adjustments that may result in complications such as shock. Some adjustment occurs with each position change, and the transfer may need to be completed over a period of time to accommodate resulting reactions. For example, it may be necessary to bring the orthopedic patient who has been lying in bed for a long period of time to a vertical position very slowly with the use of a tilt table or CircOlectric bed.

Pull-sheet transfer   Preparatory to transfer with a pull sheet, the mattress levels of the bed and stretcher must be equalized, with the bed linen folded to the side or foot of the bed.

Ideally, six persons combine efforts for this transfer, although four persons can achieve a similar result. Two persons position themselves to support the chest and abdomen; two support the pelvis and hips; one, the lower legs and feet; and one, the head, neck, and shoulders. Better leverage and body mechanics are gained if a short person kneels on the edge of the bed. The pull sheet is tightened into a hammock by folding or rolling it toward the patient's sides. Efforts to pull and lift the patient from the stretcher to the bed should be synchronized (Fig. 3-3, A).

The patient is turned to his side to remove the pull sheet. The nurses beside the bed reach across the patient, place the palms of their hands down on the posterior aspect of his shoulders, back, and hips, and roll him toward them. If immobility of the spine is desirable, his uppermost arm is held in extension on his hip, and his entire body is rolled like a log. This position of the uppermost arm prevents twisting of the torso. An alternate method of rolling the patient to his side uses the pull sheet rather than the hands. The patient is supported on his side until the pull sheet is folded or rolled tightly against his back, and the nurse tucks its edge under him by depressing the mattress slightly. Then the patient is rolled to his opposite side, completely freeing the pull sheet. Forceful removal of the pull sheet indicates disregard for the comfort and alignment of the patient and produces skin damage that becomes more apparent with time.

Three-man carry   For the three-man carry, three persons, all standing on the same side of the patient, slip their hands, palms facing up, beneath the patient (Fig. 3-3, *B*) and cradle him in their arms so that his weight rests against their chests and he faces them (Fig. 3-3, *C*).

Four-man or six-man carry

Two persons stand on each side of the patient and place their hands beneath him to form a hammock (Fig. 3-3, *D*). Two persons are added to the basic four-man carry if the patient is quite tall or heavy.

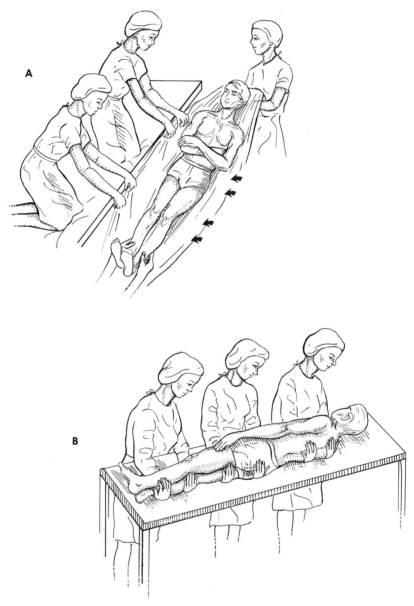

Fig. 3-3. Transfers. **A,** Pull-sheet method of transfer; arrows indicate placement of the hands of other assistants. **B,** Lifting the patient in preparation for transfer with a three-man carry.

Mechanical devices
Hydraulic lift

The hydraulic lift, also called a patient lifter or invalid lifter, enables one person to transfer a totally dependent patient with ease and safety to and from a bed, a wheelchair, a toilet, a tub, or a car. Depending upon the needs of the patient, he is supported with a pair of slings, canvas seats with or without a head support, or a stretcher. The support is placed beneath the patient and attached to the swivel bar of the lift.

Most hydraulic lifts consist of a tripod type of base on casters, a mast, a boom, a hydraulic, mechanical, or electrical pump, and a sling, harness, or stretcher. Although design varies, their operation is similar to that of the Hoyer patient lifter illustrated in Fig. 3-4.

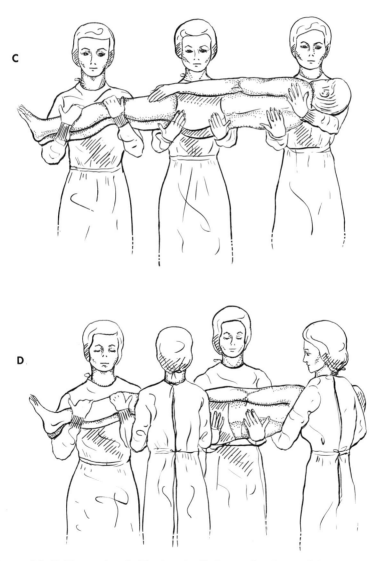

Fig. 3-3, cont'd. C, The patient is lifted and rolled onto the chests of the persons executing the three-man carry. **D,** Four-man carry.

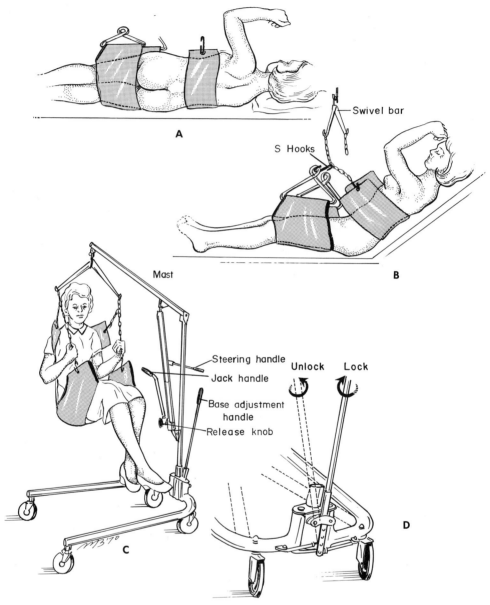

Swivel bar

S Hooks

Mast

Steering handle
Jack handle
Base adjustment
handle
Release knob

Unlock   Lock

A

B

C

D

Fig. 3-4. Hydraulic lift (illustrated after Hoyer patient lifter). **A,** Placement of slings. **B,** Attachment of slings to swivel bar. **C,** A patient in the slings is swung free of the bed. The point of adjustment has been reached. The patient will turn to face the mast before the lift is moved, **D,** View of the base. To narrow the base, the nurse unlocks the handle by rotating it counterclockwise and moving it to the left. The base is locked by turning the handle clockwise. The base is widened by unlocking the handle and moving it to the right, where it is locked in position. (Courtesy Ted Hoyer and Co., Inc., Oshkosh, Wis.)

When canvas slings are used, the nurse places the larger of the slings beneath the patient's thighs, with its lower edge above his knees. She places the smaller sling behind the small of his back by elevating the head of the bed and sliding the sling down to its place or by rolling the patient to his side, then onto the sling (Fig. 3-4, *A*). Both slings are attached to the swivel bar with S hooks that have been incorporated into the design (Fig. 3-4, *B*). The exact position of the slings must be individualized until the so-called point of adjustment is reached. This is the point at which the patient is given proper support. When the patient is lifted with proper support, he does not tip forward or backward, nor does he feel he is slipping between the slings.

After she has placed the slings, the nurse pumps the jack handle to elevate the patient. When he is sufficiently high to swing free (Fig. 3-4, *C*), she assists him to face the mast by grasping the outer edges of the swivel bar to turn him. She then turns the release knob to lower him to a sitting position. Some manual assistance may be necessary during the lowering process to guide him to the desired position.

The steering handle is used to guide the lift to the desired location. It is sometimes necessary to change the width of the base. For example, passage through a doorway requires a narrow base, while positioning the patient over a toilet requires a widened base. The narrow position should be used only if necessary. For other transfer, a slightly widened base offers more stability. To change the width of the base, the nurse unlocks the base adjustment handle by rotating it to the left (counterclockwise), then slides the handle to the left to narrow the base or to the right to widen the base. The base is locked in this position by rotating the handle to the right (clockwise) (Fig. 3-4, *D*).

Turning devices   The Stryker turning frame, the Foster reversible orthopedic bed, and the CircOlectric bed provide means of changing the patient to and from the face-lying and back-lying positions with a minimum of personnel, maximum ease, and undisturbed body alignment.

Stryker frame and Foster bed. Basic padding of the frames is similar, although the materials and fasteners may vary. Each company supplies canvas covers, mattresses, sheets, and fasteners designed to fit its product. Additional accessories are a footboard, arm supports, a utility table for diversional materials and the serving tray, and provisions for attaching traction. All frames provide openings used for normal routes of elimination. The center section of the posterior frame is removed, and the receptacle is placed within the device attached to the frame for this purpose.

Although each has distinctive features, common principles

apply in the use of all these devices. The position of the patient is stabilized similarly on all. Frequent changes of position prevent complications and facilitate nursing care. In addition, complete passivity of joints during transfer adds to patient comfort.

In the initial transfer to the posterior frame the nurse may utilize previously described transfer techniques (pages 54 to 57), or she may place a litter bearing the patient on the frame. To remove the litter without disturbing body alignment, she places the anterior frame in position and turns the patient so that the posterior frame and the litter may be removed.

Mental preparation prior to use of a turning frame helps the patient to adjust to its use. Before each maneuver, the nurse tells him which direction he will be turned and informs him of sensations likely to occur because of changes in circulation. For example, vertical change of position may produce sensations of numbness, tingling, or light-headedness. Knowledge that he is securely and comfortably sandwiched between the posterior and anterior frames helps him develop trust. Some authorities recommend that nurses involved in caring for patients on these devices experience the position transfers personally, thus increasing their sympathetic and instructional capacities.

Preparatory to lateral transfer with a Stryker turning frame or the Foster bed, the nurse places a pillow lengthwise over the patient's legs to protect the knees and stabilize the legs during transfer (Figs. 3-5, *A* and 3-6, *A*). Depending upon the size of the patient, an additional pillow may be needed. The nurse removes the pillow from the patient's head and protects the face with a face mask. Safety straps stabilize the head and prevent flexion or extension of the neck. The nurse removes arm boards and permits the patient, if he is able, to hug the frame during transfer (Fig. 3-5, *B*). If the patient is unable to do this, his arms are extended beside his body and maintained in this position with safety straps. This prevents the arms from dangling and also prevents trauma when the patient is turned. After removing the footboard of the Foster bed, two nurses place the anterior frame over the patient and secure it (Fig. 3-5, *B*). It is imperative to have two persons handle the anterior frame of the Foster bed (Fig. 3-6, *B*). The nurses also fasten the safety straps.

A nurse stands at each end of the frame, disengaging the pins that lock the frame to the base (Figs. 3-5, *C* and 3-6, *A*). Each nurse grasps the frame preparatory to rotation, one tells the patient which direction he will be turned, and together they transfer him with a synchronized turn. Preplanned placement of the nurses' hands will make this maneuver smooth.

CircOlectric bed. The CircOlectric bed has features useful in progressive rehabilitation. Because it turns the patient vertically (Fig. 3-7, *C*) and can be stopped at any point, it serves as a tilt

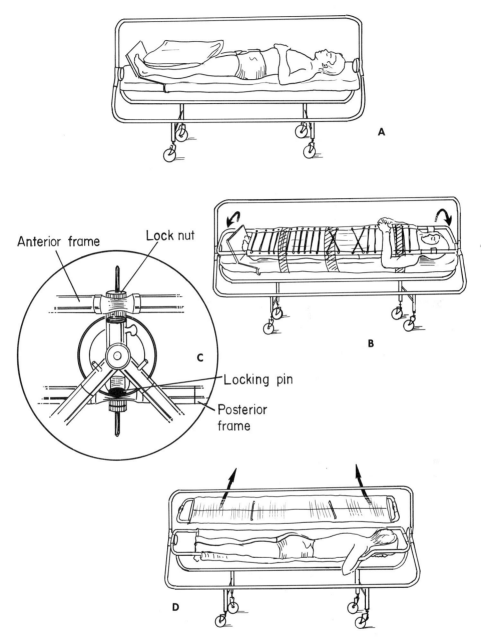

Fig. 3-5. Stryker turning frame. **A,** The top linen is removed, the pillow from the head is placed lengthwise over the legs, and the footboard is adjusted. **B,** The anterior frame is positioned with its narrow end and the face support over the face. This frame is locked securely with a knurled nut. The patient is secured with safety straps and permitted to grasp the frame. The locking pin is disengaged, and the patient is transferred laterally. **C,** End view of the turning assembly. Locknuts on each end of the frame must be tightened before the patient is turned. The locking pin at the end of the frame is pulled out, the patient is turned slightly, the locking pin is released, and the transfer is completed. **D,** After lateral transfer is completed, the posterior frame is unbolted and removed. (Courtesy Stryker Corporation, Kalamazoo, Mich.)

table. "Gatching" the posterior frame provides the same position attainable in the ordinary hospital bed; when combined with rotation in the circle frame, it brings the patient to a sitting position from which he can be easily transferred to a chair by means of slings, much as a patient is transferred with a hydraulic lift.

Preparatory to vertical transfer of the patient in a CircOlectric bed, the nurse protects the patient from unnecessary movement by positioning the footboard, placing pillows over his legs and applying the sponge rubber face mask (Fig. 3-7, *A*). She pulls the overhead frame down from its resting place on the circle frame and secures it by tightening the nut on the prepositioned

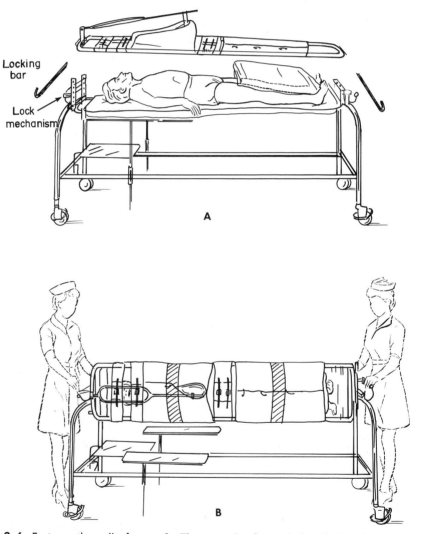

Fig. 3-6. Foster orthopedic frame. **A,** The posterior frame is installed and secured with locking bars. **B,** The lock mechanism is disengaged, and the patient is turned. Safety straps add security. Position of the nurses' hands should be planned for smooth transfer. (Courtesy Gilbert Hyda Chick Co., Oakland, Calif.)

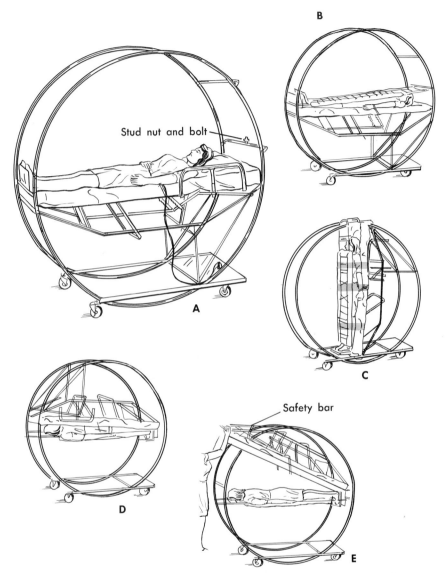

Fig. 3-7. CircOlectric bed. **A,** The patient is in back-lying position, with her hips centered at the gatch. The footboard is adjusted to prevent her from sliding downward during transfer. The pillow from her head is used to pad her legs and knees. A sponge rubber face mask is applied to protect the face. **B,** The anterior frame is installed and locked in place with a stud nut and bolt. **C,** After telling the patient which way she will turn, the nurse rotates the bed electrically. Safety straps are necessary if the patient is unable to control her arms. **D,** The posterior stud nut is removed from the head of the frame, and the safety bar is pulled forward to disengage the posterior section. **E,** The posterior section is raised high overhead and locked into the circle frame with the safety bar. (Courtesy Stryker Corporation, Kalamazoo, Mich.)

bolt (Fig. 3-7, *B*). She may then apply safety straps. After telling the patient in which direction he will turn, she moves the switch button to "face" or "back" accordingly (Fig. 3-7, *C*). After the desired level of transfer is achieved, the nurse disengages the posterior section, raises it high overhead, and locks it into the circle frame with the safety bar (Fig. 3-7, *D* and *E*).

Ambulation   Whenever feasible, early ambulation is prescribed to promote independent activity. This avoids the complications and the discouragement that are likely to accompany inactivity.

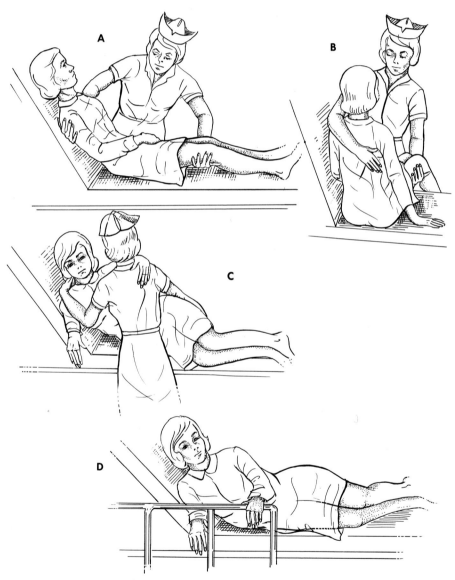

Fig. 3-8. Ambulation. **A,** With the head of the bed elevated, the nurse is preparing to pivot the patient to a sitting position. **B,** The pivot to sitting position is nearly complete. **C,** A patient receiving some assistance. **D,** Self-assisted method of sitting up.

The amount and kind of assistance needed vary. Factors such as fluid and electrolyte imbalance, inadequate nutrition, age, insecurity, limited joint motion, and paralysis result in a need for an increased amount of assistance. If necessary, the nurse helps the patient to progress through stages to independent activity. Thus, she might first assist him to sit on the edge of the bed, then to stand briefly while she assists him to a chair, next to

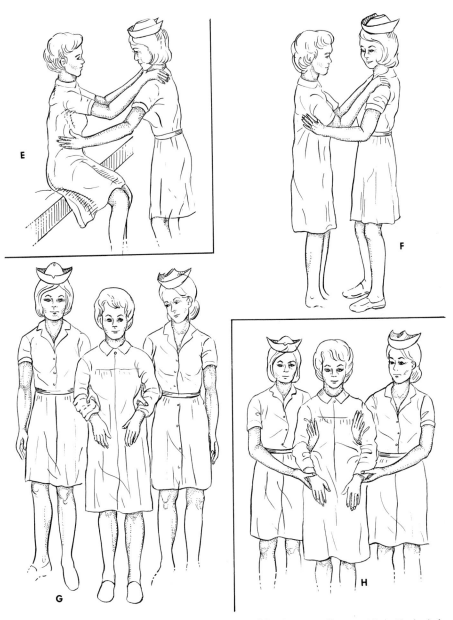

Fig. 3-8, cont'd. E, Assisting patient from edge of bed to standing position. **F,** Assisting patient to stand. Feet and knees may be braced with nurse's feet and knees for additional support. **G,** Supported ambulation. **H,** Convenient method of supported ambulation.

ambulate with necessary degrees of support, and finally to ambulate independently. She should apply supports such as arm
slings prior to ambulation. Moving the strongest part of the body
first gives the maximum support, and this, combined with effort,
increases independence. The hemiplegic would therefore transfer his uninvolved side first.

Sitting up

To assist the totally dependent patient to sit up, the nurse
elevates the head of the bed and places her left arm under his
legs and her right arm under his shoulder. Then she lifts his
shoulders slightly and simultaneously pulls his legs toward her
body, pivoting him to a sitting position (Fig. 3-8, *A* and *B*). She
permits as much self-assistance as possible. The patient in this
position can be helped to maintain it if the nurse stands facing
him, with his hands on her shoulders and her hands at his waist.

An independent method of assuming the sitting position, preferred by many patients and especially useful if an abdominal
incision is present, consists of instructing the patient to turn to
his side before sitting up. The nurse elevates the head of the
bed approximately 30°; she instructs the patient to grasp the
side rail with his uppermost arm for leverage and to push up
with his lower arm, simultaneously moving his feet toward the
edge of the bed until they hang free (Fig. 3-8, *D*). If some
assistance is needed, the patient places his upper arm on the
nurse's shoulder, and the nurse uses one arm to support his head
and neck, moving his legs with the other arm (Fig. 3-8, *C*).

Transfer from bed
to chair

To effect a transfer from the bed to a chair, the nurse places an
electric bed in low position, permitting the patient's feet to rest
on the floor, and assists him to a standing position. Depending
upon the placement of the chair, he may need only to pivot or
take one step to place his back to the chair, then seat himself
with assistance as necessary. The chair should be braced with one
foot to prevent it from slipping. The nurse does this with her
feet or by placing the chair against a wall.

If the bed cannot be lowered, the nurse supports the patient
at waist level, places his arms on her shoulders, and helps him
slip to a standing position (Fig. 3-8, *E*). Bracing his feet and
knees helps stabilize the upright position (Fig. 3-8, *F*).

Dependent
ambulation:
aids in walking

To help a patient walk, the nurse, standing at the patient's left
side, places her right arm around his waist and grasps his right
forearm with her right hand and his left forearm with her left
hand. If two nurses assist, each may place her arm so that it in-
terlocks with the patient's and may grasp his forearm for support
(Fig. 3-8, *G*). Bilateral support without clumsiness during ambulation is obtained if two nurses, standing on either side of the pa-

tient, grasp the upper arm near the axilla with the arm nearest the patient. The other hand is used to grasp the wrist (Fig. 3-8, *H*). The patient may tend to grasp the nurse's hand. However, it is important that the nurse control the points of support in order to utilize necessary leverage if the need arises.

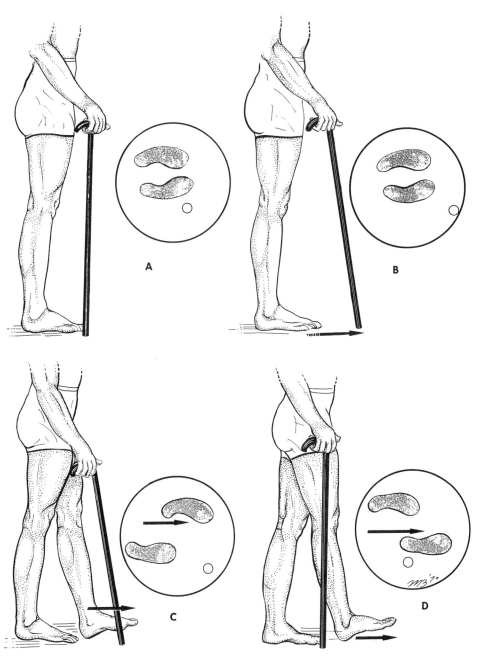

Fig. 3-9. Cane walking. **A,** The cane is positioned about 4 to 6 inches away from the toe of the uninvolved extremity. **B,** The cane is moved forward about the length of the patient's foot. **C,** The involved leg is moved forward until the toe is parallel to the cane. **D,** The uninvolved leg is moved forward until its heel is parallel to the cane.

Cane walking. To walk properly with a cane, the patient stands in normal walking position with the cane positioned about 4 to 6 inches away from the toe of the uninvolved extremity (Fig. 3-9, *A*). This prevents leaning toward the cane or having it accidentally kicked away. The patient moves the cane forward about the length of his foot (Fig. 3-9, *B*). Then he moves the

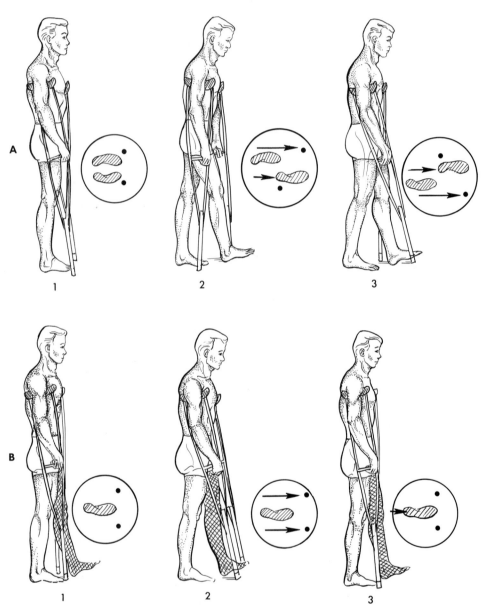

Fig. 3-10. Crutch walking. **A,** Two-point gait: **1,** position of rest; **2,** the left crutch and the right foot are advanced simultaneously; **3,** the right crutch and the left foot are advanced simultaneously. **B,** Three-point gait: **1,** weight is on the uninvolved extremity; **2,** with the weight on the uninvolved extremity, the crutches and the involved extremity are advanced; **3,** the uninvolved extremity is advanced.

involved leg forward until its toe is parallel to the cane (Fig. 3-9, *C*). He moves the uninvolved leg forward until its heel is parallel to the cane (Fig. 3-9, *D*). Alternate methods of cane walking may be used if this method is not satisfactory.

Crutch walking. As with any activity, good body alignment is essential for correct crutch walking and future rehabilitation. Holding the involved extremity in extension to prevent contracture and rotation and standing erect with the head held high and the eyes looking ahead prevent errors commonly associated with crutch walking. Supporting the weight on the hands necessitates

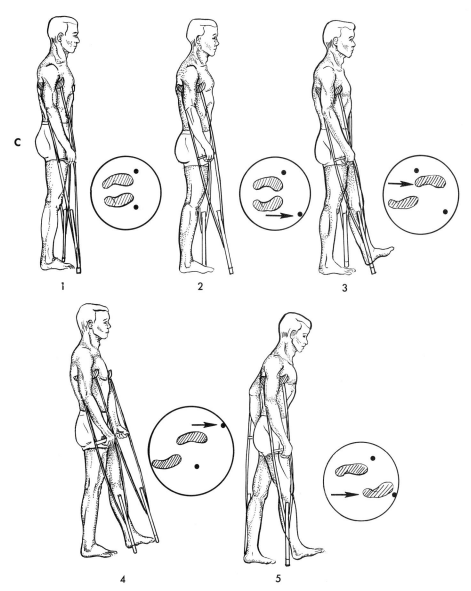

Fig. 3-10, cont'd. C, Four-point gait: **1,** position of rest, **2,** right crutch is advanced; **3,** left foot is advanced; **4,** left crutch is advanced; **5,** right foot is advanced.

keeping the elbows straight. Placing the crutches 4 to 6 inches to the side, but in front of the feet, adds stability.

Length of crutches. Numerous methods of measuring a patient for crutches are used. If the patient is able, he should stand against a wall, in a position of good posture. He must be wearing his walking shoes. Three points are used to determine the length of crutch needed: (1) a measurement from the outside of the toe of the shoe sole to a point 2 inches to the patient's side, (2) a measurement from this first point, straight forward for a distance of 6 inches, and (3) a measurement from the second point to 2 inches below the axilla. The third measurement indicates the length of crutches needed. If the patient is unable to stand, he lies on his back, arms extended at his sides, legs aligned, feet slightly apart, and his walking shoes on. A measurement taken from the axilla to a point 6 inches out from the heel represents crutch length. Evaluation of the height of the hand bar and its adjustment to individual needs are basic for preventing pressure in the axillary region.

Crutch gait is prescribed according to the kind, amount, or support required. Teaching varies with the gait and the individual.

Two-point gait. When partial weight bearing is allowed, the two-point gait increases speed. The left crutch and the right foot are advanced simultaneously. Then the right crutch and the left foot are advanced simultaneously (Fig. 3-10, *A*).

Three-point gait. When bearing the weight on one extremity is permitted, the patient may use the three-point gait. The weight is shifted to the uninvolved extremity while the crutches are advanced. Then the uninvolved extremity is advanced (Fig. 3-10, *B*). The crutches and the involved leg are moved forward at the same time. Then the uninvolved leg is moved forward. These steps are repeated.

Four-point gait. The four-point gait is slower than the two-point gait but similar to it. The right crutch is advanced, then the left foot, the left crutch, and then the right foot (Fig. 3-10, *C*).

Additional aids

Not uncommonly, prescribed levels of activity necessitate additional aids, some of which serve to prevent complications related to body position.

Finishing the edges of a cast

When a cast is thoroughly dry, unfinished edges are covered with strips of waterproof adhesive tape that have been shaped for this purpose. This procedure is called petaling the cast (Fig. 3-11). Excessive sheet wadding is trimmed from the edges of the cast, and its stockinette lining is stretched over the edges of the cast prior to petaling.

The size of the petal used varies with the size of the cast. The

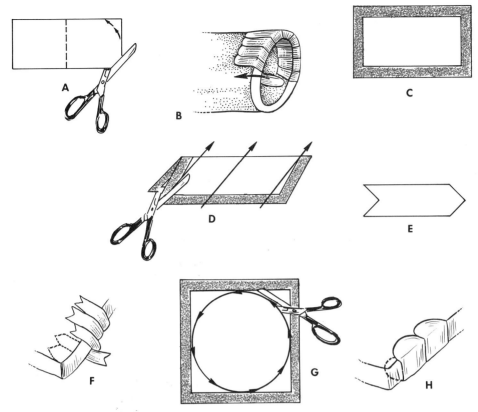

Fig. 3-11. Preparation and application of petals to the edges of a cast. **A,** The end of a piece of tape 2 inches wide and 4 inches long is rounded. **B,** The uncut end of tape is placed beneath the edge of the cast, and the petal is brought forward over the edge of the cast. Each petal overlaps the one previously applied. **C,** Tape, 2 inches wide, is placed on waxed paper. **D,** Tape and paper are folded lengthwise and cut diagonally to prepare the petal. **E,** The prepared petal. **F,** The petal is applied to the edge of the cast. **G,** A 2-inch square of tape is rounded. **H,** Application of round petals to the edge of the cast.

shape of the petal may be influenced by its size; rounded edges seem to have less tendency to curl away from the cast. The tape may be folded so that the nonadhesive sides of the tape are together, or it may be placed on waxed paper or a similar material from which it is readily separated for cutting the petals to the desired size and shape. Tape, 2 inches wide, is used for large areas, like those on a body cast, while small areas are treated with 1-inch tape.

Each petal is applied by placing one end of the petal on the inside surface of the cast, bringing the petal over the edge of the cast and smoothing its finished edges to the exterior part. Each succeeding petal overlaps the previous one by about ½ inch.

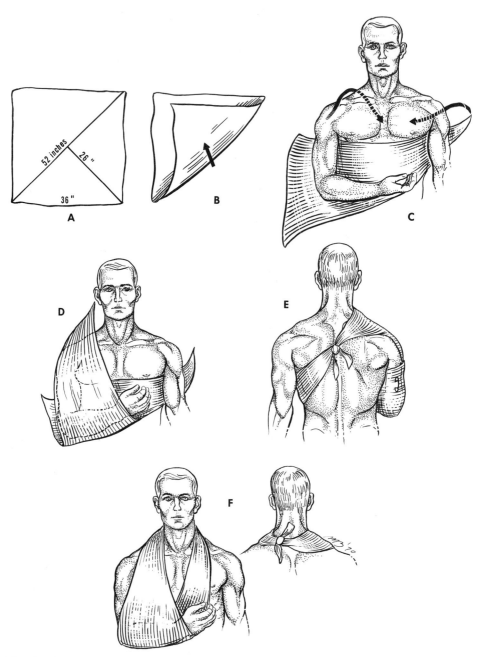

Fig. 3-12. Triangular arm sling. **A,** A square yard of material, showing the measurements of the sling. **B,** The material folded diagonally; the resulting triangle may be cut and hemmed. **C,** The apex of the triangle is placed at the elbow, with the end of the base of the triangle enclosing the arm; the arm is positioned to prevent dependent edema. **D,** Anterior view of the completed sling. **E,** Posterior view of the completed sling. The sling is pinned or knotted at the elbow to maintain position of the arm. **F,** Alternate method of applying sling.

Arm sling · · · · · A sling is used to support either the weight of a cast that has been applied to the arm or a completely dependent arm. It will, if applied correctly, elevate the hand slightly and support it, preventing edema caused by allowing the wrist and hand to hang down. It should not contribute to discomfort or poor body alignment. Fig. 3-12, *A* to *E* illustrate one method used to make and apply a triangular arm sling measuring approximately 26 by 36 by 52 inches. Another method of applying a sling is shown in Fig. 3-12, *F*.

Abdominal binder · · · · · Following surgery, an abdominal binder may be prescribed for support. Various types of binders are available, but all should be applied when the patient is in a back-lying position. They should be tightened from the most distal point upward across the abdomen and should be tucked beneath the patient for maximum support (Fig. 3-13). Care to provide even pressure and to avoid undue pressure on drainage tubes or respiratory structures is essential.

Elastic bandages · · · · · Application of elastic bandages to the legs prior to ambulation is not unlike the application of wet dressings illustrated in Chapter

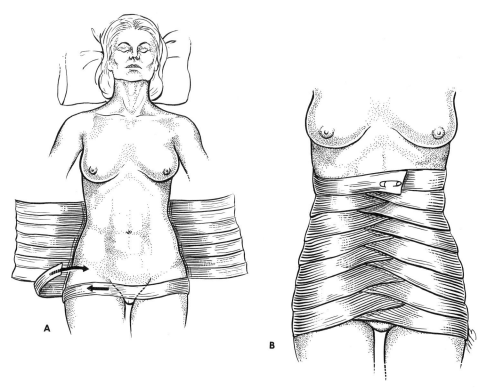

Fig. 3-13. Abdominal binder. **A,** A scultetus binder is placed beneath the patient, who is in a back-lying position. Distal tails of the binder are tightened across abdomen and tucked beneath the patient. **B,** The completed binder is fastened with a safety pin.

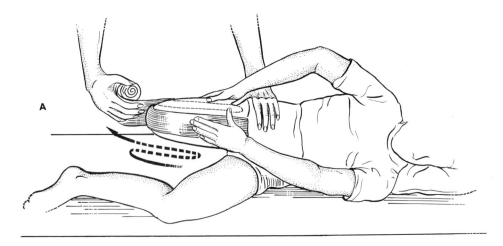

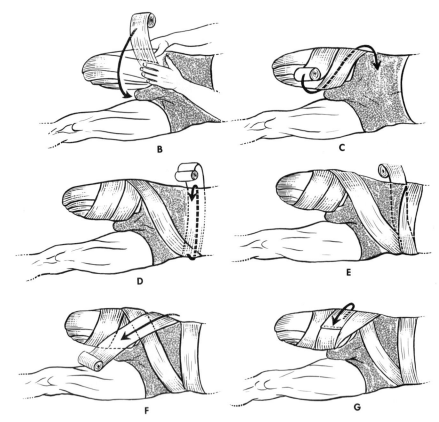

Fig. 3-14. Elastic bandage for stump shrinkage. **A,** The first turn of the bandage begins high on the front of the stump and extends across its center and to the top of the back of the stump. **B,** After making 2 to 3 turns over the end of the stump, the nurse turns the bandage for a circular spiral. **C,** Circular turns or spirals continue toward the top of the stump, then are brought across the back of the stump toward the waist. **D,** The bandage is brought across the abdomen to encircle the waist. **E,** Bandages circle the waist twice. **F,** The bandage is brought from the back of the waist to the front of the stump. **G,** The remainder of the bandage encircles the stump and is anchored in front with safety pins or tape.

6. The stretchable bandage should be sufficiently taut to provide support and increase venous return but not tight enough to produce stasis. A method of testing the tightness is to place one finger between the circular turns. If the bandage has been applied correctly, one finger will easily slip beneath the bandage as far as the first knuckle. The use of elastic stockings instead of elastic bandages requires less skill.

Preparatory to fitting an amputee with a prosthesis, the nurse may wrap the stump with an elastic bandage or apply a reducing sock. Either of these shapes the stump and supports the soft tissue, giving firmness to the stump and reducing edema.

To bandage the healed stump with compression, the nurse uses an elastic bandage. Its width is determined by the size of the stump. Frequently, a 4-inch to 6-inch width is used for the adult. The length of bandage needed also varies with the size of the individual. If more than one length of bandage is needed, sewing the two lengths of bandage together is likely to be more satisfactory than other methods of fastening. The nurse forms the bandage into a firm, even roll to facilitate its application. It must be applied with an even pressure that does not produce creasing of the skin. Pressure over the area of the healed incision is greater than that exerted at the upper portion of the stump. Frequently, each turn of bandage overlaps the previous one by about a third of the width of the bandage. Thus, if a 4-inch bandage is used, each turn overlaps the previous turn by about 1⅓ inches. Fig. 3-14 illustrates an elastic bandage being applied to a stump. The method used may be modified by using circular turns after the end of the stump has been enclosed.

Reducing sock   The physician may recommend a reducing sock of a size that will fit the stump snugly without interfering with circulation. Periodically, it is replaced with a smaller size.

Questions for discussion and exploration

1. What are some of the principles of teaching and learning that are useful in helping to prepare and carry out a plan of teaching?
2. If a patient complains of phantom pain in an extremity that has been amputated, how can you explain this phenomenon to him and at the same time provide emotional support?
3. Following amputation of his lower leg, Mr. C. insists that elevating it on a pillow would be more comfortable than his present position. How should you deal with this request?
4. When relatives of Mrs. A., 90 years of age and bedridden, confide that they feel unable to care for her at home but cannot afford the cost of care in a nursing home or in the hospital, what additional information do you need to understand their reaction? How can you help them mobilize their potentials? What community agencies can become sources of help to them?
5. Mrs. D., who is recovering after fracturing her hip, wishes to return to her walk-up apartment where she lives alone. What teaching related to ambulation does she need prior to returning home?

6. You are asked to measure Mrs. D. for crutches. What methods might be used?

7. Mrs. D. is later fitted with a cane. How would you explain, demonstrate, and teach her to walk with the cane?

8. Although Mrs. D. will be able to ambulate with a cane when she returns home, she worries that she will be unable to shop for food or clean her apartment. What community resources are available to her?

9. Due to the nature of Mr. R.'s pathophysiologic condition, the physician agrees that he can be cared for at home if the family is able to obtain a CircOlectric bed and learn to operate it and to learn to care for Mr. R. Where can the family obtain this equipment? What adjustments might need to be made in their living arrangements? Develop a plan of teaching the patient and his family about the use of the CircOlectric bed.

10. Johnny B., 8 years of age, had a fracture of his arm reduced under anesthesia. Develop a plan for teaching Johnny and his mother about the use and application of a sling and positioning of the affected arm. For what reasons should they be instructed to consult the orthopedist prior to their next appointment?

11. It is likely that Johnny will be an active lad after his dismissal from the hospital. What play activities are permissible while he is wearing a cast? Is there a plan for his taking a shower or a tub bath?

12. When Mrs. Z. is brought to her room, partially awake, following abdominal surgery, what are your responsibilities concerning transfer of Mrs. Z. from the surgical cart to her bed? What are your responsibilities to her, the relatives, and the nursing staff during the immediate postoperative period?

Selected references

American Rehabilitation Foundation (formerly Kenny Rehabilitation): Rehabilitative techniques: 1, Bed positioning and transfer procedures for hemiplegia, 1962; 2, Selected equipment useful in the hospital, home, or nursing home, 1962; 3, A procedure for passive range of motion and self-assistive exercises, Minneapolis, 1964, American Rehabilitation Foundation.

Carini, E., and Owens, G.: Neurological and neurosurgical nursing, ed. 5, St. Louis, 1970, The C. V. Mosby Co.

Grabstetter, J.: Synthetic fat helps prevent pressure sores, Amer. J. Nurs. 68:1521-1522, 1968.

Hirschberg, G. G., Levis, L., and Thomas, D.: Rehabilitation: Manual for the care of the disabled and elderly, Philadelphia, 1964, J. B. Lippincott Co.

Kelly, M. M.: Exercises for bedfast patients, Amer. J. Nurs. 66:2209-2213, 1966.

Kerr, A.: Orthopedic nursing procedure, ed. 2, New York, 1969, Springer Publishing Co., Inc.

Knocke, L.: Crutch walking, Amer. J. Nurs. 61:70-73, 1961.

Kraus, Sister R. A.: Polyurethane foam pads, Amer. J. Nurs. 65:98, 1965.

Larson, C. B., and Gould, M.: Orthopedic nursing, ed. 7, St. Louis, 1970, The C. V. Mosby Co.

Lawton, E. B.: Activities of daily living for physical rehabilitation, New York, 1963, McGraw-Hill Book Co.

Noonan, J., and Noonan, L.: Two burned patients on flotation therapy, Amer. J. Nurs. 68:316-319, 1968.

Olson, E. W.: Hazards of immobility. With: Thompson, L. F.: Effects on cardiovascular function; McCarthy, J. A.: Effects on respiratory function; Johnson, B. J.: Effects on gastrointestinal function; Edmonds, R. E.: Effects on motor function; Schroeder, L. M.: Effects on urinary function; Wade, M.: Effects on metabolic equilibrium; Wade, M.: Effects on psychosocial equilibrium, Amer. J. Nurs. 67:779-797, 1967.

Pesczynski, M.: Why old people fall, Amer. J. Nurs. 65:86-88, 1965.

Senf, H. R.: Caring for the patient in the CircOlectric bed, Amer. J. Nurs. 60:227-230, 1960.

Skinner, G.: Nursing care of a patient on a Stryker frame, Amer. J. Nurs. **46:**288-293, 1946.

Sorenson, L., and Ulrich, P. G.: Ambulation: a manual for nurses, Minneapolis, 1966, American Rehabilitation Foundation.

Toohey, P., and Larson, C. W.: Range of motion exercise: key to joint mobility, Minneapolis, 1967, American Rehabilitation Foundation.

Walike, B. C., Marmor, L., and Upshaw, M. J.: Rheumatoid arthritis, Amer. J. Nurs. **67:**1420-1426, 1967.

Chapter 4

Ventilation

Maintenance of the blood's access to oxygen is vital. If that access is inadequate, techniques that maintain ventilation may be ordered. Ventilation is the mass transport of air to and from the alveolar exchange surfaces so that carbon dioxide can be removed from the blood and be replaced by oxygen.

As air is transported from the atmosphere to the exchange surfaces, it is filtered and conditioned with heat and moisture. The level of its entry into the respiratory system affects conditioning. Gases inhaled through the nose are filtered, warmed, and moistened before reaching the exchange surfaces, while gases entering through the mouth pass less warm, moist surfaces. Gases that enter the trachea directly must be warmed and moistened by the tracheal and bronchial mucosa, which is not normally required to do this. During this process, removal of water from the mucous membranes subjects them to damage; the resulting inflammation causes increased production of secretions. These secretions tend to become viscous and may even crust, thereby impairing the sweeping action of the cilia. This may finally decrease the diameter of the bronchioles; obstruction inevitably results.

In health, certain spontaneous activities help to prevent or reverse changes that result in pulmonary complications. The use of simple nursing techniques for the same purpose must not be underrated or neglected. Following operative procedures or concurrent with reduced activity, a regimen involving periodic turning from side to side, deep breathing, and coughing may be ordered and is indeed useful. Other measures that produce alveolar expansion, change gas concentrations, and loosen and expel secretions are also used. These are forms of inhalation therapy now available in most hospitals.

Breathing exercises   Adequate explanation, early instruction, guided practice, judicious use of drugs, and incisional splinting tend to increase cooperation when breathing exercises are used. Ideally, teaching occurs some time before the actual need is present; for example, the surgical patient should be taught these exercises during the preoperative period.

For these exercises, it is desirable to assist the patient to a sitting position. If sitting up is contraindicated, the back-lying position will permit effective expansion of the lungs and effective coughing. Other positions are less effective.

The nurse encourages the patient to breathe deeply. If she holds her hands just below the costal margin, exerting firm, gentle pressure on the abdominal wall, she will feel the abdomen expand as the patient inhales. Pressing her hands firmly against this same area during exhalation may help the patient exhale more completely. This will also provide support during coughing. If the patient finds it more comfortable, he may hold a pillow or book against his abdomen (Fig. 4-1, *B*). Fig. 4-1, *C* and *D* show the use of a drawsheet to permit support of the incision and to provide pressure that assists exhalation. Fig. 4-1, *E* illustrates a method of hugging the patient to support the incision and to apply pressure that assists exhalation.

A simple breathing exercise consists of having the patient take three deep breaths by inhaling through the nose and exhaling through the mouth, slowly and gently. The patient expels a fourth breath forcefully with a cough. If an incision is involved, some method of supporting it by splinting should be used during coughing, as shown in Fig. 4-1, *A*.

A more extensive regimen consists of six series of five deep breaths, taken as described initially. Each series is followed by a short rest period. The thorax is divided into six areas. The nurse places her hand or the patient places his hand over a different area for each series of breaths, and the nurse directs the patient to concentrate on breathing against the hand, causing it to move (Fig. 4-2). At the conclusion of each series, the nurse encourages the patient to expel secretions from the lower respiratory tract with a forceful cough.

If the patient is unable to breathe deeply and cough effectively, the nurse may be able to achieve comparable results by

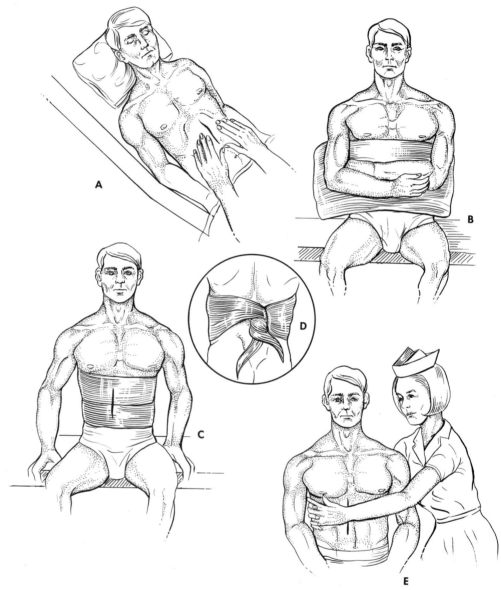

Fig. 4-1. Methods of splinting incisions. **A,** Manual splinting of incision. The nurse's hands exert firm, gentle pressure on the abdominal wall. The pressure is directed slightly toward the incision. **B,** A pillow pressed against the incisional area offers moderate support during coughing. **C,** Anterior view of the drawsheet folded into thirds and tightened smoothly over the incisional area. **D,** Posterior view of the drawsheet, showing the method of tightening it. The twisted ends are directly opposite the incision. **E,** Hugging the patient in this manner permits support of the incision as well as pressure that assists exhalation.

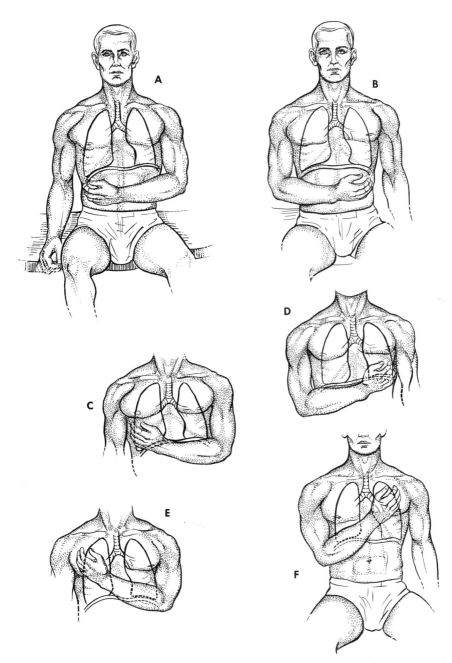

Fig. 4-2. Breathing exercises to encourage lung expansion. The nurse directs the patient to concentrate on moving the prepositioned hand with each series of deep breaths. **A,** The left hand is placed over the right side of the diaphragm. **B,** The right hand is placed over the left side of the diaphragm. **C,** The left hand is placed above the base of the right lung. **D,** The right hand is placed on the area above the base of the left lung. **E,** The left hand is placed over the apex of the right lung, with the fingers lying in the depression above the clavicle. **F,** The right hand is positioned over the apex of the left lung.

commanding him to "sniff" with his nose until he feels his lungs are as full of air as possible. The patient may use several short, deep, staccato coughs instead of one forceful cough to expel secretions.

Postural drainage   Postural drainage is the use of positioning to drain secretions from segments of the lungs and bronchi. Coughing will expel secretions that reach the trachea. Effectiveness of postural drainage depends on positioning that allows gravity to drain the secretions, liquefaction of secretions, ciliary action, and effective breathing. Secretions are liquefied by adequate hydration, humidification of gases, and the use of certain drugs. Drugs may be prescribed to dilate the bronchi also. These adjuncts must precede postural drainage if the effectiveness of this technique is to be increased.

During drainage, the nurse may use cupping and vibration to dislodge and mobilize secretions. Percussion or cupping involves rhythmic percussion of the area with the nurse's hands held in a cupped position and the fingers and thumb held together in a manner that traps air between the nurse's hands and the patient's chest. It is begun gently and increased in forceful-

---

Fig. 4-3. Postural drainage. Selected positions used to promote drainage from various parts of the lungs. Pillows are used to promote maximum comfort and relaxation. The nurse should place a pillow between the legs with the knee of the uppermost leg resting on the pillow, and pillows should be used to support the back when the patient is placed in a side-lying position. The nurse uses additional pillows to position the arms and may use pillows to achieve the desired angle of head down inclination if the bed cannot be adjusted for this purpose. After the patient has been in a position for the desired length of time and before he is changed from that position, the nurse should encourage him to breathe deeply and to cough effectively. **A,** Posterior segments of both lower lobes. The nurse should flex the patient's knees slightly and support them with a pillow to achieve a relaxed position. The head down angle of inclination is altered according to the patient's tolerance. **B,** Right middle lobe. The nurse positions the patient on his left side with the thorax tilted slightly backward, the buttocks elevated, the lower extremities flexed, the left arm abducted and flexed, the right arm resting on the bed or on pillows, and the head supported with a pillow. The head down angle of inclination is altered according to the patient's tolerance. **C,** Lingular segment of the left upper lobe. The nurse positions the patient on his right side with the thorax tilted somewhat backward, the buttocks elevated at the apex of the bed, the lower extremities flexed, the right arm abducted and flexed, and the left arm resting on the bed or on pillows. The head down angle of inclination is altered according to the patient's tolerance. **D,** Left lateral segment of the left lower lobe. The nurse places the patient on his right side, buttocks elevated, lower extremities flexed, right arm flexed, and the hand placed under the pillow to support the head. The left arm is abducted and flexed so that its palm and fingers rest on the head of the bed. The inclination of the head down angle varies with the tolerance of the patient.

ness as the patient tolerates increased percussion. Cupping should never be done over breast tissue because this causes discomfort and serves no useful purpose. Vibration is done by placing one's hands over the affected area and shaking from one's shoulders, thus shaking the area and mobilizing secretions. This shaking is comparable to the type of shaking one does when one chills.

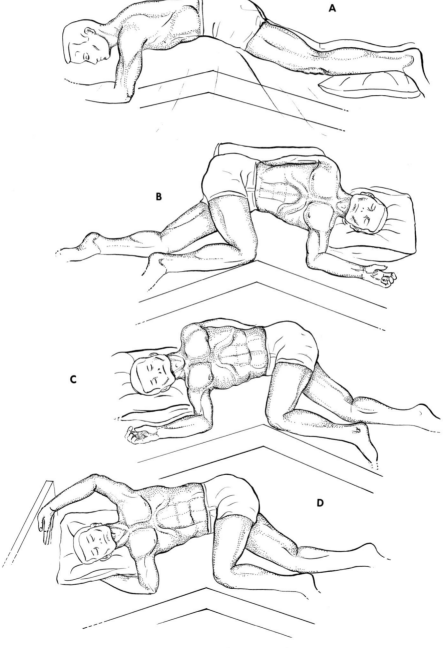

Fig. 4-3. For legend see opposite page.

Continued.

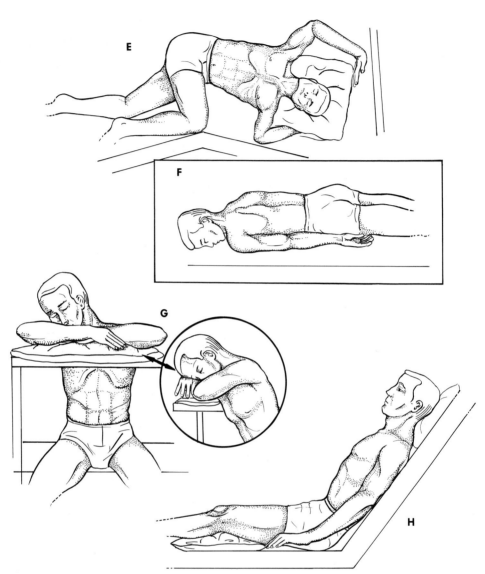

Fig. 4-3, cont'd. E, Lateral segment of the right lower lobe. The nurse places the patient on his left side with his hips elevated, the lower extremities flexed, the left arm flexed, and the hand placed under the pillow. The right hand rests on the head of the bed, and the head is supported with a pillow. The angle of head-down inclination varies with the patient's tolerance. **F,** Superior segment of the right lower lobe. The nurse places the patient in a prone position on a bed that is absolutely flat. This position places the bronchus from the superior segment of the right lower lobe at a nearly 90° angle to the floor. **G,** Posterior portion of both upper lobes. The patient is seated, his feet are supported, the shoulders are rotated anteriorly, and the arms are flexed. The arms may be rested on a pillow placed on the table as shown, or the elbows may be rested on the thighs. **H,** Anterior portions of both upper lobes. The patient is positioned with his back leaning backward at about a 45° angle, and the upper extremities are relaxed. This position can also be achieved by having the patient lean backward while sitting on the edge of the bed if someone is available to support him in this position.

Following postural drainage, percussion, and vibration, the nurse helps the patient, if he has been in a head down position, to a position favorable for effective coughing. Percussion and vibration should always be followed by breathing deeply at least three times and coughing deeply at least twice.

Head injuries and certain cardiac conditions contraindicate the use of head down positioning. Severe dyspnea does not necessarily contraindicate the use of a head down position, but the patient must not be left unattended during such positioning. His tolerance to a head down position will need to be developed gradually, starting with a minute or less and increasing the length of time as tolerated. The physician must be consulted to be certain that he wants the patient to have chest physical therapy if the patient has active hemoptysis, possible cerebral hemorrhage, cancerous lesions, or lung abscesses.

The nurse begins postural drainage at the patient's level of cooperation. Therefore, positioning may begin on a level surface with the degree of tipping the head down increased each time until the patient can tolerate full Trendelenburg positioning. The patient who is unconscious, severely dyspneic, producing more than a normal amount of secretions, or has a decreased cough reflex must never be left alone during postural drainage. Equipment for removing secretions with suction must be available if there is any evidence that the patient may be unable to expel secretions.

The physician identifies the areas to be drained with the aid of x-ray and bronchographic examination. The nurse individualizes positioning for each patient in a manner planned to promote relaxation. Properly placed pillows will enhance relaxation, promote drainage, help the patient maintain the desired position, and protect him from injury. Regardless of the positions used, the patient's spine should be as straight as possible to allow maximum expansion of the lungs. Because the patient's tolerance to a given position and the number of areas being drained vary, the time used for a given position will vary also. As a guide, one position may be used for a few minutes or for as long as a half hour.

Following postural drainage or chest physical therapy, the patient should breathe deeply at least three times and then cough effectively at least two times. Because secretions leave an unpleasant taste and feeling in the mouth, oral hygiene is important. Such therapy should be planned to precede meals and sleep. This seems to reduce nausea and vomiting that could cause aspiration of stomach contents into the lungs.

Fig. 4-3 illustrates some basic positions used for postural drainage. The nurse places the bed in Trendelenburg position if the patient can tolerate a head down position. The means by which this is accomplished depends upon the design of the bed.

It is important that the patient understand what is expected of him during chest physiotherapy. The nurse teaches this to the patient verbally and by example. The areas that the nurse must consider include the following:

1. Relaxation is of utmost importance.
2. One must breathe in through the nose to humidify and moisten the inhaled air.
3. Exhalation takes place through pursed lips as though one is whistling or saying, "Oh."
4. One must concentrate on the area on which the hands are placed.
5. The surgical incision must be supported during coughing.

The nurse must also spend adequate time in teaching the patient and his family as well as in motivating them if chest therapy is to be continued at home. The exact regime planned will vary with the patient's condition. For example, the nurse might tell the patient with bronchitis to cough after awaking in the morning if his chest feels rattly, then to breathe deeply three times, in through the nose and out through pursed lips, and, finally, to take another deep breath and cough deeply. The nurse would instruct him to carry out this same regime prior to meals and at bedtime.

Inhalation therapy

The physician evaluates the individual's need for and response to inhalation therapy. He prescribes what the gas concentration should be, how it is to be administered, and whether the treatment is to be continuous or intermittent. Table 4-1 shows oxygen concentrations possible with various equipment. Each general type of equipment has qualities that make it more desirable for some cases than for others.

Table 4-1

Oxygen concentrations possible with various equipment

Equipment	Approximate percentage concentration of oxygen delivered
Mask	
Rebreathing	90-100*
Nonrebreathing	40-100
Nasal cannula	30- 45
Face tent	30- 40
Oxygen tent	30- 40
Bennett respirator	40 to 100
Bird® respirator	40 or 100

*A percentage concentration of 100 indicates that the patient receives the gas delivered without outside air dilution; this gas is usually 99.7% oxygen.

Oxygen Regardless of the technique of oxygen administration used, the nurse must give the patient and his family some explanation, stressing the fact that the purpose of such therapy is to prevent damage. This will combat the mistaken belief that oxygen is given only to the dying.

Precautionary measures to ensure the patient's safety must accompany the administration of oxygen. Materials that produce static electricity, sparks, or flame are dangerous. Therefore, alcohol rubs are prohibited when an oxygen tent is in use, wool blankets are not permitted within the tent, and either a mechanical extension is attached to the electric call signal or a hand bell is substituted. Matches, ashtrays, cigarettes, and candles should not be permitted in the room. If oil or related materials are used, personnel must be trained to cleanse their hands thoroughly before operating gas therapy equipment.

Signs cautioning visitors and personnel that oxygen is in use and that smoking or other flames are prohibited must be displayed conspicuously. Direct communication that further emphasizes these precautions is recommended.

Oxygen masks. High concentrations of oxygen can be administered by mask. Essentially, the mask used will be either a partial rebreathing mask (Fig. 4-4, *A*) or a nonrebreathing mask (Fig. 4-4, *B* to *D*). The clinical technique involved is similar for both. If humidification of the oxygen is prescribed, the nurse prepares the humidifier by filling it to the designated level with distilled water. She attaches the mask to an oxygen supply and adjusts the flow as prescribed, often at 6 to 8 L. per minute. It is unusual for the flow to be greater than 12 L. per minute. During the short period after the mask is first applied, the patient may breathe more rapidly than usual. It is advisable to increase the flow to 10 to 12 L. per minute during this time, and then readjust the flow to the prescribed level when a normal breathing rate is resumed.

The oxygen must be flowing before the mask is fitted to the face. For the fitting, it is helpful if the nurse places the mask in the patient's hand and then places her hand over his (Fig. 4-5, *A*). By doing so she permits the patient to control the mask until he becomes accustomed to it. She places the mask over the bridge of his nose first, then over his mouth (Fig. 4-5, *B*). When the patient is accustomed to the feel of the mask, she places the retaining straps around the patient's head (Fig. 4-5, *C*) and adjusts them until the mask fits snugly, but not tightly, against the face (Fig. 4-5, *D*).

Observation to ensure that the mask is fitted correctly and that the patient is breathing properly is essential. The reservoir bag will expand and collapse with normal breathing (Fig. 4-5, *C* and *D*). If the bag collapses completely, the oxygen flow

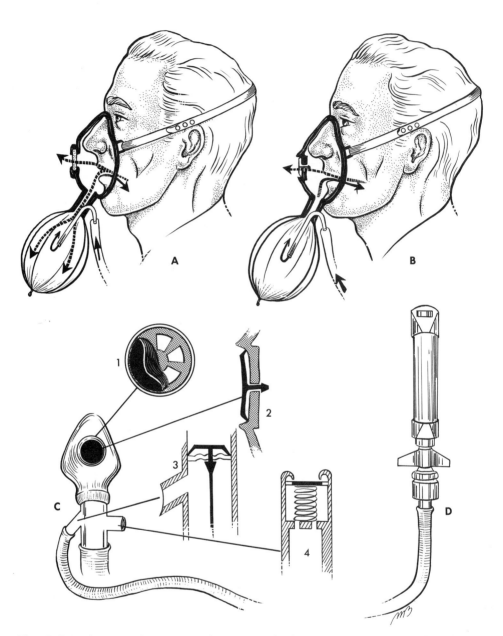

Fig. 4-4. Basic types of oxygen masks. **A,** Partial rebreathing mask. At end of inhalation oxygen is flowing into the reservoir bag, and exhaled gases also flow into reservoir bag until it is filled. If oxygen flow is sufficient to fill the reservoir bag immediately, no exhaled gas will flow into the bag. **B,** Nonrebreathing mask. Construction of the mask prevents exhalation into the reservoir bag. **C,** Front view of a nonrebreathing mask, showing construction of the valves: **1,** front view of exhalation valve; **2,** side view of exhalation valve; **3,** one-way inhalation valve construction permits oxygen to flow into the reservoir bag but prevents exhalation into the bag; **4,** safety valve permitting inhalation of air, if malfunction occurs. **D,** A preset valve attached to the oxygen inlet determines the concentration of oxygen.

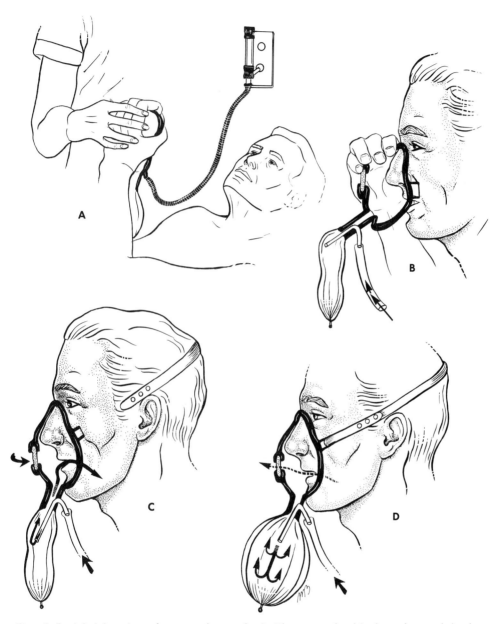

Fig. 4-5. Administration of oxygen by mask. **A,** The nurse should place the mask in the patient's hand and then place her hand over his. This permits the patient to control the mask until he becomes accustomed to it. Oxygen flow is set at 10 to 12 L. per minute during initial fitting. **B,** The narrow part of the mask is placed over the bridge of the nose. The mask is then brought over the mouth. **C,** Retaining straps are fastened after the patient has become accustomed to the feel of the mask. The reservoir bag collapses with inspiration; however, complete collapse indicates a need to increase oxygen flow. **D,** During exhalation the reservoir bag expands. When the patient is accustomed to breathing through the mask, oxygen flow is reduced as prescribed, often to 6 to 8 L. per minute.

needs to be increased. The nurse should correct leakage around the mask by repositioning it.

If the mask is used for prolonged therapy, the nurse should remove it periodically, wash and powder it lightly, or use a new disposable mask if one is available. Care of the facial skin must be meticulous if its healthy condition is to be preserved. Commonly, the mask and skin should be cared for every hour or two.

Nasal cannula. The nasal cannula may be used if the patient breathes through his nose. He must be discouraged from mouth breathing, for this dilutes the gas concentration with room air. The setting of the flowmeter determines the concentration of oxygen delivered.

The cannula is connected to a source of oxygen, the flow of the gas is set as prescribed (often at 4 to 5 L. per minute), the cannula is placed, and the retaining straps are fastened (Fig. 4-6). Higher flows of oxygen are quite uncomfortable and are

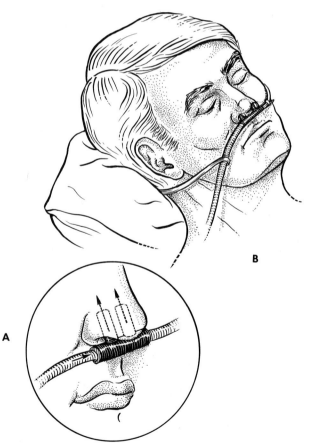

Fig. 4-6. Nasal cannula. **A,** A cross section showing insertion of cannula. Oxygen flow is set at a rate of 4 to 5 L. per minute. **B,** The cannula is held in place with retaining straps.

rarely used. The use of humidification should be related to patient comfort. The nasal cannula may be cleansed as necessary. If areas of irritation are present, a water-soluble lubricant or an anesthetic agent may be used for the patient's comfort.

Nasal catheter. The nasal catheter is used to administer oxygen nasopharyngeally. No additional benefit is gained from oropharyngeal placement; in fact, it stimulates the gag reflex. Initially, the nurse places the catheter oropharyngeally as a method of determining actual placement; however, it should be withdrawn 1 to 2 cm. (½ to 1 inch).

To approximate the depth to which the catheter should be inserted, the nurse measures the distance between the tragus of the ear and the external nares (Fig. 4-7, A). She marks this point on the catheter and uses it as a guide when she rotates the catheter between her thumb and forefinger to determine its natural droop (Fig. 4-7, B). The catheter is inserted in such a way that its curvature follows that of the nasopharyngeal passage (Fig. 4-7, C).

Prior to insertion, the nurse should test the catheter for patency and lubricate it. It is suggested that petroleum jelly or a noninflammable lubricant such as silicone grease be applied sparingly in order to avoid trauma to the mucosa during removal of the catheter. Water-soluble lubricants will not serve this purpose. **However, any oily material must be completely removed from the hands before the oxygen regulator is touched.** This includes such substances as mineral oil, petroleum jelly, and glycerin.

After the catheter is inserted, the nurse checks its exact placement visually. When the tip of the catheter is seen behind the uvula (Fig. 4-7, D), it is withdrawn about 1 cm., or approximately ½ inch (Fig. 4-7, E). The flow of oxygen is then regulated as prescribed. This may range up to 6 L. per minute. Flow rates above this are uncomfortable. As has been emphasized, humidification of gas for nasal catheters is essential. Frequent observations are necessary to determine that the catheter is patent. If the patient seems comfortable and the catheter is working well, cleansing is not indicated. Crust formation around the catheter or occlusion of its lumen indicates that the catheter should be changed.

Face tent. The face tent can be used to supply oxygen or mist. If it is used only to increase concentrations of oxygen, it is connected to the oxygen supply with small-bore tubing. If it is used to supply mist, a large-bore tubing must be used (Fig. 4-8). Also, the humidifier must be filled with distilled water, and the volume of mist produced is checked visually.

Prior to application, the flow of oxygen is regulated as prescribed. This usually ranges between 5 and 8 L. per minute.

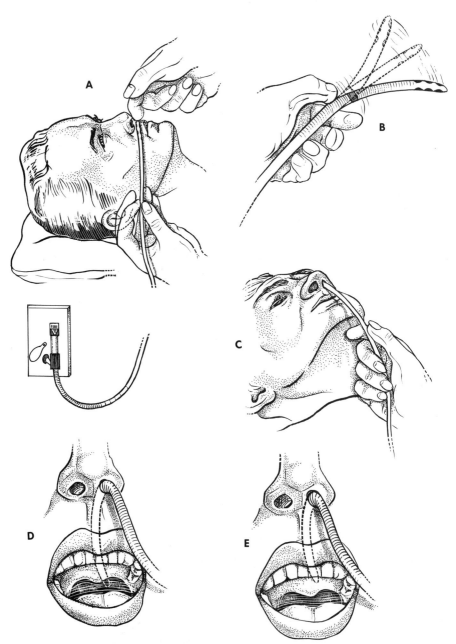

Fig. 4-7. Nasal catheter. **A,** Approximating the distance the catheter will be inserted by measuring the distance between the tragus of the ear and the external nares. **B,** Tape may be used to mark the predetermined distance of insertion. The catheter is rotated between the thumb and forefinger to find its natural droop. **C,** The catheter, lubricated with silicone grease, is inserted so that its curvature follows that of the nasopharyngeal passage. **D,** The tip of the catheter is seen behind the uvula. **E,** The catheter is withdrawn about 1 cm. (½ inch) to obtain correct placement.

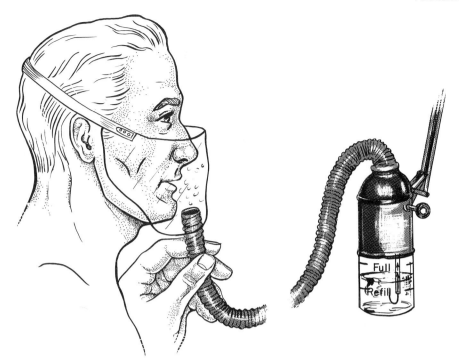

Fig. 4-8. Face tent. When the purpose of the tent is to supply mist, large-bore tubing and a humidifier are used. When its purpose is only to supply oxygen, small-bore tubing replaces large-bore tubing. (Courtesy Mist②gen, Oakland, Calif.).

The principles of applying the face tent are similar to those of applying masks. However, fitting presents no problem. The patient may prefer to hold the appliance in place. This permits its easy removal. Once the patient is accustomed to it, the nurse may adjust the retaining straps as desired.

Oxygen tent. The use of oxygen tents has decreased markedly in hospitals that have modern air conditioning. Occasionally, oxygen tents are used for patients who are too restless or are unable to cooperate in the use of other methods of administering oxygen or humidification. As stated previously, the patient needs reassurance and must be told its purpose before he is placed in an oxygen tent. The nurse covers the part of the mattress that will be within the tent with rubber, plastic, or other material that oxygen cannot penetrate readily.

The tent is placed near the head of the bed (Fig. 4-9, *A*). If piped oxygen is not available, the placement of the cylinder of oxygen should be planned so that it does not interfere with nursing care.

The nurse assists the patient to a comfortable position. Often a semisitting position is desirable. She folds the top linen to waist level unless the tent has a full, bed size canopy, turns on the air conditioner of the machine, and sets the temperature

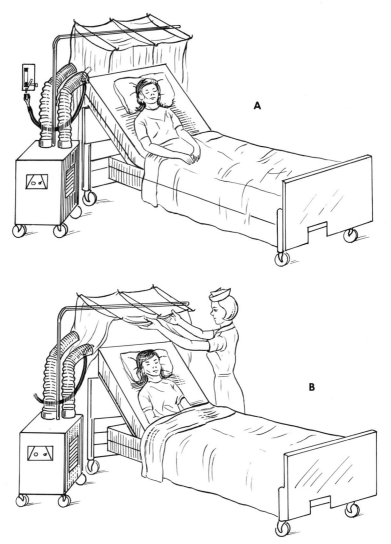

Fig. 4-9. Oxygen tent. **A,** The tent is placed near the head of the bed with its canopy draped behind the mattress. Oxygen flow is set at 10 to 12 L. per minute, the machine's air conditioner is turned on, and temperature is set at 70° F. (21.1° C.). **B,** The canopy is lifted over the patient, and the back of the canopy is tucked under the head of the mattress.

control, usually at 70° F. The temperature is altered for comfort, but it is not usually changed more than 10°. There is no need to cover the patient's ears or to enclose his shoulders with a blanket. If he complains of being too cool, the nurse should reset the temperature control. The flow of oxygen is usually set at 10 to 12 L. per minute.

After the nurse lifts the canopy carefully over the patient and tucks its skirt under the top and sides of the mattress, she arranges the lower edge around the thighs to minimize escape of oxygen (Fig. 4-9, *B* to *D*). Placing a folded bath blanket over

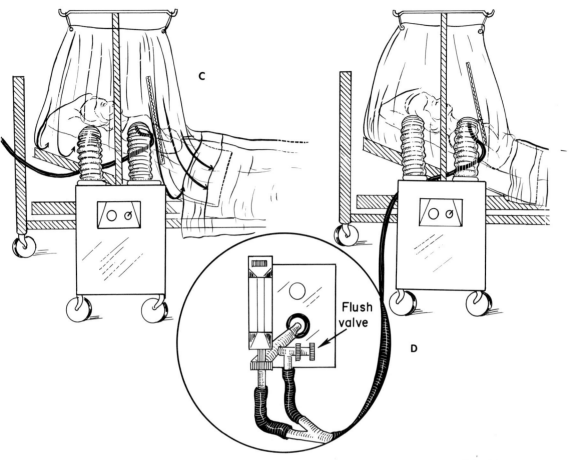

Fig. 4-9, cont'd. C, The sides of the canopy are tucked beneath the mattress, and the lower edge is arranged to conform to the patient's body. **D,** Linen that secures the lower edge of the canopy conforms to the body. The tent should billow when it is flushed with oxygen. The highest possible flow of oxygen should be continued for at least 1 minute.

the lower edge of the tent skirt and tucking it under the mattress will further secure the canopy. The top linen will serve the same purpose.

Initially, the nurse flushes the tent with oxygen for a specified period of time (Fig. 4-9, *D*). Because the flushing process varies with equipment, it is suggested that she open the flowmeter fully. If this causes the tent to billow, that is, bulge outward, the nurse should continue full flow for at least one full minute. If the tent does not billow, the nurse should check it for leakage by determining that the zippered openings are closed and that the canopy has been properly secured by tucking it smoothly beneath the mattress.

Each time care is given through the zippered openings, the nurse should flush the tent with oxygen for at least one full minute. For extensive care, the nurse moves the skirt of the canopy to the upper chest of the patient. After this, or after the tent has been removed for a time, the nurse should flush it as initially specified.

Determining oxygen concentrations   When the patient is receiving oxygen-enriched gases, the oxygen content of the gases delivered is measured to ensure correct concentration initially and at frequent intervals until the desired concentration is reached—then at prescribed intervals, commonly three times a day.

An oxygen analyzer is used to determine oxygen concentrations. Several designs are available. Some operate on either of two principles: (1) that the magnetic susceptibility of oxygen produces changes in a magnetic field or (2) that the thermal conductivity of the atmosphere varies with the amount of oxygen present. A third type operates on the principle that when oxygen is consumed by an electrochemical fuel cell, an electric current is generated in proportion to the amount of oxygen consumed.

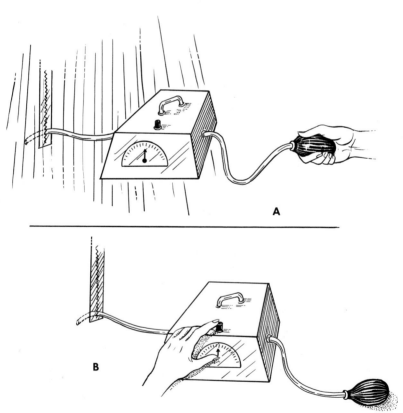

Fig. 4-10. Determining oxygen concentrations. **A,** With the oxygen analyzer held horizontally and the sampling tube inserted well within the tent, the bulb is squeezed a prescribed number of times to aspirate a sample. **B,** The switch button on the analyzer is depressed until the reading stabilizes.

Analyzers operated by magnetic susceptibility or thermal conductivity. The accuracy of analyzers operating on the first two principles may be influenced by the relative humidity, the temperature, the gas mixture sampled, the technique of obtaining the sample, and the position in which the analyzer is held. Usually, a horizontal position is necessary. Silica gel crystals used to alter the relative humidity of the sample must be checked for color changes prior to the operation of the analyzer. Because the color change indicating excess moisture in the crystals varies with the particular analyzer, the manufacturer's directions should be consulted for details of use and proper care of this equipment. Analyzers operated by thermal conductivity should be used to measure oxygen-nitrogen mixtures only.

To determine oxygen concentrations within a tent, the nurse inserts the sampling tube of the analyzer through an opening in the tent. Some tents contain a special opening for this purpose; the zipper opening may be used and may be preferable if mist production is used within the tent. The nurse places the end of the sampling tube well within the tent and distal to the source of mist because moisture tends to increase the need for maintenance of the analyzer. The nurse withdraws the sample with an aspirator, which consists of a rubber bulb attached to tubing. Compressing and releasing the bulb alternately a prescribed number of times allows its full expansion (Fig. 4-10, *A*). Following aspiration, it is necessary to depress the switch button until the reading on the scale stabilizes (Fig. 4-10, *B*). A second reading is then taken.

Analyzers operated by generation of an electric current. The oxygen analyzer that operates on the principle of an electric current being generated by a fuel cell in proportion to the amount of oxygen available can be used to determine oxygen content in an oxygen-enriched atmosphere or it can be fitted with adaptors to sample oxygen content of gases delivered by a ventilator. It differs from the analyzers described previously in that it is unaffected by relative humidity, ordinary temperature ranges, and the position in which it is held (Fig. 4-11). Maintenance involves changing the fuel cell. For details of this, consult the manufacturer's directions.

Determining accuracy of readings obtained by oxygen analyzers. Testing samples of room air and pure oxygen indicates whether the equipment is functioning properly, for atmospheric air contains 20.9% oxygen. The scales of all analyzers are calibrated from 0% to 100% oxygen. When determining oxygen content of gases being delivered to the patient, a second reading should be taken. Duplicate readings are of value in determining the stability of gas concentrations. The reading obtained is compared to the prescribed oxygen concentration, and the oxygen

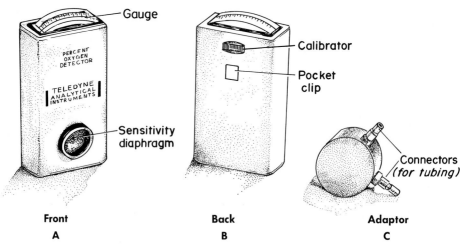

Fig. 4-11. Teledyne percent oxygen detector. **A,** Anterior view of the Teledyne percent oxygen detector showing the gauge and sensitivity diaphragm. The analyzer can be placed within any oxygen-enriched atmosphere to determine oxygen content. A reading can be taken within 30 seconds. **B,** Back view of the analyzer. The calibration button is used to calibrate the analyzer by turning the button until the pointer on the gauge matches the red line on the gauge. Calibration is done in room air. **C,** An adaptor can be placed over the sensitivity diaphragm and connected to tubes to sample oxygen content of gases being delivered by ventilators. (Courtesy The Harris Calorific Co., Cleveland, Ohio.)

flow is regulated accordingly. Erratic readings may indicate malfunction of the equipment, the presence of environmental factors that alter its accuracy, or improper technique.

Other gases

Carbon dioxide. A mixture of 5% carbon dioxide in oxygen may be prescribed for its pharmacologic effects on blood vessels, to eliminate volatile substances from the body, or to stimulate respiration. The nurse administers it intermittently and for relatively short periods of time, often 5 to 15 minutes. When carbon dioxide is used to dilate the cerebral blood vessels, it is necessary to use drugs to control response of the respiratory center. The nurse should administer the gas mixture by mask, using a technique similar to that described for oxygen masks.

Helium. A mixture of 80% helium and 20% oxygen reduces the work of breathing. When this mixture is used to relieve symptoms of asthma, the physician may prescribe its further dilution with additional oxygen. This gaseous mixture should always be administered by mask.

Humidity

Humidity of inspired gases can be improved as follows:
1. It can be increased approximately 10% with room vaporizers that disperse water vapor into the atmosphere or with a bubbler placed in the oxygen flowline.
2. It can be increased 90% with cool mist generators.

3. It can be increased 100% with heated mist generators when mists are delivered with a face tent or mask.

Room vaporizers. Adequate humidification can be obtained without boiling water. However, vaporizers that boil water to produce humidification are still in use. They are dangerous, and precautionary measures to prevent thermal injury must be observed. The vaporizer must be placed so that the vapor is projected from a safe distance—the distance required varies with the design of the equipment. In addition, placement of the vaporizer should be planned to prevent accidental contact with the vaporizer itself. This becomes extremely important when the nurse is dealing with children.

If the humidity of the air is to be increased appreciably by this means, the nurse should close the doors and windows of the room during therapy. Occasionally a croup tent is used to confine the vapor.

When the hot water vaporizer is used, the nurse should be aware that loss of body heat may be interfered with and that the patient may therefore develop a fever.

Inline humidifiers. Incorporating a mist generator or humidifier into the flowline of equipment for administration of compressed air or oxygen provides increased humidity. Heating the gas increases its capacity for transporting moisture. This is accomplished best by heating the water through which the gas passes. Therefore, in clinical practice, a heating element may be used in conjunction with an inline humidifier. If cool mist is desired, either the unit is not connected to electricity or a unit without a heating element is used.

The nurse should fill the reservoir with sterile distilled water. She should consult the manufacturer's directions to learn the method of filling a particular design of humidifier. This reservoir must be kept in an upright position so that it will function properly. If it is tipped, water may enter the delivery tube and block the flow of mist. Similarly, water may collect in the delivery tube as the result of condensation. If this occurs, the nurse should correct the position of the humidifier and remove the water from the delivery tube by draining it.

The flow of the compressed gas is adjusted to produce a steady flow of mist; with piped oxygen, a flow of 6 to 8 L. per minute is used. If mist is not produced, the equipment may need cleaning. The manufacturer's directions should be consulted, because the exact method of cleaning varies with the equipment used.

Nebulization of drugs

Certain drugs may be administered by inhalation. For this process, a nebulizer may be placed in the oxygen flowline. A nebulizer is inadequate for humidification purposes; therefore, if humidification is necessary, a large humidifier must also be incorporated into the flowline with the nebulizer.

The nurse should prepare the nebulizer by detaching it from its connection and placing the prescribed amount and kind of drug and diluent into it. She should replace the nebulizer in the line and check nebulization. Production of aerosol is related to the flow of oxygen.

Hand nebulizer. The nurse should connect the hand nebulizer to one extension of a Y tube supplied with oxygen. If the nebulizer is fitted with stoppers, the nurse should remove them. Then she should place the drug in the nebulizer and add a diluent, if it has been prescribed. She should turn on the flow of oxygen, usually to 4 L. per minute.

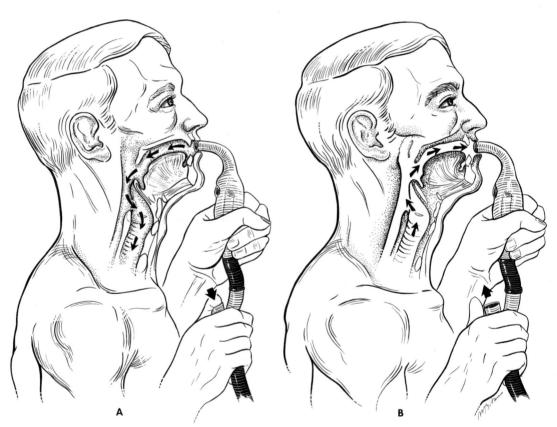

A   B

Fig. 4-12. Use of a hand nebulizer. **A,** After the drug is placed in the nebulizer, oxygen flow is set at 4 L. per minute, and the end of the nebulizer is placed in the patient's mouth. His lips must not close tightly around the nebulizer, and the small opening in the nebulizer should not be occluded. During inspiration, he occludes the free end of the Y tube to nebulize the drug. **B,** During exhalation, he removes his thumb from the end of the Y tube. Unless he does so, some drug will be wasted. If he desires, he may remove the nebulizer from his mouth during exhalation.

The patient is asked to place the free end of the nebulizer in his mouth. He must not close his lips tightly over the end of the nebulizer; rather he should be encouraged to keep his mouth open. Next, the nurse should ask the patient to occlude the free end of the Y tube with his thumb during inspiration. This routes the oxygen through the nebulizer and converts the drug to an aerosol. The nurse must encourage the patient to inhale when he occludes the free end of the Y tube (Fig. 4-12, *A*) and to remove his thumb from the Y tube when he exhales (Fig. 4-12, *B*). The patient should not swallow the drug, for doing so defeats the purpose of the therapy and may cause discomfort. If a supply of oxygen is not available, an air compressor can be used. Some nebulizers can be fitted with a bulb that the patient compresses manually to force air past the drug to produce an aerosol.

Positive pressure breathing units
Assisted ventilation

In response to inspiration, positive pressure breathing units deliver compressed gas into the airway under positive pressure until a preset pressure is reached. This is followed by passive exhalation through a valve that can be moved close to the patient. The resulting respiration is called *intermittent positive pressure breathing, inspiratory,* commonly abbreviated IPPB. Because the flow of gas is triggered by inspiration, the process is also termed assisted ventilation.

Use of IPPB units

Use of the IPPB units involves the combined efforts of the physician, inhalation therapy technician, and nurse. Initially, the physician or inhalation therapy technician adjusts the control settings to the needs of the patient. Indiscriminate manipulation of the controls is dangerous and should be prevented. After the controls are adjusted, the nurse should check them visually and observe the pressure indicator to make certain that the unit is functioning properly.

Prior to using the unit, the technician attaches a test lung to it to check the controls and to make certain that the unit is functioning properly. The test lung can also be used to demonstrate how the machine will help the patient breathe with less effort.

During the final preparation of the equipment, additional explanation is given, and the respiratory rate and rhythm of the patient are assessed. This information is used as a basis for determining whether the pressure selected is helpful to the patient. When the unit is applied to the patient, a decrease in respiratory rate means that the tidal volume is increased and that the patient is receiving assistance. If the respiratory rate increases, the pressure must be increased.

Observation of the pressure gauges during therapy is useful

in determining that the unit is functioning properly and that the patient is breathing with the machine. Prior to inspiration, the needle on the breathing gauge rests on zero. With inspiratory effort, the needle will show negative pressure of one unit or less; then it should move into the positive pressure zone as the unit switches on and gas flows into the airway. At this point, the patient can and should relax and let the machine fill his lungs. The needle on the breathing gauge will continue to rise steadily until the control set is reached. Then the unit switches off and permits passive exhalation. Deviation from this pattern suggests that the patient is not breathing with the machine or that the settings need to be changed.

If, on inspiration, the needle on the breathing gauge moves farther than one unit into the negative pressure zone, the patient is exerting excessive inspiratory effort. To correct this, the following measures should be carried out in this order:

1. Increase the pressure, which increases the tidal volume, thus improving the patient's ventilation.
2. Increase the flow in an attempt to meet the patient's demand for oxygen.
3. Urge the patient to cease inspiratory effort as soon as he feels gas beginning to flow into his airway.

If the unit does not switch on with inspiratory effort, its sensitivity is probably insufficient. If the unit has a special sensitivity control, readjust it to give the desired result. It must be emphasized that air should not be allowed to escape through the mouth or nose, or the unit will not switch off at the end of inspiration. If the patient finds it difficult to occlude his nose voluntarily when he is using a mouthpiece, apply a noseclip to prevent the escape of air through his nose. The patient must mold his lips around the mouthpiece. However, he should not clench the mouthpiece tightly between his teeth as though biting it, for this may permit air to flow around the mouthpiece or may even obstruct the flow.

If the unit switches off prematurely, the patient may be blowing into the mouthpiece before his lungs are filled with gas. He must be encouraged to let the machine fill his lungs completely and must be reassured that the unit will switch off automatically.

Pressure settings. Most units give little or no assistance if the pressure is less than 10 cm. of water. Pressure above this may be prescribed. The physician's prescription is, of course, limited by the capability of the machine.

Gas concentrations. IPPB units can be operated with compressed air or oxygen. When the latter is used, either 40% or 100% concentration is available with the Bird® medical respirator, and a 40% to 100% concentration is available with the Bennett therapy unit.

Humidity. When the mouthpiece is used, humidification is desirable; when a tracheostomy is present, humidification is essential. When a mask is used, the inhaled gas may or may not be humidified, depending upon the condition being treated.

Use of the nebulizer. Preparation of the solution to be nebulized must be in accordance with the physician's prescription. Usually the prescribed drug is diluted with a suitable agent. If the drug is inhaled more rapidly than prescribed or if it is not completely used within a specified period of time, the physician should be consulted. The nurse must assess the physiologic response to the drug and initiate nursing action that is appropriate. Permitting unused medications to remain in the nebulizer between treatments is dangerous. Not only does this predispose to inaccurate dosage, but also some drugs act as culture media for microorganisms; others may deteriorate and even produce toxic materials.

Specific units used for assisted ventilation

Of the available positive pressure units, the Retec Model N-30, the hand-E-vent II, one model of the Bennett IPPB therapy unit, and one model of the Bird® medical respirator are illustrated. The manufacturer's directions should be consulted for detailed information concerning the assembly, operation, and use of these and other models.

Retec Model N-30. This unit has no moving parts; operation depends upon the flow of gases through confined passages. It can be attached to piped or tank oxygen or to a compressed air source, and it will cycle automatically unless excessive leakage occurs. When aerosol production is desired, a nebulizer can be attached to the inlet. Pressure under which gas is delivered to the patient depends upon the flow rate of the gas. Usually the flow rate is set between 6 and 10 L. per minute when the nebulizer is not incorporated into the system. It is set between 10 and 15 L. per minute when the nebulizer is incorporated into the system. These settings deliver gas under an inspiratory pressure between 10 and 20 cm. of water.

If the patient is breathing with this unit, he is seated comfortably, seals his lips around the mouthpiece, inhales until his lungs feel comfortably full, then exhales. The machine will cycle off when the preset pressure is reached and will cause exhalation on its own, also. Removal of the mouthpiece is neither desirable nor necessary for exhalation. The device is designed so that the desired gas and nebulized material can flow only into the lungs, and exhaled gases flow only away from the lungs through the exhaust part of the machine. If the machine is cycling automatically, the patient can voluntarily override its cycle. Fig. 4-13 illustrates Retec Model N-30.

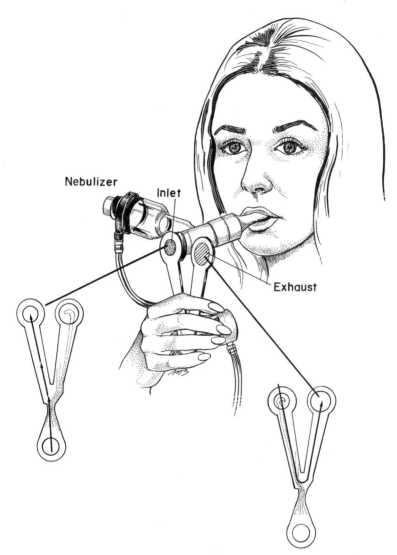

Nebulizer

Inlet

Exhaust

Fig. 4-13. Retec Model N-30. The prescribed medication and diluent are placed in the nebulizer. The flow of gas is set between 10 and 15 L. per minute. Arrows show the direction of gas flow during inhalation and exhalation. Intermittent manual occlusion of the exhaust port is used to control the rate of respiration as desired. (Courtesy Retec Development Laboratory, Portland, Ore.)

The hand-E-vent II. This unit can be connected to compressed air, an air pump, piped or tank oxygen. If a relief valve is used with a compressor, the maximum amount of pressure delivered at the mouthpiece is fixed at 20 cm. of water. When a compressor with a needle valve and gauge or compressed air or oxygen fitted with a regulator valve is used, the maximum amount of pressure delivered to the mouthpiece can be preset. The pressure to be delivered to the patient is set by occluding the porthole and opening the needle valve by rotating the control knob until the prescribed pressure registers on the gauge. The gauge is cali-

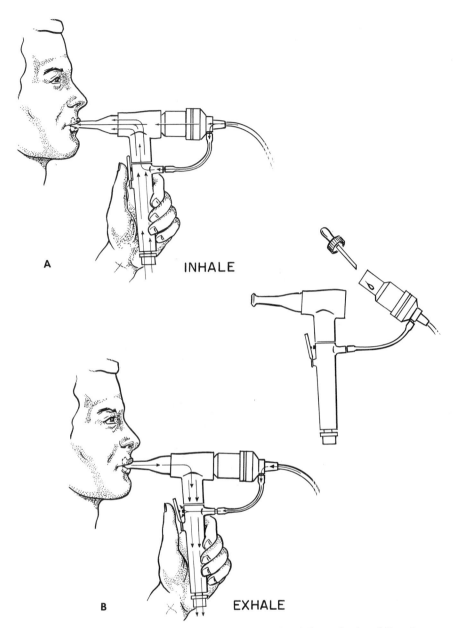

Fig. 4-14. Use of the hand-E-vent II. **A,** The nebulizer is removed from the hand-E-vent, and medication or distilled water is added as prescribed. The thumb is placed over the porthole during inhalation. **B,** The thumb is removed from the porthole during exhalation. (Courtesy Ohio Medical Products, Division of Air Reduction Co., Inc., Madison, Wis.)

brated in centimeters of water. The pressure prescribed is often between 10 and 15 cm. of water. The manufacturer's directions should be consulted for details regarding the use of pressure gauges and valves and for adjusting the pressure.

During use, the hand-E-vent II should be held in a horizontal position to ensure maximum nebulization and to avoid spillage.

If the patient is too ill to cooperate in the use of the hand-E-vent II, another IPPB device may be indicated. Patients who are sufficiently strong to sit up and who are able to cooperate can usually learn to use this device and may continue its use at home, as prescribed by the physician.

Teaching the patient to use the hand-E-vent II involves teaching him to prepare the nebulizer as prescribed by the physician, having him learn to seal his lips around the mouthpiece and to inhale with the nasal passages occluded by the palate or a nose-clip. Once the patient has learned that he can inhale and exhale through the handle of the machine without removing the mouthpiece from his mouth, he is ready to begin inhalation with positive pressure on inspiration. To do this, he occludes the hole in the handle of the hand-E-vent II and breathes in slowly until his lungs feel comfortably full (Fig. 4-14, *A*). To exhale, he removes his thumb from the porthole and exhales through the mouthpiece and, therefore, through the handle of the machine (Fig. 4-14, *B*). He repeats this procedure for the prescribed length of time, usually about 15 to 20 minutes.

Bennett therapy unit (Model TV-2P). The unit is connected to compressed oxygen with a regulator, to piped oxygen, or to compressed air. Prescribed medication or distilled water is placed into the bowl of the nebulizer (Fig. 4-15, *A*). After the prepared nebulizer has been replaced in the circuit, the oxygen to the nebulizer is turned on until a fine spray is produced (Fig. 4-15, *B*). If the humidifier has a heater (Fig. 4-15, *C*) and heat is prescribed, it must be connected to a source of electricity. Fig. 4-15, *D* describes regulation of production of mist with the flow of oxygen to the nebulizer. Set controls as prescribed by the physician (Fig. 4-16).

Initially, the therapist adjusts the oxygen flow to the nebulizer to produce a steady flow of mist. If the tube leading to the nebulizer pops off the connection, the oxygen flow to this point is too great and should be reduced. Failure of the nebulizer to function properly may also be related to loose connections. Tapping the side of the nebulizer will cause medication clinging to its walls to fall to the bottom so that it can be nebulized.

After assisting the patient to a comfortable position, preferably a sitting or semisitting position, the oxygen flow is turned on and the mouthpiece or mask is applied. The nurse should observe to determine that the patient is breathing with the unit and that it is functioning properly. (See also pages 101 and 102.)

Bird® medical respirator (Mark 7). The controls are set in the following order, beginning at the right side of the unit. The pressure control (Fig. 4-17, *A*) is set. Next, the oxygen (40% or pure O_2) concentration is selected. If 40% oxygen is desired, the air-mix control (Fig. 4-17, *B*) is pulled out. The expiratory timer

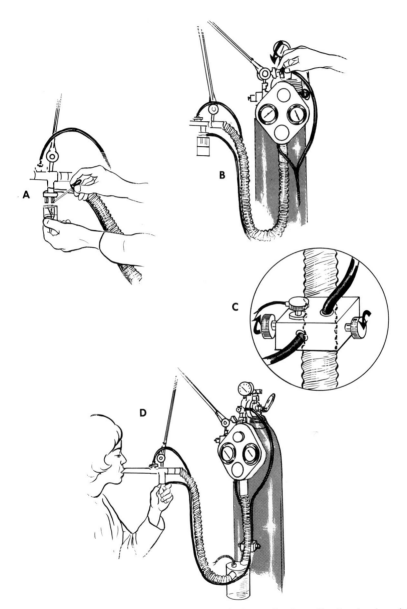

Fig. 4-15. Bennett therapy unit (Model TV-2P). **A,** Prescribed medication is placed into the bowl of the nebulizer. **B,** After the prepared nebulizer has been replaced in the circuit, the oxygen to the nebulizer is turned on (arrow) until a fine spray is produced. **C,** Valves when the heated mist unit is used. To regulate production of mist with the flow of oxygen to the nebulizer, the valve on the left side is closed, and the valve on the right side is opened, as shown by arrows. **D,** After the unit has been connected to oxygen, the nebulizer has been prepared, and controls have been set, it is applied to the patient. (Courtesy Bennett Respiration Products, Inc., Santa Monica, Calif.)

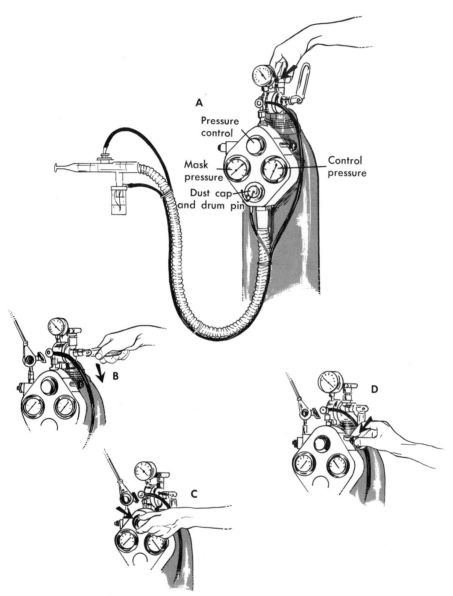

Fig. 4-16. Bennett therapy unit (Model TV-2P). **A,** After the unit has been connected to oxygen, the cylinder valve (arrow) is opened fully. If piped oxygen is used, the unit is connected directly to the outlet. A flowmeter is not used. **B,** The shutoff lever is pulled down completely to turn on the flow of oxygen. **C,** The control pressure is turned until the prescribed pressure is reached on the pressure control gauge. **D,** The oxygen concentration is selected. Pushing the lever in gives 40% oxygen; pulling the lever out as far as possible gives 100% oxygen. (Courtesy Bennett Respiration Products, Inc., Santa Monica, Calif.)

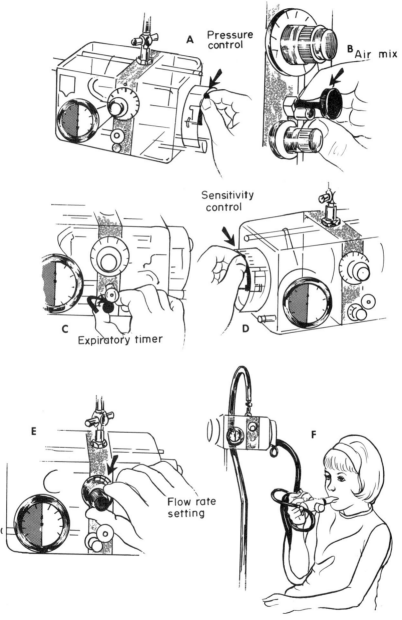

Fig. 4-17. Bird® medical respirator (Mark 7). **A,** The pressure control is set as prescribed. **B,** The air mix control is pulled out if 40% oxygen is prescribed. If pure oxygen is needed, this control is pushed all the way in. **C,** The expiratory timer is turned off. **D,** The sensitivity control is set. **E,** The flow rate setting is adjusted. **F,** The unit is applied to the patient. (Courtesy Bird Corporation, Richmond, Calif.)

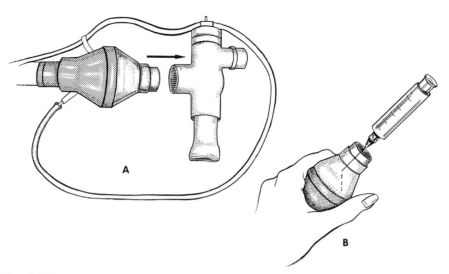

Fig. 4-18. Preparation of the nebulizer on the Bird® medical respirator. **A,** The nebulizer is disconnected from the mouthpiece and exhalation valve. **B,** Medication is placed in the nebulizer, which is then replaced within the breathing circuit. (Courtesy Bird Corporation, Richmond, Calif.)

(Fig. 4-17, *C*) is then turned off, the sensitivity control (Fig. 4-17, *D*) is set, and the flow rate (Fig. 4-17, *E*) is adjusted. These settings serve as reference points only. The physician must assess the individual's ventilatory needs and must alter the settings accordingly. A starting point of 15 is suggested by the manufacturer for the pressure, sensitivity, and inspiratory flow rate settings. After this unit is connected to compressed oxygen, the controls are set, the humidifier and nebulizer (Fig. 4-18) are prepared, and the unit is applied to the patient (Fig. 4-17, *F*). (For further elaboration, see "Use of IPPB Units," page 101.)

Resuscitation with
IPPB Units

If inspiratory efforts are not present, IPPB units can be used as resuscitators. The patient is positioned as described for mouth-to-mouth resuscitation (Chapter 1, pages 4 to 9), either an airway is inserted (Fig. 4, *A* and *B*) or the jaw is supported to relieve obstruction by the tongue (Figs. 1-2 to 1-4), and the mask is fitted snugly over the mouth and nose. Pressure should be set at 25 cm. of water or above.

The inspiratory phase is actuated by triggering the unit manually. On Bennett therapy units, the drum pin is flicked upward to initiate inspiratory flow (Fig. 4-19). With the Bird® medical respirator, the control rod in the center of the sensitivity ring is pushed quickly toward the center of the machine. This rod must be released immediately if the unit is to function as desired (Fig. 4-20).

If the mask is used for any extended length of time, air will

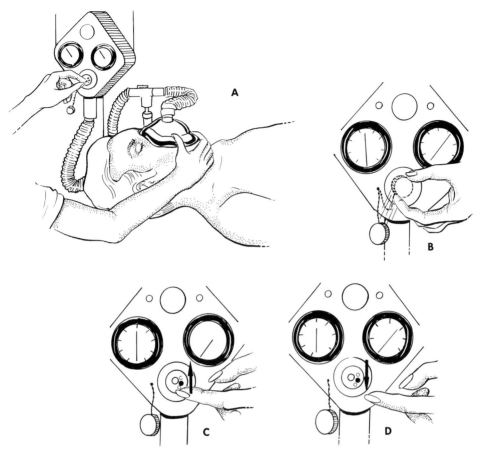

Fig. 4-19. Resuscitation with Bennett therapy unit. **A,** The patient is positioned to maintain patency of the airway, the mask is applied, and resuscitation is begun. **B,** Removal of the dust cap to expose the drum pin. **C,** The drum pin is flicked upward to initiate inspiratory flow. **D,** The finger is removed from the drum pin immediately. (Courtesy Bennett Respiration Products, Inc., Santa Monica, Calif.)

flow into the stomach and must be removed. Remove the air by gastric intubation or by external pressure on the epigastric region. Dangers that accompany the latter method are discussed in Chapter 1, pages 9 and 10. This problem is avoided when the units are used with a tracheostomy or tracheal tube.

Whenever resuscitation is necessary, the physician is notified immediately.

Controlled respiration. When the patient is unable to initiate inspiration, IPPB units equipped with automatic cycling devices can be used as respirators. The decision to cycle the machine automatically, thus controlling respiration completely, involves a medical diagnosis. Therefore, only the physician decides whether controlled respiration is indicated.

Constant vigilance is indicated when automatic cycling is

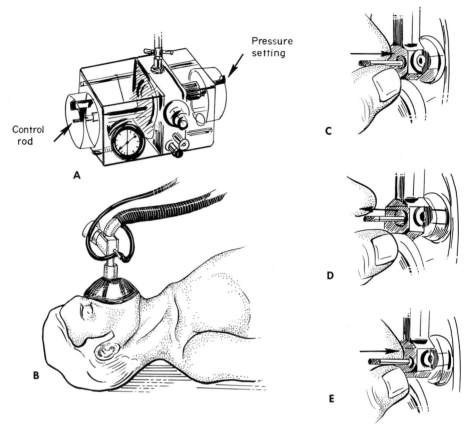

Fig. 4-20. Resuscitation with the Bird® medical respirator. **A,** The control rod used to initiate inspiration is located within the sensitivity ring. Pressure is set at 25 cm. of water. **B,** Patency of airway is maintained with positioning and an artificial airway. The mask is applied. **C,** The control rod is pushed quickly toward the center of the ring. **D,** The control rod must be released immediately. **E,** Following passive exhalation, the control rod is again pushed toward the center of the machine to start another inspiration. (Courtesy Bird Corporation, Richmond, Calif.)

used. The nurse should know that the characteristic sound of the unit cycling indicates only that the machine is operating, and she should realize the importance of observation to determine whether the patient is receiving the desired benefits. Methods of measuring expired volume are available. Also, various alarm systems may be incorporated into special units. When these are used, the nurse must find out how they work and must be familiar with the alarm system. If for any reason the mask or adaptor is displaced or the airway is occluded, the purpose of the therapy is thwarted and life is jeopardized.

If the unit is capable of exerting negative pressure during expiration, close supervision is mandatory. Misguided application of negative pressure can be dangerous.

Periodic deep inspirations (sighing). With controlled ventilation, periodic deep inspirations or sighs tend to prevent atelectasis. When these are prescribed, they can be accomplished with the described IPPB units as follows:

1. With the Bennett therapy unit, at prescribed intervals for a prescribed number of breaths, turn the pressure control (Fig. 4-16, *C*) fully clockwise, giving high pressure.
2. With the Bird® medical respirator, push the control rod in and hold it until the prescribed pressure is reached (Fig. 4-20, *C*). At this point, the control rod must be released immediately (Fig. 4-20, *E*). This action is repeated for the prescribed number of breaths.

Care of the temporary tracheostomy

A temporary tracheostomy may be necessary to preserve life. When the patient has a tracheostomy, humidification of inspired oxygen is essential, infection must be prevented, and secretions must be removed by a catheter introduced into the airway for aspiration. In addition, the inner cannula of the tracheostomy tube is removed periodically for cleaning. If either the catheter or the inner cannula is handled carelessly, large numbers of microorganisms will be introduced, and this introduction of pathogens can result in overwhelming infection. The described technique is aimed toward preventing such an outcome.

For suctioning the tracheostomy a suction apparatus fitted with a Y connector is necessary. Sterile supplies include a catheter, a basin containing hydrogen peroxide or another cleansing agent, a basin of sterile water, a tracheal tube brush, disposable gloves, and an external dressing. The diameter of the catheter used should be considerably smaller than that of the tracheostomy tube. For example, a No. 16 French catheter is used with a No. 3 tracheostomy tube.

After washing her hands, the nurse opens the tray and places the appropriate portion of the catheter on the Y connection. She then gloves the hand that she uses to introduce the sterile catheter (Fig. 4-21, *A*). Although some references state that the catheter should not be introduced more than 4 to 5 inches, or the length of the cannula, when secretions are a problem it should be advanced farther. This method of removing secretions from the tracheobronchial tree is also referred to as deep suction.

Tracheobronchial suction

To direct the catheter into the right main bronchus for tracheobronchial suction, the nurse turns the patient's chest slightly to the right and his head to his far left (Fig. 4-21, *A*). To suction the left bronchus, she reverses that position (Fig. 4-21, *D*). She observes the catheter to be certain that it curves toward and passes into the left bronchus. She does not apply suction until she has passed the catheter as far as possible without force. As she withdraws it, she rotates it continuously and applies suction (Fig. 4-21, *B*). When a collection of mucus is contacted, she

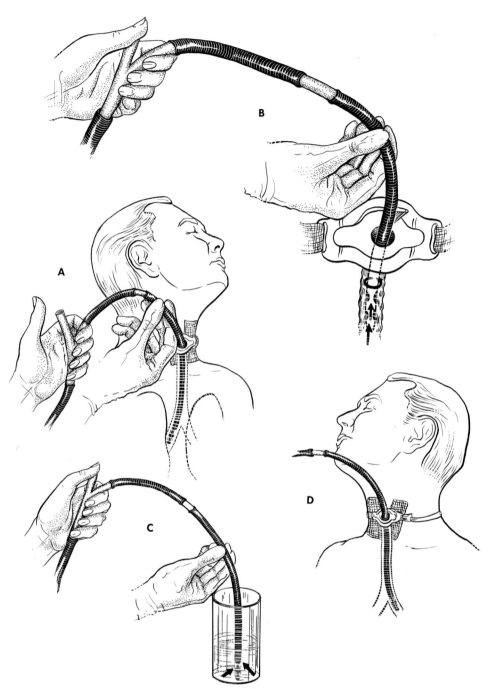

Fig. 4-21. Tracheobronchial suction. **A,** If the catheter is to be directed into the right main bronchus, the patient's chest is turned slightly to the right, and his head is turned to the far left. **B,** The nurse gloves the hand used to introduce the sterile catheter. Suction is not applied until the catheter has been introduced. As the catheter is withdrawn, it is continuously rotated while suction is applied. **C,** Sterile water is aspirated through the catheter, with attention given to the amount of mucus removed. **D,** The catheter is directed into the left main bronchus, and aspiration is repeated.

moves the catheter back and forth until the mucus is aspirated. She repeats this process until the catheter is completely withdrawn. Then she aspirates sterile water through the catheter, giving attention to the relative amount of mucus removed (Fig. 4-21, *C*). This process is repeated until the water appears clear following aspiration. However, the catheter must not remain in the airway for more than 3 to 5 seconds during any single aspira-

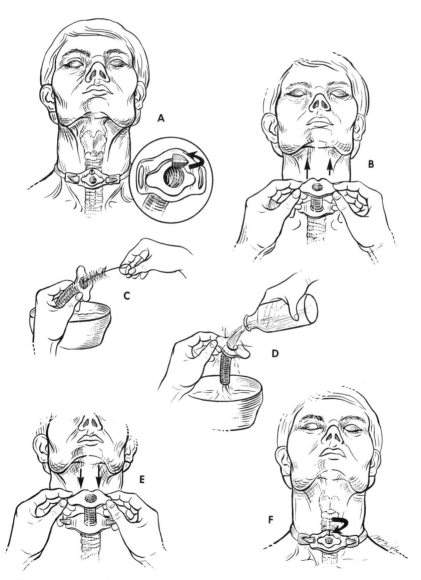

Fig. 4-22. Care of the inner cannula. **A,** The turn key is unlocked in preparation for removal of the inner cannula. The inset shows turning the key to unlocked position. **B,** The inner cannula is removed. **C,** Cannula is cleansed with brush and cleansing agent. **D,** Cannula is rinsed thoroughly with sterile water. **E,** Cannula is replaced. **F,** Turn key is moved to locking position.

tion. This same catheter is used throughout a single series of tracheobronchial aspirations unless it is contaminated. However, the next time secretions need to be removed, another sterile catheter is used.

Care of the cannula

When the secretions have been aspirated from the airway, the nurse removes the inner cannula (Fig. 4-22, *A* and *B*) and places it in a basin of solution for cleaning. The solution used varies. Hydrogen peroxide is helpful in loosening secretions; however, soap and water or other mild agents may be used. The inner cannula is brushed until it is completely clean when it is subjected to visual inspection (Fig. 4-22, *C*). Following this inspection the cannula is rinsed thoroughly with sterile water (Fig. 4-22, *D*). It is then replaced in the outer cannula and locked in place (Fig. 4-22, *E* and *F*).

Some plastic tubes have no inner cannula but possess built-in cuffs. Minimal inflation of these cuffs prevents leakage around the tube. The technique of inflation varies with the type of cuff or cuffed tube. It is necessary to deflate single cuffs from time to time. The more critically ill the patient, the more important it is to keep the cuff minimally inflated so that periods of deflation can be kept to a minimum. No hard-and-fast rules can be given for the prevention of damage to the trachea.

Inflation of cuffed tracheostomy tubes

When a tracheostomy tube is used for controlled ventilation, the nurse removes the inner cannula and fits the outer cannula with an adaptor that connects to the ventilator. The outer cannula and some single plastic tracheostomy tubes are surrounded by a single or a double inflatable cuff. The cuff can be inflated to seal the space between the tube and the trachea. If the tube has only one cuff, it is deflated for 5 minutes of every hour in order to avoid trauma to the trachea; if the tube has a double cuff, inflation of the two cuffs is alternated.

During initial inflation of the cuff, the tracheostomy tube is connected to the IPPB machine. Leakage between the trachea and the tube produces a gurgling sound. The person inflating the tube must listen to this sound carefully. The cuff is inflated with air until the gurgling sound just barely disappears. The amount of air needed to inflate the cuff varies but is often less than 5 ml. The method of inflating the cuff varies some with the design of the tubing used for inflation. In some the end of the syringe filled with air is inserted directly into the tubing; in others a syringe fitted with a needle must be used. After the cuff has been inflated, the inflation tubing must be sealed or clamped. This varies with the design, also.

The cuff should be deflated every hour. Prior to or at the time of deflation, secretions that have collected above the cuff must be removed by suctioning. This can be accomplished by placing the patient in Trendelenburg position for a few minutes to drain the secretions by gravity and then removing them with a catheter attached to suction. If a second or double cuff is present, it is inflated when the other cuff is deflated.

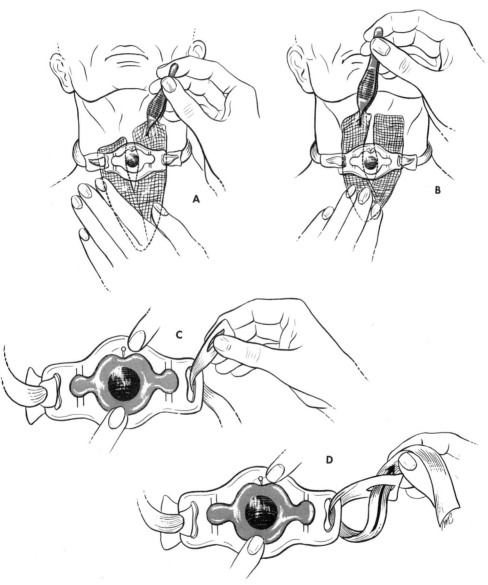

Fig. 4-23. Tracheostomy dressings and tie tapes. **A,** A prepared bib dressing is placed beneath the tie tapes and beneath the flange of the tube. **B,** Forceps are useful in positioning the dressing. **C,** An assistant holds the outer cannula to prevent its dislodgment when tie tapes are changed. Prepared tape is slipped through the opening in the flange of the outer cannula. **D,** The method of securing tape through the opening in the flange. Following this, the tapes are securely tied together with a knot at one side of the neck.

*Tracheostomy
dressings*

A bib dressing, fashioned by folding a 4-inch by 8-inch piece of gauze lengthwise and then into a V shape, or by splitting a 4-inch by 4-inch or 4-inch by 8-inch gauze dressing to approximately 1½ inches, is placed beneath the tie tapes and beneath the flange of the tube (Fig. 4-23, *A* and *B*). This protects the wound and the surrounding skin.

*Changing the tie
tapes*

The physician or the nursing coordinator usually assumes the responsibility for changing soiled tie tapes. During this procedure an assistant should hold the outer cannula securely but gently (Fig. 4-23, *C*), for manipulation or pressure will stimulate coughing, the force of which may dislodge the tube.

To change tapes the nurse will need two strips of twill tape, ⅜ inch wide and 15 inches long. The end that will be fastened to the flange of the tube is slit horizontally, about an inch from the end of the tube. After the tapes are fastened to the tube (Fig. 4-23, *D*), they must be knotted securely. Placing the knot to one side of the neck is desirable.

*Dislodgment of the
tube*

If the outer cannula becomes dislodged, an infrequent but serious occurrence, the nurse can maintain the airway by inserting a tracheal dilator or a sterile curved clamp into the stoma and spreading the incision apart. The physician will insert a sterile tracheostomy tube, which should be readily available. To do this, he lays aside the inner cannula and places the obturator within the outer cannula. After lubricating the tip of the obturator he slips the unit quickly into place. He immediately removes the obturator and attaches tie tapes to hold the outer cannula in place.

*Questions for
discussion and
exploration*

1. What natural methods do we normally use for humidifying inspired air?
2. Discuss the artificial methods for humidifying inspired gases, the advantages and disadvantages of each, and the relative importance of humidification depending on the anatomic point at which gases are delivered to the patient.
3. Mr. J. is scheduled to have abdominal surgery tomorrow. What will you teach him about deep breathing, turning, and coughing? What methods will you use to teach him?
4. If, during the postoperative period, Mr. J. is to receive oxygen by mask, what information must you know? What approach will enable him and his family to accept this therapy?
5. If a patient receives oxygen by nasal cannula, what factors will influence its effectiveness in delivering the percentage of oxygen prescribed? Why must he be encouraged to breathe through his nose?
6. If Mr. S. needs humidified gases, the physician might order mist with oxygen to be delivered to Mr. S. via a face tent. How can you troubleshoot the equipment used when it seems not to be working well?
7. For what reason might a nasal catheter be used? How often does it need to be changed? What effects will the catheter have on the mucous membrane lining the nose if it is lubricated with a water-soluble lubricant and remains in place for several days?

8. Compare the flow rates used for a cannula, catheter, face tent, and face mask. How can you know if the prescribed flow rate is adequate?

9. What are the inherent dangers in using pure oxygen, pure helium, or a high percentage of carbon dioxide for inhalation therapy?

10. Mrs. R. asks your opinion about a room vaporizer that she plans to purchase for use with her preschool children. What factors can you help her consider prior to making a selection?

11. Discuss the qualities of drugs used in your hospital for inhalation therapy. Would drugs with an oil base be prescribed? Why should the nebulizer be cleansed following use? Why must the nurse administering drugs by inhalation therapy know the side effects, toxic effects, and expected effects of drugs that are inhaled? Can you determine a common denominator for dosage of drugs given by this method?

12. If you are to assist a patient in learning to use an IPPB device effectively, what must you be able to explain to him as reasons for this therapy? How will you know if he is using the device correctly? If he uses it improperly, how can you help him learn to breathe properly with the device? What sort of emotional support should you be able to give him?

13. As you turn on the Bennett IPPB therapy unit and the patient begins to use it, a tube pops off and nebulization of the drug ceases. How can you correct this problem?

14. If one continues to aspirate tracheal secretions for an extended period of time, what is likely to happen to the patient that may necessitate emergency action? Why?

15. What are the differences in resuscitating someone with various IPPB devices?

16. Why should a mask being used with an IPPB machine to resuscitate be replaced with a tracheostomy or endotracheal tube as soon as possible?

17. Patients and the families of patients who have tracheostomies need a great deal of emotional support. How can you provide this? Compare the different reactions that can be anticipated if the tracheostomy is done as an emergency procedure to those expected if the patient and his family are told beforehand that a tracheostomy is necessary.

18. Why do you suppose that the use of sterile rather than clean technique for tracheostomy care is gaining increasing favor by many authorities in respiratory care?

19. If you note an unpleasant odor that seems related to soiled tie tapes on a tracheostomy tube, what action can you take? What precautions must be used in changing the tie tapes?

20. If a patient is to leave the hospital with a tracheostomy tube in place, what teaching would be needed? What supplies should be available to the patient at home?

21. If a patient has a permanent tracheostomy, how can he or she protect the fenestration so that foreign materials will not be inhaled and the opening will not be apparent? Consider the possibilities for men, women, and children.

22. If you learn that relatives are crying for unknown reasons and you are able to elicit from them that they feel their relative is dying because he is receiving oxygen, how can you help them? How might this situation have been prevented if oxygen therapy were simply a part of the therapeutic plan?

Selected references   Adler, R. H., and Brodie, S. L.: Postoperative rebreathing aid, Amer. J. Nurs. **68**:1287-1289, 1968.

Bendixen, H. H., Egbert, L. D., Hedley-Whyte, J., Laver, M. B., and Pontoppidan, H.: Respiratory care, St. Louis, 1965, The C. V. Mosby Co.

Betson, C.: Blood gases, Amer. J. Nurs. **68**:1010-1012, 1968.

Burgess, A. M.: A comparison of common methods of oxygen therapy for bed patients, Amer. J. Nurs. **65**:96-99, 1965.

Burns, H. L.: A pure fluid cycling valve for use in breathing equipment, Inhalation Therapy **69**:11-19, 1969.

Cherniak, R. M.: Care of tracheostomy, Canad. Anaesth Soc. J. **12**:386-397, 1965.

Eastwood, D., and Mabrey, J. K.: Suction and the maintenance of an airway, Amer. J. Nurs. **53**:552-553, 1953.

Egan, D. F.: Fundamentals of inhalation therapy, St. Louis, 1969, The C. V. Mosby Co.

Flatter, P. A.: Hazards of oxygen therapy, Amer. J. Nurs. **68**:80-84, 1968.

Fordham, M. E.: Cardiovascular surgical nursing, New York, 1962, The Macmillan Co.

Geis, D. P., and Lambertz, S. E.: Acute respiratory infections in young children, Amer. J. Nurs. **68**:294-297, 1968.

Hadley, F., and Bordicks, K. J.: Respiratory difficulty: causes and care, Amer. J. Nurs. **62**:64-67, 1962.

Hanamey, R.: Teaching patients breathing and coughing techniques, Nurs. Outlook **13**:58-59, 1965.

Helming, M., editor: Nursing in respiratory disease, Nurs. Clin. N. Amer. **68**:381-487, 1968.

Kurihara, M.: Postural drainage, clapping and vibrating, Amer. J. Nurs. **65**:76-79, 1965.

Kurihara, M.: Assessment and maintenance of adequate respiration, Nurs. Clin. N. Amer. **68**:65-76, 1968.

Nett, L. M., and Petty, T. L.: A new IPPB device for bronchial hygiene, Amer. J. Nurs. **68**:2570-2571, 1968.

Physiotherapy for medical and surgical thoracic conditions, London, 1967, Physiotherapy Department, Brompton Hospital.

Pitorak, E. F.: Laryngectomy, Amer. J. Nurs. **68**:780-786, 1968.

Rae, N. M.: Caring for patients following open heart surgery, Amer. J. Nurs. **63**:77-82, 1963.

Robinson, F. N.: Nursing care of the patient with pulmonary emphysema, Amer. J. Nurs. **63**:92-96, 1963.

Seedor, M.: Therapy with oxygen and other gases: a programmed unit in fundamentals of nursing, Philadelphia, 1966, J. B. Lippincott Co.

Shafer, K. N., Sawyer, J. R., McCluskey, A. M., and Phipps, W. H.: Medical-surgical nursing, ed. 5, St. Louis, 1971, The C. V. Mosby Co.

Sovie, M., and Israel, J.: Use of the cuffed tracheostomy tube, Amer. J. Nurs. **67**:1854-1856, 1967.

Totman, L. E., and Lehman, R. H.: Tracheostomy care, Amer. J. Nurs. **64**:96-99, 1964.

Chapter 5

Administration of drugs

Interpretation and implementation of orders for drug therapy utilize considerable knowledge of the patient, the drug, and the plan of therapy. Knowledge of the nature of the drug, the usual range of dosage, dosage forms, methods and techniques of administration, expected effects, and symptoms of overdosage offers guidance. Reliable sources of information should be consulted whenever necessary. In addition, the reason the patient is receiving the drug, any history of previous drug reactions—including allergy and idiosyncrasy—and information transmitted by the physician should be used if the acceptance of drug therapy is to be promoted. Frequently, the physician discusses the plan of therapy with the patient and his family. It is always wise to know what the patient has been told and his interpretation of this information. Special circumstances may restrict the information given to the patient. Such restriction precludes discussion of the therapy in these instances.

Clinical response to the therapy is used to alter drug therapy. For this reason, drugs are withheld prior to certain laboratory tests and in the presence of significant physiologic reactions. For example, morphine is withheld if the respirations are 12 or less per minute, and oral drugs are withheld if the swallowing reflex is absent or persistent vomiting is present. Knowledge of these circumstances is used to guide the decision to consult the physician for further orders.

Thoughtful consideration of the patient's comfort will influence his acceptance of the therapy. The nurse should assist him to assume a comfortable position that is compatible with his condition and the method of planned administration and should give him a brief, though not frightening, explanation of what is to be done and what is expected of him. Unless it is contraindicated, she should offer a brief explanation of the purpose of the medication and of effects that might otherwise prove frightening. For example, the surgical patient who has epilepsy may be relieved to know that the injection he is receiving contains medication to control this condition, and a patient is less likely to be worried by discoloration of the sputum, stool, or urine if he has been forewarned. If the drug depresses the central nervous system appreciably, necessary limitations of activity should be explained and emphasized.

The patient's record should include notations concerning the drug and dose given, the method of administration, and the reaction to therapy. Additional records will be required if the drug is being investigated. Compliance with state and federal drug legislation necessitates additional records for certain drugs. These include narcotics and other habit-forming drugs.

Legally, the physician's order should state the preparation, dose, and method and frequency of administration. It may also contain additional directions. In all cases, the order is to be used intelligently, and the physician is to be consulted if a change in the order appears to be indicated.

The nurse may transcribe the order to a medication card, also called an identification card. Although these vary in form, they usually contain the full name of the patient, hospital room number, name of the drug, dose, times and method of administration, date the order was written, date the order expires when this is known, and initials of the person transcribing the order. This information should be rechecked prior to the preparation of each subsequent dose and should be used to identify the dose while it is being transported to the patient. In addition, the card serves to identify the room number and the patient.

Frequently, the exact times of administration become a nursing responsibility. Establishment of these times should be planned to provide for consistency and to promote the purpose of the therapy. Table 5-1 is planned to avoid meals served at 7:30 A.M., 11:30 A.M., and 5:30 P.M. A few drugs should be administered at mealtime, and sleep may need to be interrupted in order to maintain the blood level of certain drugs. No time is stated in the table for medications given at the hour of sleep, since this time is individualized, though it is frequently between 10 and 10:30 P.M.

Table 5-1

Suggested times for drug therapy*

Abbreviation	Interpretation	Time of administration
a.c.	before meals	7-11-5
b.i.d.	twice a day	9-7
p.c.	after meals	9-1-7
p.r.n.	whenever necessary	dose may be repeated according to stated time interval
q.d.	every day	9 a.m.
q.h.	every hour	7-8-9-10, etc.
q. 2 h.	every 2 hours	7-9-11, etc.
q. 3 h.	every 3 hours	6-9-12-3, etc.
q. 4 h.	every 4 hours	8-12-4-8
q. 6 h.	every 6 hours	6-12-6-12
q.i.d.	four times a day	9-1-4-7
si op. sit.	if necessary	
stat.	immediately	

*These are the suggested hours for drug administration if meals are served at 7:30, 11:30, and 5:30.

A stock supply or an individual supply of medication is dispensed by the pharmacist and stored in a medication locker unless the patient is permitted to take the medication as the need arises. In this case, the physician may permit the medication to be left at the bedside.

Preparation of the single dose may involve mathematical computation, which becomes the nurse's responsibility. The use of prepackaged single doses of drugs tends to conserve nursing time and provides· identification of the drug and the dose during transport. The name of the drug and the dose are printed on the wrapper of strip-packaged drugs; therefore, the wrapper is left intact until the drug has been taken to the bedside and is about to be administered. Before preparing or administering a drug, the hands should be as clean as possible. (See section entitled "Hand Washing" in Chapter 2.)

After preparing the individual dose, the nurse is ready to administer the drug. She must take precautions to identify the drug and the patient by comparing the information on the medication card with the information found at the door, the bedside, and the identification bracelet. In addition, she should state the patient's name or ask him to state his name. The latter is useful when it is uncertain that the patient understands the nurse. If the patient is to continue taking the drug at home, it is important to teach him when and how to take it and also to give him information concerning adverse effects that should cause him to contact his physician. Teaching should begin early. It is helpful if written instructions to which the patient may refer are given to him.

Oral, sublingual, and buccal administration

The preparation of doses for oral, sublingual, and buccal administration is similar. Guidelines, such as checking the label when the drug is removed from the shelf, before it is placed into the medication cup, and again when the stock medication is being returned to the shelf, are useful in making certain that the correct drug and dose are prepared. If the medication is individually packaged, the wrapper enclosing it is imprinted with identifying information and should remain intact during transport to the bedside. Medications should be removed from a bottle without contact with the medication itself. Liquid preparations are measured into a calibrated medicine glass or with calibrated medicine droppers. For the former, the bottom of the meniscus rests on the calibration line. Manipulating the cover of the container enables the nurse to remove solid dosage forms without touching them.

Unless contraindicated, the patient should swallow oral medications with sufficient water to lubricate solid forms as well as to dissolve and dilute the drug. The nurse should give drugs that are harmful to the teeth to the patient through a straw. She should disguise, as necessary, preparations with a disagreeable taste. However, she should avoid the use of foods if possible. If the patient is unable to swallow a solid medication, the nurse should ask for permission to use a more suitable form.

Sublingual administration of drugs consists of placing the tablet beneath the patient's tongue and instructing him to retain it in this location until it has dissolved (Fig. 5-1, A). Buccal administration of drugs involves placing the tablet between the cheek and the teeth until it dissolves (Fig. 5-1, B).

Inhalation

A few drugs are available in single, fragile ampules, also called pearls, which are sheathed in a loosely woven cloth covering (Fig. 5-2, A). These are crushed at the bedside (Fig. 5-2, B), and the saturated cloth is held near the patient's face so that he inhales the released vapor as it is passed back and forth (Fig. 5-2, C). Drugs such as amyl nitrite and spirits of ammonia act quickly, and overdosage is prevented by permitting only 2 to 3 inhalations per dose. Inhalation of nebulized drugs is discussed in Chapter 4, pages 99 to 101, 103 to 107, and 109 to 110.

Eyedrops and ointments

Care to instill the correct strength, amount, and drug into the correct eye is essential. The following abbreviations are com-

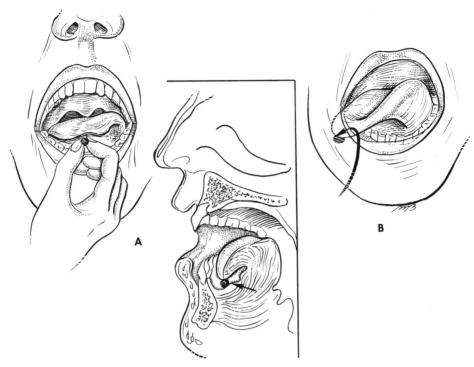

Fig. 5-1. Oral medications. **A,** Sublingual administration. **B,** Buccal administration.

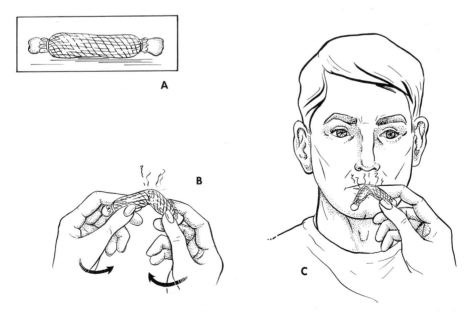

Fig. 5-2. Inhalation of vapors. **A,** A fragile ampule sheathed in loosely woven cloth. **B,** Crushing the ampule releases vapor. **C,** The saturated cloth is held near the patient's face for inhalation of vapor.

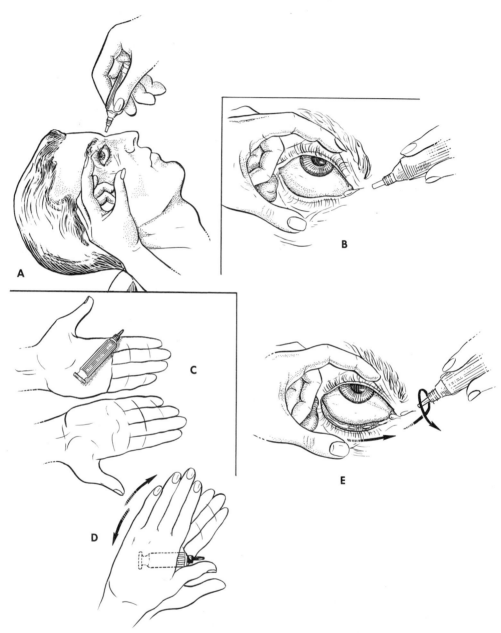

Fig. 5-3. Eyedrops and ointments. **A,** The nurse positions the patient and exposes the cul de sac. **B,** She places drops in the lower cul de sac. The approach to the eye assists the patient in rotating his eye away from the point of instillation. **C,** The nurse warms the ointment by holding the tube in the hand. **D,** She rolls the tube between the palms of the hands to hasten the warming process. **E,** She squeezes ointment from the tube into the cul de sac, rotating the tube rapidly to detach ointment from it. A cotton pledget held in the hand that retracts the lower lid is used to absorb excess drug.

monly used to designate the eye to be treated: O.D., right eye; O.S., left eye; and O.U., both eyes. Prescribed strengths are necessarily dilute. Frequently, a strength of less than 1% is used, although a few drugs may be used in a strength as high as 10%. Prior to instillation, the drug should be at room temperature and should be examined for signs of deterioration. Ointment dispensed in small tubes can be warmed by holding the tube in the hand for a few minutes (Fig. 5-3, *C* and *D*). Cloudiness or precipitation almost always represents deterioration. If the nurse observes this, she should return the drug to the pharmacy and obtain a new supply.

The nurse should position the patient comfortably, either in a back-lying position with his face directed upward or in a sitting position with his head supported as necessary to maintain a chin-up position. With a drop dispenser, either a medicine dropper or a dropper bottle, held in one hand, the nurse exposes the cul-de-sac by gently retracting the tissue proximal to the lower eyelid. She instructs the patient to look up, thereby rotating the eye upward and removing the sensitive cornea from the point of instillation. If she approaches the eye from above its inner angle, she thereby helps the patient to rotate his eye upward. She should not allow the dispenser to touch the eye nor let the medication fall on the cornea, for this produces a reflex squeezing-together of the eyelids that can damage recent surgical repair. A cotton pledget held in the hand that retracts the lower lid is used to absorb excess drug (Fig. 5-3, *A*, *B*, and *E*), or, if indicated, to remove excess drug. For this, the eye may be wiped gently from the inner to the outer canthus, that is, from the nose to the outside of the eye. When both eyes are medicated, clean pledgets should be used for each eye. This reduces the possibility of transferring organisms from one eye to the other.

Eardrops

Occasionally, instillation of eardrops is prescribed. To instill drops, the nurse asks the patient to turn his head to the side so that the ear being treated faces upward. She then manipulates the external ear gently to expose the orifice of the external canal and drops the medicine against the internal wall of the canal (Fig. 5-4). Gentle retraction of the external ear is directionally upward and posteriorly in a child and downward and posteriorly in an adult.

Nose drops

Infrequently, nasal instillations are prescribed. When drops are to be instilled, the nurse tilts the patient's head backward by elevating his shoulders with pillows. Then she instills the drops (Fig. 5-5). Unless doing so is contraindicated, the patient may lower his head over the edge of the bed, or, if he

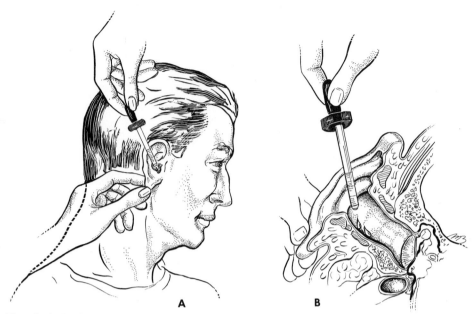

Fig. 5-4. Eardrops. **A,** The nurse asks the patient to turn his head to the side so that the ear being treated faces upward. She then manipulates the external ear gently to expose the external canal. **B,** The nurse directs the medication toward the internal wall of the canal.

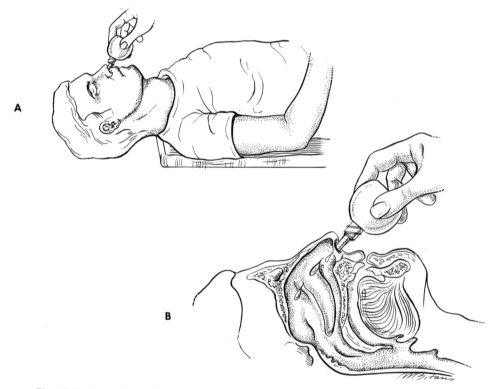

Fig. 5-5. Nose drops. **A,** The patient's head is tilted backward by elevating his shoulders. **B,** Cross section showing instillation of drops.

is in a sitting position, he may hyperextend his neck. If a nasal spray is prescribed, the patient is placed in a sitting position. Expectoration of medicine that enters the pharynx following instillation is desirable.

Genitourinary tract instillations

Prior to instilling medications into the genitourinary tract, the nurse assists the patient to a back-lying position with her legs flexed, and partially adducted (Fig. 5-6, *A*). A lithotomy position or a modified Sims' position may be used, if preferred. A drape is arranged so that the area is exposed. After washing her hands, putting on sterile gloves, and cleansing the area, the nurse locates the orifice and administers the drug. Every effort must be made to prevent introduction of organisms into the urethra and bladder.

Knowledge that a prescribed drug is likely to discolor clothing is useful in guiding the patient's choice of clothing following this treatment; sanitary pads may be provided to protect clothing from permanent staining.

Bladder

Catheterization precedes instillation of medications into the bladder. Catheterization is described in Chapter 10 and illustrated in Fig. 10-2. After the bladder has been drained, the catheter is kept in place, and a sterile funnel through which

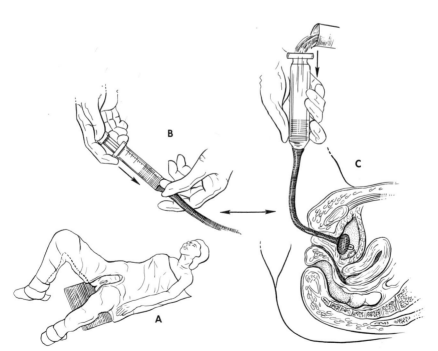

Fig. 5-6. Bladder instillation. **A,** Position of the patient. **B,** Medication may be instilled through the catheter with a syringe, or, **C,** it may be poured into a funnel attached to the catheter.

the medication can be poured is connected to it (Fig. 5-6, C). Although the drug can be injected with a syringe, the nurse must do this very slowly and gently. The rate at which the injection is done should approximate the time required for the medication to flow into the bladder by gravity. The nurse can control this by rotating the plunger of the

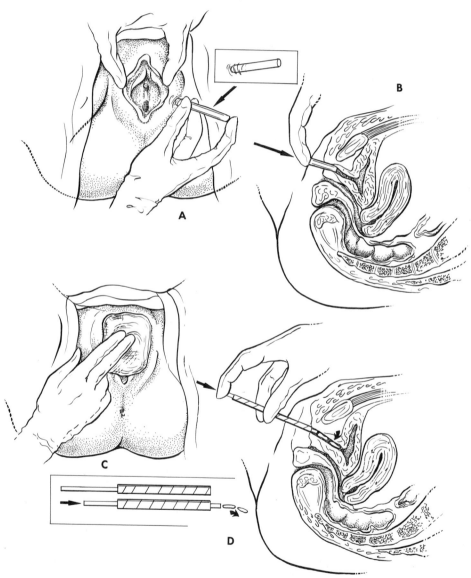

Fig. 5-7. Urethral suppositories. **A,** The nurse inserts a lubricated suppository into the urethra, observing sterile precautions. **B,** Cross section showing insertion of the suppository. **C,** The nurse holds a sterile sponge against the meatus until spasms subside. **D,** The nurse inserts a suppository supplied in an applicator by pushing it through the applicator with the plunger. Inset shows suppository supplied in an applicator.

syringe rather than by pushing the plunger forward (Fig. 5-6, *B*). The nurse then withdraws the catheter and applies pressure to the meatus with a soft sterile sponge. The patient should be instructed to retain the medicine for the designated period of time, frequently 20 to 30 minutes.

Urethra   Often, the nurse administers a urethral suppository immediately following bladder instillation. If the suppository alone is ordered, the nurse would prepare and drape the patient as for bladder instillation immediately after the patient has emptied her bladder. After cleansing the meatus and adjacent areas, the nurse lubricates the tip of the suppository with water or a water-soluble lubricant and inserts it into the urethra (Fig. 5-7, *A* and *B*). Immediately after inserting the suppository, the nurse applies firm pressure to the meatus with a sterile sponge until the suppository melts or spasms subside (Fig. 5-7, *C*), frequently about 10 minutes. The patient should be instructed to refrain from voiding for 15 to 30 minutes if possible, because voiding will remove the medication. Fig. 5-7, *D* shows the insertion of a suppository supplied in an applicator.

Vagina   The patient should void prior to vaginal instillation and should maintain a recumbent position following the instillation. This must be explained to the ambulatory patient. Ideally, she should be told about it sometime prior to instillation so that she can plan her activities accordingly. The nurse wears a glove on the hand that is used to expose the orifice. If the medication is inserted manually, she wears gloves on both hands. Unless otherwise specified, clean technique is permissible.

Vaginal applicators are filled with medicated creams and jellies directly from a tube (Fig. 5-8, *A*). The nurse inserts the filled applicator into the vagina to a depth of 1½ to 2 inches (Fig. 5-8, *B*). As she pushes the plunger forward, depositing the medication, she in turn withdraws the applicator itself (Fig. 5-8, *C*). Immediately after use, the reusable applicator is disassembled and washed. Initial rinsing with cold water removes protein without causing coagulation. Disposable applicators are available.

Special devices for insertion of vaginal tablets are available (Fig. 5-8, *D* and *E*), or the nurse may insert a suppository by grasping it between her thumb and forefinger and then pushing it into the vagina until it is deposited near the posterior aspect of the cervix (Fig. 5-8, *F*).

Rectal instillations   To administer a rectal instillation, the nurse, after assisting the patient to a comfortable side-lying position with the lower leg extended and the upper leg flexed, retracts the upper buttock to expose the anal area (Fig. 5-9, *A*). After unwrapping the suppository (Fig. 5-9, *B*), she may lubricate it with a water-soluble lubricant. Some suppositories are self-lubricating. When inserting the suppository, the nurse should either protect her thumb and forefinger with finger cots or wear a glove (Fig. 5-9, *C* and *D*). The suppository is pushed forward until it

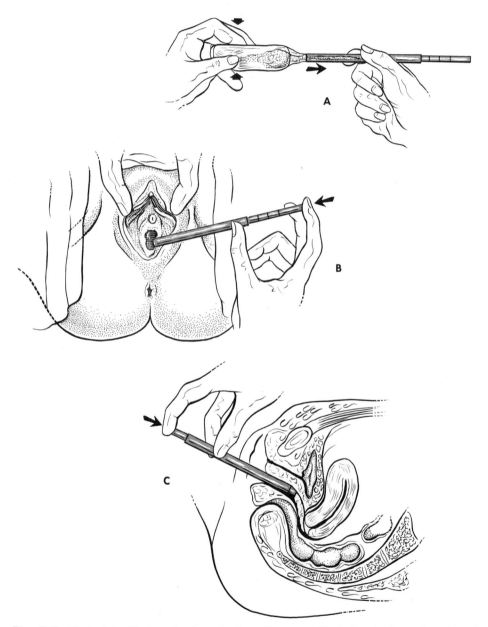

Fig. 5-8. Vaginal instillation. **A,** A vaginal applicator is filled directly from the tube of medication. **B,** The nurse inserts the applicator into the vagina. As she pushes the plunger forward, medication is deposited, **C,** and she withdraws the applicator.

passes the anal sphincter. The administration of medicated enemas is prescribed occasionally. Fig. 9-1 shows the administration of a disposable enema. The purpose of the rectal instillation and the length of time it is to be retained should be explained to the patient.

Injection   The prevention of infection must accompany administration of drugs by injection. Both the equipment and the drug must be sterile. After the site for injection has been selected, the nurse cleanses an area about 2 inches square, usually with 70% alcohol, benzalkonium chloride, or benzine. Cleansing with a circular motion proceeds from the center of the site outward.

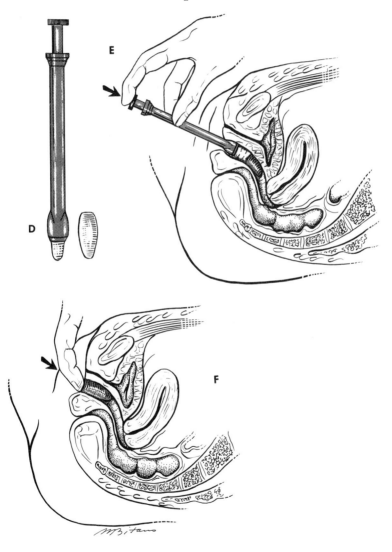

Fig. 5-8, cont'd. D, A device for inserting vaginal tablets. **E,** After insertion of the device, the tablet is deposited by pushing the plunger forward. **F,** The nurse may insert a suppository manually, using the index finger to position it.

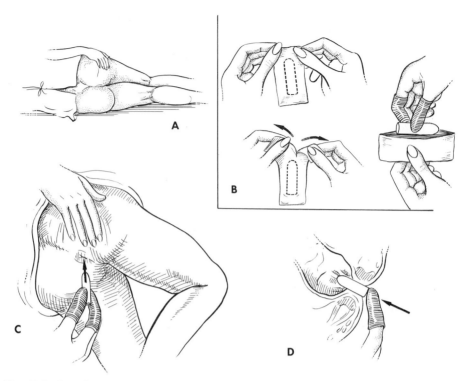

Fig. 5-9. Rectal suppositories. **A,** Position of the patient. **B,** The nurse opens the wrapper containing the suppository and removes it. **C,** The nurse inserts the suppository. **D,** Cross section showing insertion of the suppository. The suppository will be advanced beyond the anal sphincter.

Disposable equipment reduces transmission of pathogens. This is essential if causative organisms of certain diseases such as viral hepatitis are present.

The preparation of the syringe and needle varies with the method of packaging. Individually packaged needles and syringes can be attached to each other without removing the needle from its container. Prefilled syringes may be supplied in a completely assembled state, or various degrees of assembling may be necessary. Some drugs are supplied in cartridges (Fig. 5-10). Labeling on these provides additional identification of the drug and the dose. The manufacturer usually supplies directions concerning the assembly of equipment.

Selection of the needle

The nurse selects needle size according to the desired depth of insertion and the viscosity of the drug that must pass through the needle. The length of the needle is relative to the depth of tissue that must be penetrated. A longer needle is used for deep intramuscular injections than for subcutaneous injections; a longer needle is needed for obese patients than for those who are thin. A viscous drug requires a needle with a large

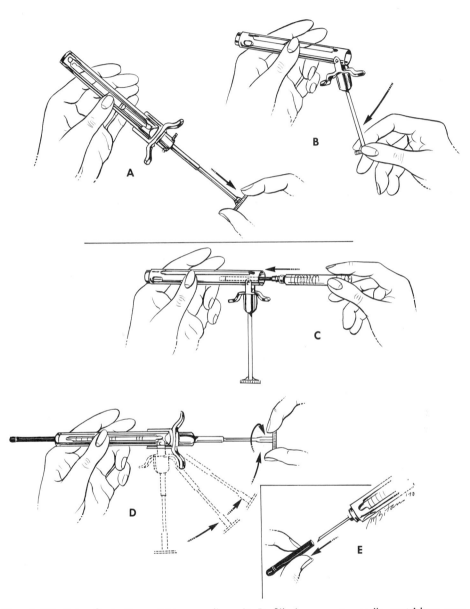

Fig. 5-10. Tubex® sterile cartridge-needle unit. Prefilled or empty sterile cartridges may be used. Following assembly, the prefilled cartridge is ready to be injected; the prescribed dose must be drawn into an empty cartridge from a vial or an ampule. **A,** The nurse holds the barrel of the syringe in one hand and pulls back the plunger. **B,** She pulls the plunger downward until it locks at a right angle to the barrel. **C,** The nurse inserts a sterile cartridge into the barrel, needle end first. **D,** She swings the plunger into place and turns the end of the plunger until it is fitted tightly onto the threaded end of the cartridge. **E,** The nurse removes the sheath from the needle prior to injection. (Courtesy Wyeth Laboratories, Philadelphia, Pa.)

bore, while a drug of waterlike consistency passes easily through a small needle without clogging. The bore, or inside diameter of the needle, increases in size as the gauge number becomes smaller. Thus, a 13-gauge needle has a large bore and a 27-gauge needle has a small bore. As a guide, the size commonly used for subcutaneous injection is 2 cm. (¾ inch) long and 24 or 25 gauge; for intramuscular injection a needle 1 to 2 inches long and 19 to 22 gauge is selected.

Selection of the syringe

The volume of drug to be injected influences the choice of syringe according to its size and calibration. Measurement of a small dose is most accurate if the syringe is of small diameter. For many injections, a 2-ml. syringe calibrated in minims as well as milliliters (cubic centimeters) is used; a 1-ml. tuberculin syringe calibrated in minims is used for very small doses; and syringes calibrated in units are used for administration of insulin. In the latter case, the syringe should be calibrated with the same number of units per milliliter as the insulin preparation.

Preparation of the dose

Unless prefilled syringes are used, the nurse must withdraw the dose from a sealed container. Throughout preparation, she must avoid contamination of the drug by keeping sterile the needle, the inside of the syringe, and the part of the plunger that will be enclosed by the barrel of the syringe. In addition, she must measure the dose accurately.

Vial. If the drug is dispensed in a vial, the nurse cleanses the rubber stopper with an antiseptic sponge prior to introducing the needle (Fig. 5-11, *A*). The antiseptic usually used is 70% alcohol. She withdraws the plunger of the syringe until the tip of the plunger rests on the calibration that indicates the amount of solution needed (Fig. 5-11, *B*). She inserts the needle, previously attached to the syringe, through the center of the rubber stopper and pushes the plunger forward, introducing a volume of air equal to the volume of solution that she is to withdraw (Fig. 5-11, *C* and *D*). This increases the pressure within the vial, facilitating withdrawal of the dose. She then inverts the vial and syringe and withdraws the designated dose (Fig. 5-11, *E*). After preparing the dose, she sheaths the needle within a sterile protector in order to transport it to the patient care center. A sterile package containing an alcohol sponge will serve this purpose if the needle is not supplied in an individual sterile wrapper (Fig. 5-11, *F*).

If two drugs are to be mixed in one syringe, every precaution must be taken to prevent contamination of one drug with the other. For example, when a mixture of insulin preparations is desired, the nurse injects a volume of air equal to the dose into the vial of modified insulin and withdraws the needle; she repeats this procedure with the unmodified preparation, that is, regular insulin. Following this she withdraws the desired amount of unmodified insulin and then withdraws the modified insulin. Next, air is drawn into the syringe, and it is tipped or rotated vertically so that the air bubble moves back

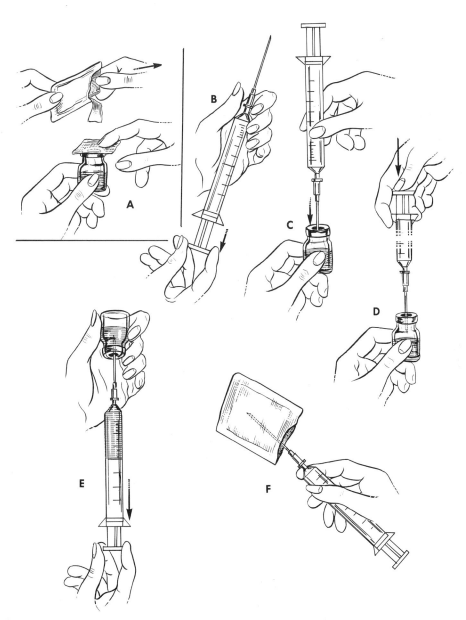

Fig. 5-11. Preparation of a dose from a vial. **A,** The nurse cleanses the rubber stopper with an alcohol sponge. **B,** She draws air equal to the prescribed dose into the syringe. **C,** She inserts the needle into the vial. **D,** The air is injected into the vial. **E,** She inverts the vial to withdraw solution. **F,** She sheathes the needle in a sterile wrapper for transport.

and forth, mixing the solution. This should be done slowly and gently.

The pharmacist dispenses in crystalline form drugs that deteriorate rapidly after being placed in solution. Immediately prior to use the nurse mixes them with the amount and kind of diluent

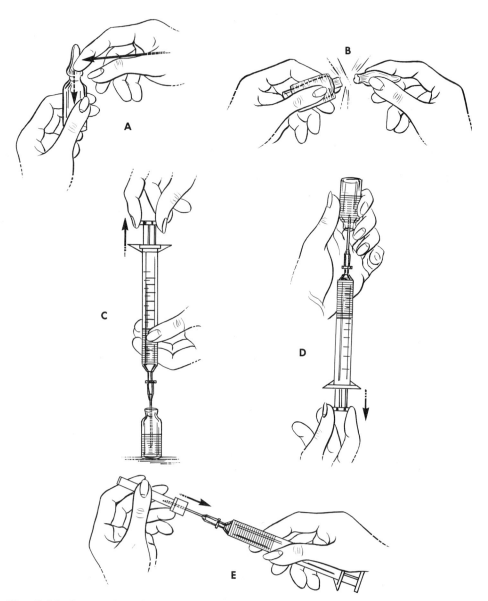

Fig. 5-12. Preparation of a dose from an ampule. **A,** Tapping the top of the ampule causes solution to collect in the body of the ampule. **B,** The nurse opens the ampule by exerting pressure with the thumb and forefinger placed on each side of the constriction. **C,** If the needle is sufficiently long, the drug may be withdrawn without inverting the ampule. **D,** When a short needle is used, the nurse inverts the ampule. **E,** She sheathes the needle in a sterile container during transport.

recommended by the manufacturer. Occasionally, some agitation is necessary to dissolve the solid particles. Rolling the vial back and forth between the palms of the hands mixes the solution without producing air bubbles that interfere with accurate measurement. Repeatedly withdrawing the solution and reinjecting it forcefully against particles adhering to the wall of the vial tend to hasten solution, although repeated withdrawal and reinjection produce froth.

Ampule. Before breaking a hermetically sealed ampule, the nurse taps the apex of the ampule, causing solution trapped by the constriction in the neck of the ampule to flow into the body of the ampule (Fig. 5-12, *A*). If the ampule is not designed with a break line, she forms one by drawing a file across the constriction several times. She uses the same method to remove the top of the ampule that has been filed as she uses to break an ampule with a ready-break line (Fig. 5-12, *B*). It is advisable to protect the hands during the breaking of the ampule by enclosing the area of the break line in alcohol sponges, pledgets, or gauze. Wiping the neck of the ampule with an antiseptic before breaking it will help in removing any external contamination.

If the needle the nurse uses to withdraw the drug is sufficiently long, she need not invert the ampule; however, she should not permit the needle to touch contaminated parts of the ampule (Fig. 5-12, *C*). If she inverts the ampule to withdraw the solution (Fig. 5-12, *D*), she must use care to prevent contamination of the needle by her hands. She must avoid injecting air into the ampule because this displaces the drug, causing it to drip from the ampule and resulting in its loss. Unused solution should be discarded. The needle is sheathed in a sterile container during transport (Fig. 5-12, *E*).

Subcutaneous injection

The sites most frequently used for subcutaneous injection are the upper arms and thighs, although other areas such as the abdomen may also be used (Fig. 5-13, *A*). If repeated injections are given, the nurse should rotate the site of injection so that each succeeding injection is about 2 inches away from the previous site. A definite plan for rotating sites of injection and a record of the site injected is necessary.

After preparing the drug, the nurse cleanses the site and grasps the area between her thumb and forefinger to tense it (Fig. 5-15, *B*). She then inserts the needle at about a 45° to 60° angle, piercing the skin quickly and advancing the needle steadily to minimize pain. After aspirating to determine that the needle has not inadvertently entered a blood vessel (Fig. 5-13, *C*), she injects the drug slowly (Fig. 5-13, *D*). To do this, she changes the position of her hands, taking care not to increase

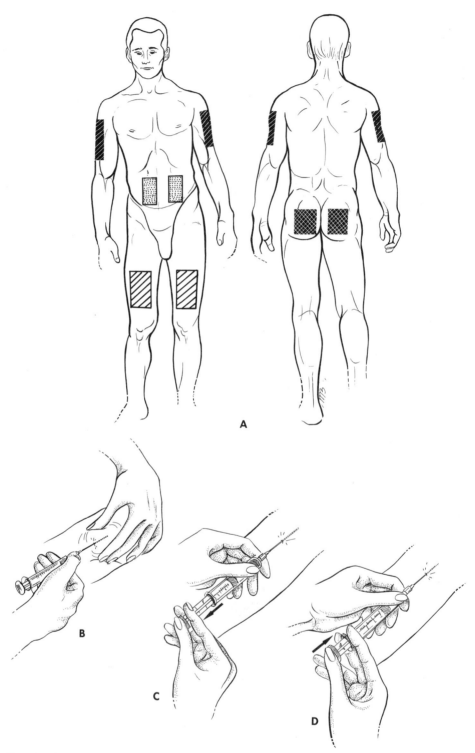

Fig. 5-13. Subcutaneous injection. **A,** Possible sites for injection. **B,** A method of tensing tissue during insertion of the needle; the area is cleansed just before the tissue is tensed. **C,** Following insertion of the needle, the nurse withdraws the plunger slightly to determine that the needle is not located within a vessel. **D,** She injects the drug by pushing the plunger forward.

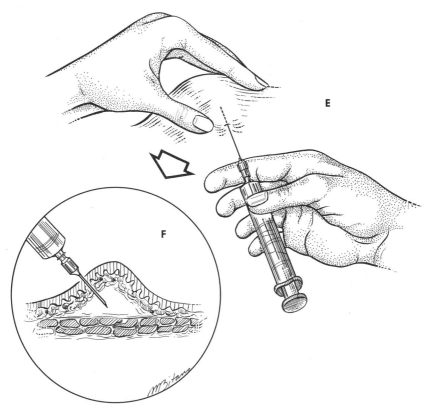

Fig. 5-13, cont'd. E, The method of tensing tissues that is used for injection of irritating drugs such as insulin. **F,** Cross section showing relationship of the needle to the tissues.

the patient's discomfort by moving the needle. When she has injected the drug, she withdraws the needle and massages the area with a sterile alcohol sponge.

If the drug to be injected is known to irritate the tissues, a modified technique is used to ensure deposition of the drug in the deep subcutaneous tissues. The tissue overlying the injection site is grasped with the thumb and forefinger to form an elevated roll (Fig. 5-13, *E*). After the site is cleansed, the needle is inserted before the hold on the tissue is relaxed. Opinions vary as to the angle at which the needle should be inserted. Often it is inserted at a right angle to the thumb when insulin is being injected (Fig. 5-13, *F*), but it may be inserted perpendicular to the tissue mass when drugs such as emetine hydrochloride or sodium heparin injection are being administered.

Intramuscular
injection

Selection of sites. Selection of sites for intramuscular injection frequently includes gluteal tissues, and, less often, the thighs and the upper arm. Various methods of selecting the site of injection have been described and may be used.

Posterior gluteal area. When the injection is to be given into the posterior gluteal area, the nurse can obtain maximum relaxation of the muscles by correctly positioning the patient. Ideally, the patient lies on his abdomen with his toes pointed inward (Fig. 5-14, *A*). The nurse may place a pillow beneath the lower legs to add to the comfort of this position. The arms may dangle over the edge of the table, or the patient may extend

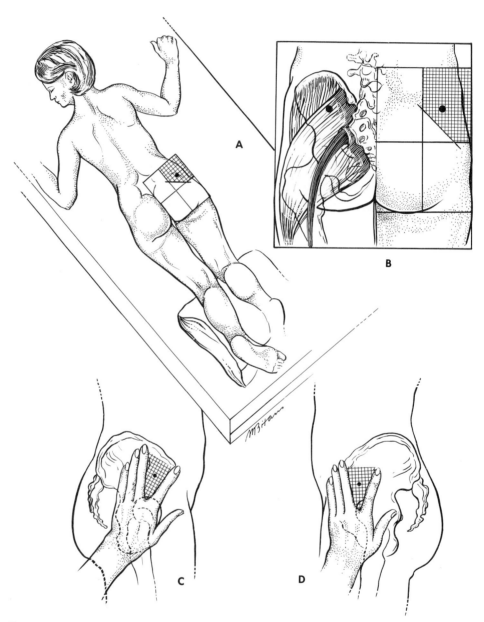

Fig. 5-14. Sites for intramuscular injection. **A,** Position of the patient when the posterior gluteal area is used. **B,** Diagram showing the anatomy of the posterior gluteal area and the method of finding the injection site. The large dot indicates the site of injection. **C,** Location of the site for injection into the right ventrogluteal area. **D,** Location of the site for injection into the left ventrogluteal area.

them at his side. When this position is uncomfortable or impossible, the patient may lie on his side with the lower leg extended and the upper leg flexed. The injection is given in the gluteal area of the uppermost side. It is inadvisable for the patient to stand during injection because this tends to increase

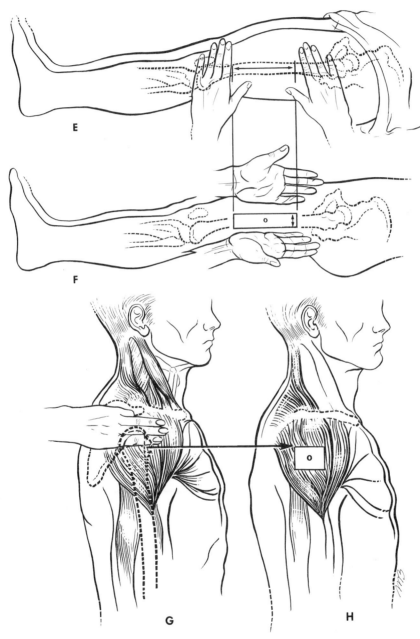

Fig. 5-14, cont'd. E, Location of length of the boundary for injection into the vastus lateralis. **F,** Location of breadth of the boundary for injection into the vastus lateralis. **G,** Location of the site for injection into the deltoid is two to three fingerbreadths below the acromion process. **H,** Injection should be made above the groove inferior to the deltoid.

tenseness of the muscles and permits a tensing reaction when the needle is inserted or the drug injected. Increased discomfort, plus the possibility of needle breakage in a muscular person, results from the increased muscular tension. Both the face-lying and the side-lying positions prevent the patient from seeing the approach of the needle. This is said to be of psychologic benefit.

The gluteal area is exposed and divided into quadrants. This area must not be equated with the buttocks. Instead, the anatomic area is determined by careful palpation of the landmarks. The gluteal area is bounded by the iliac crest, the anterior iliac spine, the inferior gluteal fold, and the division between the buttocks (Fig. 5-14, *B*). If, upon palpation, gross deformity of the skeletal structures appears to exist, the clinical specialist's or the physician's assistance in locating a safe site for injection should be sought. After the gluteal area has been outlined, it is divided into four quadrants with intersecting vertical and horizontal lines.

The nurse then gives the injection in the upper outer quadrant. To be certain that this area has been identified correctly so that the sciatic nerve is well removed from the point of injection, the nurse draws a line from the posterior superior iliac crest to the head of the femur (Fig. 5-14, *B*). Injection lateral and superior to this line will be within the gluteal mass and will not traumatize the sciatic nerve.

Ventrogluteal site. Another site for intramuscular injection is the ventrogluteal site. This location is preferred for intramuscular injection in children and is recommended by some physicians for injection in adults. Major vessels and nerves are not found in this area if it is outlined properly.

The nurse places the patient in either a back-lying or face-lying position for use of this site. The area is located by either of three methods. If the right ventrogluteal site is to be used, the nurse places the tip of the index finger of the left hand on the anterior superior iliac spine and presses the left hand on the hip, with the tips of the fingers pointing toward the patient's head. She spreads the index and middle fingers as far apart as possible, thus forming a V (Fig. 5-14, *C*). Injection is made between these two fingers and below the iliac crest. If the left ventrogluteal area is used, the nurse places the middle finger on the anterior superior iliac crest and moves the index finger away from it to form the V (Fig. 5-14, *D*). Another method of locating this site involves drawing imaginary lines from the anterior and posterior edges of the iliac crest to the greater trochanter. These lines also form a triangle within which the injection is given.

Vastus lateralis. The patient may assume a back-lying, face-lying, or sitting position when the vastus lateralis area is used. The nurse marks the area for injection by a distance of a hand-breadth below the head of the greater trochanter and a hand-breadth above the knee (Fig. 5-14, *E*), the midanterior thigh, and the midlateral thigh (Fig. 5-14, *F*). She inserts the needle to a depth of 1 inch.

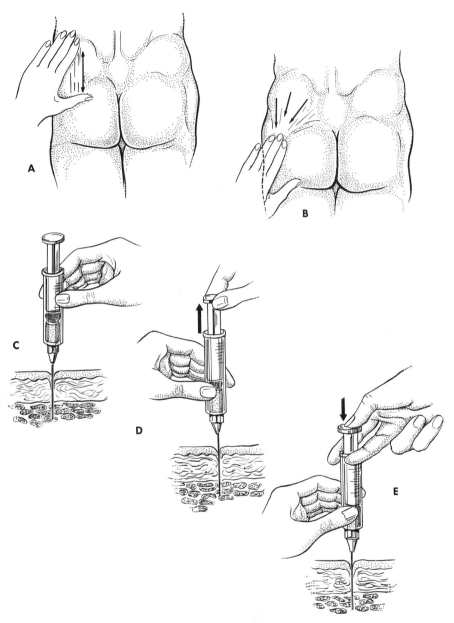

Fig. 5-15. Technique of intramuscular injection. **A,** One method of stretching the tissues. **B,** An alternate method of stretching the tissues. **C,** The nurse inserts the needle at a right angle to the tissues. **D,** She withdraws the plunger slightly to make certain that the needle is not located within a blood vessel. **E,** The nurse injects the solution. Note the air bubble at the top of the solution that is forced through to clear the shaft of the needle of residual drug.

Deltoid area. Injection into the deltoid area is likely to produce more pain than at other sites of intramuscular injection. The area cannot be exposed satisfactorily by rolling up a sleeve; the gown or shirt should be removed. Injection should be 2 to 3 fingerbreadths below the acromion process (Fig. 5-14, *G*) and above the groove inferior to the deltoid (Fig. 5-14, *H*). Injection into the middle or lower third of the upper arm is avoided because it might injure the radial nerve.

Technique of intramuscular injection. After the site has been selected and cleansed, the tissue is stretched, reducing the amount of subcutaneous fat that must be penetrated and ensuring penetration into the muscle. Pressure exerted in opposite directions with the thumb and forefinger will serve this purpose (Fig. 5-15, *A*). Another method, sometimes referred to as the Z track technique, involves pulling the tissue in one direction only, so that an outline of a Z is formed (Fig. 5-15, *B*). This slides the layer of subcutaneous tissue to one side during the injection. When it is released following the injection, the tissue slides back into position. This prevents the medication from flowing into the upper layers of tissue and promotes absorption of the drug.

The nurse introduces the needle through the skin at a 90° angle with a quick thrust and then advances it as necessary. She should not introduce it as far as the hub. She withdraws the plunger slightly to be certain that the needle has not been placed within a blood vessel. She injects the solution slowly, followed by a small bubble of air previously drawn into the syringe (Fig. 5-15, *C* to *E*). The air is used to clear the shaft of the needle or drug that could theoretically be deposited in the overlying tissues as the needle is withdrawn. Following the injection, the nurse should massage the site.

Massaging the site of injection for a minimum of 30 to 60 seconds reduces pain, discoloration, and induration. Massage is contraindicated by the nature of certain preparations, particularly those containing heavy metals. The manufacturer's brochure should identify this contraindication. If capillary bleeding occurs when the needle is withdrawn, the nurse should apply direct pressure to the site with a sterile sponge until the bleeding stops. Patients appreciate an explanation of why the nurse is applying pressure or massaging the area. These measures reduce physical and mental discomfort to the patient and help maintain the tissues in a healthy state, thus preserving a maximum area into which future injections can be given.

Questions for discussion and exploration

1. When you bring a capsule to Mrs. R., she says, "Oh, the doctor must have ordered a new drug for me!" If you are not aware that this is a new drug for Mrs. R., what might her comment indicate? What might you say if you know that this is a new drug for her?

2. In order to disguise the bitter taste of codeine you place the tablet inside a gelatin capsule. Mrs. T. takes the capsule but telephones the supervisor to report that she cannot sleep because the nurse gave her the wrong pain medication. How might you have prevented this situation from developing?

3. Mrs. G. finds it impossible to swallow capsules and complains about the bitter-tasting particles of the drug lodging beneath her dentures when she chews the capsules. What possible alterations can be made in the method of administration that will make taking the drug more pleasant? What facts must you know in order to make your decision?

4. Mr. N. refuses to take his sleeping medication at the time you bring it to him. He tells you to set it on his bedside table and he will take it when he is ready to go to sleep. You are extremely busy caring for six other patients who need considerable nursing care. How should you respond to his request?

5. When you bring an injection to Mrs. C.'s room, she begins to cry and tearfully says, "Not another injection. I just can't take another one." How can this individual be helped? The drug is an antibiotic.

6. Miss Y. shows you a large black and blue area near her hip where she says she was given an injection. She tells you it hurts so much that she cannot walk and that the person who gave her the injection shouldn't be allowed to ever give another to anyone. How can you safely respond to her and what can you do to make her more comfortable? What records and reports need to be made?

7. Miss Q., aged 14, has been admitted to the hospital for control of her diabetes. Prepare a teaching plan that you might use to help her learn how to measure, administer, and store her insulin. What points must be emphasized in relation to insulin dosage, measurement, and diet?

8. Miss Y.'s mother needs to know when and how to administer glucagon. Although the opportunity to administer this drug to her son never arises during his hospitalization, what must Mrs. Y. be taught and how?

9. Mr. Z. will be maintained on psychotherapeutic drugs following his dismissal from the psychiatric unit. What must he and his family know about the drugs that he is taking? If Mrs. Z. comments that she wonders how they'll manage because Mr. Z. has always been reluctant to take any medicine, even aspirin, what is she indicating and what are your responsibilities?

10. Mrs. S. is to continue treatment of vaginitis at home with the aid of a daily medicated suppository. What knowledge, understanding, and planning does she need?

11. You are asked to instill a liquid drug preparation into Mrs. G.'s bladder. Mrs. G. has an indwelling catheter in place. How would you carry out this technique, maintaining the sterility of the bladder and making certain that the drug is retained for a period of 20 minutes?

12. Mr. K. is in the terminal phases of cancer of the spine and is receiving injections of dihydromorphinone (Dilaudid) and promethazine hydrochloride (Phenergan) every 2 to 3 hours. His muscles have wasted and are lumpy from previous injections. The promethazine hydrochloride is supplied in sterile cartridge (Tubex), but the dihydromorphinone must be withdrawn from a vial. What possible sites might you use for giving both drugs? What additional factors might be considered that could promote comfort?

Selected references

Bergersen, B. S., and Krug, E. E.: Pharmacology in nursing, ed. 11, St. Louis, 1969, The C. V. Mosby Co.

Brodie, D. C.: Trends in pharmaceutical education, Amer. J. Nurs. **68:** 948-951, 1968.

Coates, F. C., and Fabrykant, M.: An insulin injection technique for preventing skin reactions, Amer. J. Nurs. **65:**127-128, 1965.

Gordon, D. M.: The inflamed eye, Amer. J. Nurs. **64:**113-117, 1964.

Hanson, D. J.: Intramuscular injection injuries and complications, Amer. J. Nurs. **63**:99-101, 1963.

Kern, M. S.: New ideas about drug systems, Amer. J. Nurs. **68**:1251-1253, 1968.

Pitel, M., and Wemett, M.: The intramuscular injection, Amer. J. Nurs. **64**:104-109, 1964.

Saunders, W. H., Havener, W. H., Fair, G. I., and Hickey, J. T.: Nursing care in eye, ear, nose, and throat disorders, ed. 2, St. Louis, 1968, The C. V. Mosby Co.

Schwartau, N., and Sturdavant, M.: A system of packaging and dispensing drugs in single doses, Amer. J. Pharm. **61**:542-559, 1961.

Shaffer, J. H., and Sweet, L. C.: Allergic reactions to drugs, Amer. J. Nurs. **65**:100-103, 1965.

Watkins, J. D., and Moss, F. T.: Confusion in the management of diabetes, Amer. J. Nurs. **69**:521-524, 1969.

Wempe, B. M.: The new and the old intramuscular injection sites, Amer. J. Nurs. **61**:56-57, 1961.

Zitnik, R.: First, you take a grapefruit, Amer. J. Nurs. **68**:1285-1286, 1968.

Chapter 6

Application of topical medications

Instructions concerning the kind, strength, and form of topical medications and frequency, area, and method of their application are obtained by the nurse from the physician's orders. After the necessary dressings, equipment, and drug preparations have been assembled, the medication may be applied.

Contact with the patient during treatment gives the nurse the opportunity to demonstrate her acceptance of him and his condition. In most instances, the use of gloves 'and· other devices that suggest self-protection should be avoided. Self-protection should be practiced if the condition being treated is contagious, if the drug is likely to be harmful to the nurse, or if the medication possesses a disagreeable odor that is difficult to remove. Transparent plastic aprons are sometimes used to prevent staining of the nurse's uniform.

A cheerful, tactful, and understanding approach is essential. The patient and his relatives are concerned about his appearance and the prolonged period of treatment required. Anxiety related to the discomfort of pruritus, insomnia, anorexia, and decreased ability to function normally adds to their burdens. Any method that helps gain the acceptance and cooperation of the patient, his relatives, and his employer is of value. Teaching the patient how to live successfully with his condition should be reinforced at every opportunity. Instructions should be given carefully, and learning should be evaluated objectively. If treatment is to continue at home, clearly written instructions that can be understood easily should be provided. Impatience leads to a temptation to overtreat or to use home remedies, producing disastrous results. The intense desire to scratch when itching occurs must be diverted if healing is to occur. Use of antihistamine, sedative, tranquilizing, and other systemic drugs, as prescribed, helps the patient to cope with problems that may seem to be insurmountable.

An understanding of the principles of physiology will help the nurse promote the patient's comfort. Knowledge that itching increases when the capillary bed dilates indicates careful and conscientious control of factors that influence this mechanism. Regulation of the temperature of the environment will be affected by humidity, activity of the patient, and method used for the application of drugs. Thus the use of wet dressings frequently dictates the need to increase the temperature of the environment. Knowledge that constriction, friction, heat, and perspiration increase itching will guide the selection and use of fabrics for dressings and clothing.

External medications are usually stored in medication lockers. Appropriately labeled individual trays will facilitate their storage and transport, and lining the trays with paper protectors will minimize the effort needed to keep them clean.

The physician may prescribe the use of more than one form of treatment. For example, ultraviolet light therapy may be ordered to follow the removal of ointment with oil, a therapeutic bath may be ordered to precede the application of ointments, or a prescription may be given to enclose in wet dressings a skin area to which lotion has been applied. Various other combinations of treatments may also be prescribed. When a combination of treatments is prescribed, sequence and timing are crucial for obtaining maximum therapeutic results. For example, ointments must be applied immediately following the bath; if time elapses, dryness, itching, and irritation occur. These delay the healing process.

Ointments

Ointments serve as a vehicle for therapeutic drugs, a protective coating, lubrication, and softener of the skin.

After the nurse has assisted the patient in removing the necessary clothing and in assuming the desired position, she places a small amount of ointment in one of her hands. Then she spreads it to the inner aspects of both hands by gently drawing them across each other. This action not only places an equal amount of ointment on both hands but also warms it, thus facilitating even application of a thin coating that will protect the skin surface from contact with air. Heavy applications of

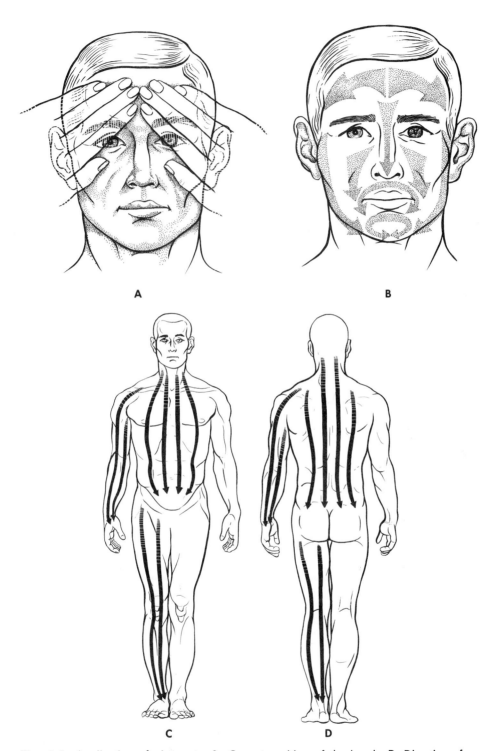

Fig. 6-1. Application of ointments. **A,** Correct position of the hands. **B,** Direction of application to the face. **C,** Direction of application to the anterior surface of the body. **D,** Direction of application to the posterior surface of the body.

ointments tend to cake onto the skin, producing irritation. Removal of heavily applied ointments requires vigorous efforts, also irritating and damaging to the skin.

In applying the ointment, long, smooth strokes that follow the direction of hair growth are used. Short, uncoordinated strokes accompanied by insufficient or excessive pressure, as well as rubbing or repetitious stroking, tend to increase itching and should be avoided. Rubbing or repetitious stroking should also be avoided to prevent introduction of the ointment into the hair follicles. The nurse begins each stroke by placing her hands on the area to be treated in such a way that they meet and act as a single unit, with the flat portion of the hands used to deposit a film of ointment on the body surface (Fig. 6-1, *A*).

It is important that the nursing plan provide for a consistent technique in the application of ointments and that the nurse who applies the medication teach by example, explanations, and repeated instructions any patient who is to participate in his own treatment.

Following treatment, the ointment is kept in contact with the body surface by dressings. Loosely fitted cotton pajamas, laundered to remove fillers that may prove irritating to the condition being treated, fulfill the requirements of a satisfactory dressing and may be worn for 3 days without laundering. White cotton stockings and gloves or tubular gauze may be used to keep ointments in contact with the skin. Paper scuffs, available commercially, or scuffs made of toweling can be worn on the feet.

The usual schedule of treatment provides for 2 to 3 applications of ointment daily. If dryness occurs, additional ointment applications may be indicated.

Upon completion of an ointment application, the nurse should cleanse her hands by wiping them with a paper towel before using soap and water.

Applying ointment to face

Application of ointment to small areas of the face requires use of the flat portion of the fingers. Use of the fingertips for the application of topical medications is contraindicated because it may cause abrasions that would predispose the skin to infection even though the nails are closely trimmed. Treatment of the face is begun at the midline, with both hands used simultaneously to apply the ointment. Direction of application to facial areas is shown in Fig. 6-1, *B*.

Applying ointment to trunk and extremities

In applying ointment to the trunk, the nurse should begin the first stroke at the midline. If the entire anterior surface of the trunk is to be treated, the nurse begins this stroke under the chin and extends to the genital area (Fig. 6-1, *C*). She begins the second stroke at the uppermost point of treatment adjacent to either side of the area to which the ointment was applied by the first stroke. This outward pattern is repeated until the anterior surface is treated. The same pattern is used to treat the posterior surface of the trunk, with the initial stroke beginning at the hairline (Fig. 6-1, *D*). The extremities are treated in a similar fashion. Usually two strokes are needed to treat each extremity, although this will vary, depending on the size of the extremity. The patient wears a loin cloth, which allows all areas of the body to be treated except the genital area. He is usually permitted to apply medication to the genitalia after receiving instructions from the nurse.

Although the position of the patient is only of relative importance in the application of ointment to the trunk and extremities, having him stand erect seems to facilitate treatment. In addition, the patient is usually quite pleased not to have his bed unnecessarily soiled by the medication.

Heavy ointments

Heavy ointments such as Lassar's paste are intended for heavy application. Spreading is more readily accomplished if the nurse uses a wooden spatula. The direction of application follows the direction of hair growth whenever possible.

Removal of ointments, crusts, scales, and dried secretions

The nurse may remove excess or dried ointment and crusts, scales, and dried secretions with a nonirritating solvent. An oil of the cottonseed type is a satisfactory solvent for most oil-base ointments. Other oils, such as mineral, olive, and castor oils, will serve this purpose; however, expense, odor, and ease of removing the oil itself should be evaluated carefully.

The nurse pours some oil into her hands and lubricates them by rubbing them together. Then she smooths oil onto the body area to be cleansed, using the same strokes described for the application of ointment. (See pages 150 to 153 and Fig. 6-1.) When large areas are to be oiled, the patient may stand on the floor, which should be protected with paper mats. Liberal amounts of oil should be used, and the entire procedure should be repeated many times to ensure easy and complete removal of the ointment. Rubbing produces irritation and damage to the skin and is contraindicated.

Excess oil and ointment are removed by gentle wiping of the area with a soft cloth. Gauze that has been washed to remove fillers is also satisfactory. Again, the same directional strokes described previously are used. This method of removing ointments leaves on the skin a residual film of oil that is removed by the therapeutic bath, and it may also be used to help remove scales, crusts, and dried secretions.

Trial application of ointments

The physician may test the feasibility of using a specific ointment by requesting a trial application to a small area. The size of the area used is about 1½ inches in diameter. He may specify the site to be used, usually the abdomen or the inner aspect of the forearm. In this trial application to a small area of the body, the same principles as those used for applying ointment to a large area of the body hold true.

If stock supplies are being used, the nurse may wish to place a small amount of the specified ointment on a wooden spatula or tongue blade, place the ointment-laden end inside a waxed envelope, and record identifying information on the portion extending from the envelope. If waxed envelopes are unavailable, sandwich bags may be substituted.

Lotions
Lotions are used to protect and soothe the skin. The lotion may be prescribed for the purpose of lubrication, cooling, drying, or relieving itching. Due to the nature of the ingredients found in many lotions, application near the eyes and the mucous membranes is usually contraindicated.

Prior to application, the nurse must shake most lotions until it is obvious that the solution is thoroughly mixed. If the lotion does not mix well within a reasonable period of time, the nurse should assume that it is defective and should obtain a new supply.

The nurse should apply lotions gently and frequently and permit them to dry thoroughly before the treated area is covered with dressings or pajamas. Cotton or rayon pledgets should not be used to apply lotions because the fibers tend to absorb the solute or drug, leaving primarily the solvent in contact with the area being treated. Painting the lotion onto the skin with a paintbrush has been described by various authorities. However, applying the lotion with a gentle patting or stroking motion of the hands permits control of the amount and kind of pressure used. This method appears to aid in preventing increased sensations of itching. If the lotion prescribed is quite watery, the nurse may wish to apply it with soft gauze that does not contain fillers. The lotion should not be permitted to form a thick layer on the skin because this is irritating and reduces evaporation. The direction of application of lotion is the same as that for ointments (Fig. 6-1, *B* to *D*). Lotions are applied at the prescribed time intervals.

Dressings
Wet dressings
Various types of wet dressings may be prescribed to reduce inflammation, edema, and pruritus. In addition, they may be used to cleanse the skin and to treat infection. Prior to the application of wet dressings, it may be necessary to place a dry, sterile dressing over ulcerated or denuded areas. Such a dressing should be of nonirritating material. Dressings that do not adhere readily to lesions are preferred.

Although the solutions prescribed are not always the same, they are usually very dilute. A solution that is too concentrated will produce flare of the skin condition rather than the desired resolution. The nurse diluting the solution must know whether sterile, tap, or distilled water is to be used. She warms the diluted solution to the desired temperature, usually 95° to 98° F.,

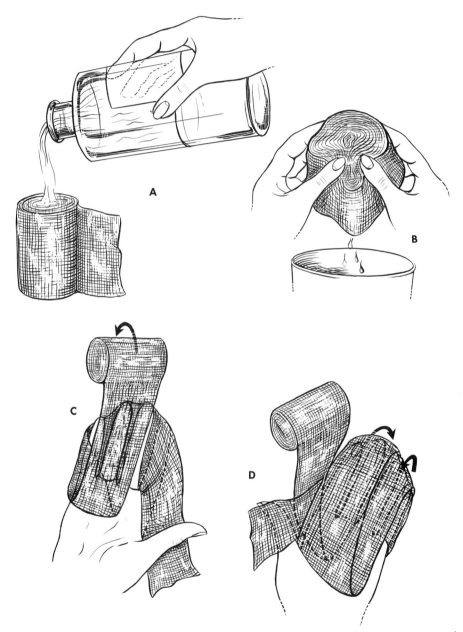

Fig. 6-2. Application of wet dressings to the upper extremity. **A,** The nurse saturates the gauze thoroughly with warm solution. **B,** She compresses the gauze between her hands to remove excess solution. Then she interweaves gauze between the patient's fingers, **C,** covering his fingertips with folds of gauze, **D.**

Continued.

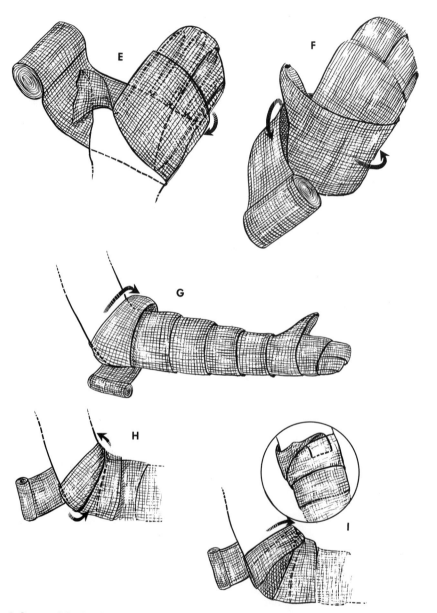

Fig. 6-2, cont'd. E, The nurse anchors the gauze that covers the fingertips with a circular turn of bandage. **F,** She encircles the thumb with gauze and encloses the forearm with circular turns of bandage. **G,** Then she places a circular turn of gauze around the elbow. **H,** With a circular turn of bandage, she anchors the lower edge of the gauze enclosing the elbow. **I,** She anchors the upper edge of gauze enclosing the elbow, encircles the remaining portion of the extremity with gauze, and tucks the free end of the gauze under the last circular turn to anchor the bandage.

and pours it over the dressing (Fig. 6-2, *A*), which has been previously placed in a suitable container. After the dressing has been saturated with the solution, it is compressed between the hands to free it of excess moisture (Fig. 6-2, *B*). Although it should be thoroughly and uniformly wet, it should not drip. A dressing that contains the correct amount of solution will sound "swishy" when it is compressed or squeezed, but moisture will not drip from it. During application of the dressing, which utilizes techniques of bandaging, the nurse should exercise care to place them smoothly and gently and to prevent contact between skin surfaces. She should apply wet dressings slightly loose, since they shrink a bit as moisture evaporates from them.

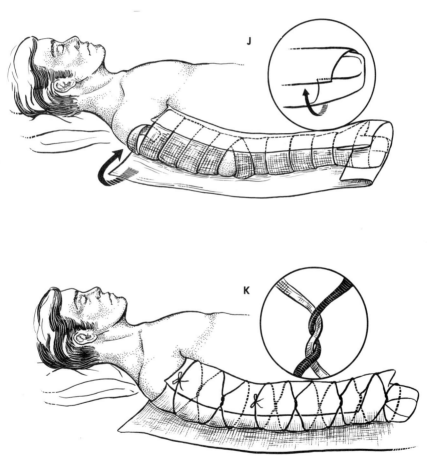

Fig. 6-2, cont'd. J, The nurse encloses the dressed extremity in a Turkish towel or a double layer of cotton flannel. Note envelope folds over the hand, which permit the patient to retain some grasping motion between his thumb and fingers. **K,** She secures the cloth covering with ties, which may be fashioned from strips of roller bandage. The tie is placed around the tips and the base of the fingers to preserve the action of the thumb and to avoid bony prominences. The inset shows the method of twisting ties to permit their rapid application and removal. A protector placed under the extremity keeps the linen dry.

Because evaporation of the solution produces cooling, the patient must be kept warm. Not only must the room temperature be well regulated and drafts eliminated, but the bed linen should be kept as free of moisture as possible. Placing plastic sheeting covered with a pillowcase under the part being treated and a cradle over the part will help keep both the bottom and top linen free of moisture. Measures to prevent chilling must be increased proportionately as increased body surface area is enclosed in wet dressings.

The nurse removes, remoistens, and reapplies the dressing periodically. If continuous wet dressings are ordered, she repeats the procedure every 3 hours. If the dressings dry more rapidly, she usually removes and remoistens them more frequently. As the moisture evaporates, the concentration of the drug contacting the skin increases. This may aggravate the condition unless the dressings are removed while still moist and resoaked thoroughly before being reapplied. The nurse must moisten the dressing thoroughly if it is to be warmed adequately. Application of additional solution to the dressings with a syringe prevents the nurse from observing the reaction of the skin to the prescribed treatment. In addition, it can, unless it is skillfully done, cause maceration of the skin due to excess moisture and increased concentration of the solution. Enclosing a wet dressing in moistureproof materials, although sometimes desirable, results in the retention of body heat and moisture, which tends to result in maceration of the tissues, irritation of the skin, and folliculitis.

Application to extremities. To dress an entire extremity, the nurse first interweaves the gauze between the patient's fingers (Fig. 6-2, *C*), then places it over the ends of the fingers (Fig. 6-2, *D*), enclosing them completely, and finally applies it with circular turns. With the first circular turn she anchors the folds placed over the fingers (Fig. 6-2, *E*). She wraps the thumb in a manner that allows it to move independently, permitting the patient to retain a pinching movement between the thumb and forefinger so that he can accomplish a number of activities (Fig. 6-2, *F*). She then continues circular wrapping of the dressing until it reaches the elbow. At this point, she takes care to preserve movement of the joint (Fig. 6-2, *G* to *I*). She secures the completed bandage by tucking the free end under the last circular turn (Fig. 6-2, *I, inset*).

If the dressing is to be enclosed with a dry outer covering, Turkish towels or a double layer of cotton flannel may be used (Fig. 6-2, *J*). The nurse may secure this outer covering with the aid of ties fashioned from lengths of roller bandage 1 inch wide. Care should be taken to avoid placing knots or ties over joints (Fig. 6-2, *K*). Application and removal of the ties are

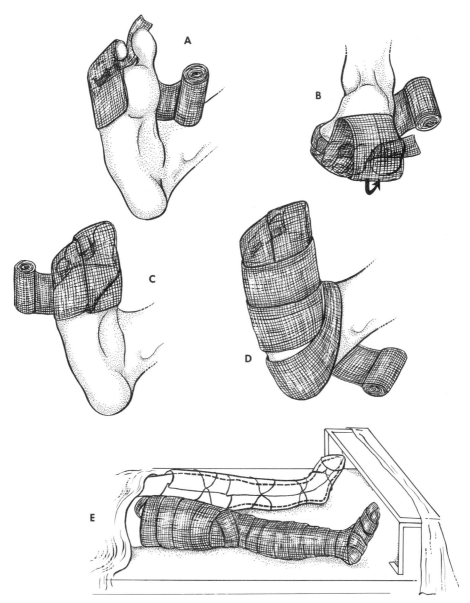

Fig. 6-3. Application of wet dressings to the lower extremity. **A,** The nurse weaves the dressing between the patient's toes. She folds the dressing over the toes, **B,** using a circular turn of dressing to anchor the folds that cover the toes, **C. D,** The nurse encloses the foot with circular turns of bandage. Edges of the gauze enclosing the heel are anchored with circular turns of bandage, permitting freedom of joint motion. **E,** The nurse also encloses the extremity with circular turns of bandage. Note the method of enclosing the heel and knee to permit freedom of movement. The left extremity is shown enclosed in outer wrappings. A cradle keeps the top linen free of moisture.

expedited if they are twisted rather than looped (Fig. 6-2, *K, inset*). The use of metal fasteners is to be avoided because, it is believed, they may contribute to further irritation of the skin.

The application of wet dressings to the lower extremities is similar and is illustrated in Fig. 6-3.

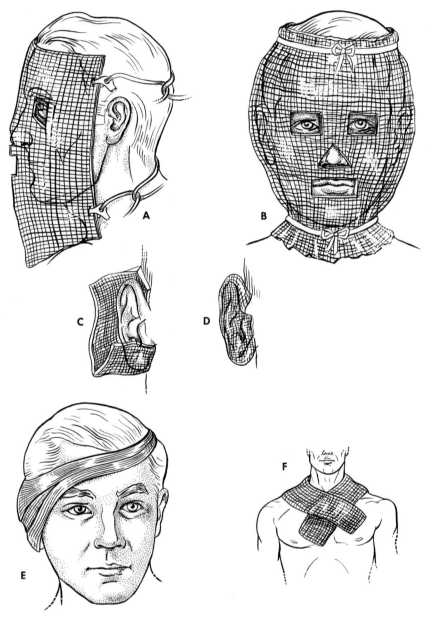

Fig. 6-4. Application of face, ear, and neck dressings. **A,** Method of securing a treated face mask posteriorly. **B,** Anterior view of the completed face mask. Anchoring the ties with bows facilitates removal. **C,** A dressing placed around the external ear. **D,** The dressing is tucked into depressions in and around the external ear. **E,** A bandage to secure the dressing on the ear. **F,** Wet dressing placed on the neck. A dry towel placed over this dressing may be secured with a safety pin. The pin must not contact the skin, however.

Application to other parts of body. The nurse may apply wet dressings to the face, ears, eyes, neck, head, trunk, axilla, groin, and perineum. Their application is guided by the same concepts and principles discussed previously. Preparation of the solution, moistening of the dressing, and reapplication are carried out in a similar manner.

The nurse applies the face mask in such a way that the patient can see, breathe, and drink without undue difficulty. She ties it over the forehead and beneath the chin (Fig. 6-4, *A* and

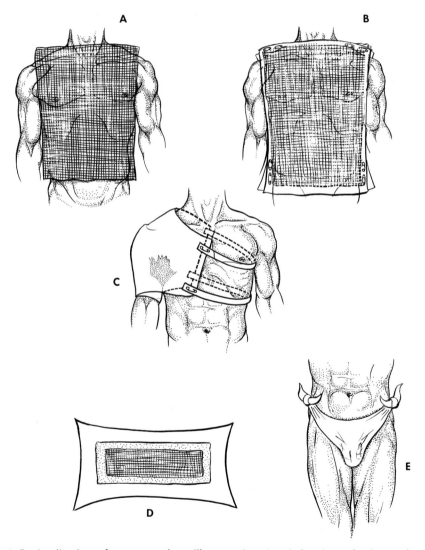

Fig. 6-5. Application of upper trunk, axillary, and perineal dressings. **A,** A wet dressing applied to the upper trunk. **B,** A method of anchoring a dressing applied to the upper trunk and covered with dry material. **C,** A method of anchoring a dressing applied to the axilla, utilizing a towel, roller bandage, and safety pins. **D,** A prepared perineal dressing is placed on a folded Turkish towel on a drape or four thicknesses of flannel. **E,** Completed perineal dressing tied in place.

B). She applies ear dressings carefully to keep the medication in contact with all parts of the ear. She should use gentle pressure to press the dressing into the depressions and crevices in and around the outer ear (Fig. 6-4, *C* and *D*). Ear dressings can be held in place with a bandage (Fig. 6-4, *E*). Depending upon the condition of the patient, eye dressings may also be secured with bandages. Neck dressings are applied in the way a neck scarf is put on (Fig. 6-4, *F*) and are covered with a dry dressing.

Dressings applied to the trunk will remain stationary if the nurse places towels or layers of cotton flannel over the dressings and fastens them with safety pins at the shoulder line and on both sides of the body (Fig. 6-5, *A* and *B*). Dressings applied to the axilla are kept in place with a device fashioned from a towel and roller bandage (Fig. 6-5, *C*). Dressings applied to the groin and perineum are kept in contact with the area being treated with the aid of a cloth that looks like a giant-sized bikini. Usually four thicknesses of flannel or a folded Turkish towel is placed between the wet dressing and the "bikini" (Fig. 6-5, *D*). The "bikini" can be tied in place (Fig. 6-5, *E*). The nurse may use other methods of securing dressings, depending largely on her ingenuity.

Occlusive dressings   The nurse may use occlusive dressings after the prescribed medication has been applied to the area. These may consist of a thin sheet of plastic material fastened with transparent adhesive tape. The dressing should be sealed in an effort to prevent evaporation of moisture. Plastic gloves or plastic booties are practical for the hands and feet. After the nurse positions the glove or bootie, she tapes the upper part to prevent the entry of air.

Lengths and widths   The lengths and widths of dressings needed for specific anatomic
of dressings   parts are shown in Table 6-1. The face mask may be prepared from 28 by 24 mesh, grade 50 gauze that is 36 inches wide. A 3-yard length of the dressing, which comes folded, is opened, folded into thirds, and then folded lengthwise to the desired size (12 inches by 12 inches). This will result in approximately 24 thicknesses of gauze. Commonly, 20 by 12 mesh, 8-ply, grade 10 gauze is used for the extremities and the trunk. Although gauze applied to the trunk and perineum contains 16 folds or is 16 ply, a similar effect is achieved on the extremity by using 8-ply gauze, since the dressing is applied in such a way that each circular turn overlaps the previous circular turn by about half the width of the gauze. Dressings applied to the neck, upper trunk, groin, and perineum may be prepared from 20 by 12 mesh, 5-ply gauze. Folding it into thirds achieves the neces-

Table 6-1

Lengths and widths of dressings for specific parts of body

Anatomic part	Length of dressing (yards)	Width of dressing (inches)
Arm (hand to shoulder)	5	4
Axilla	2½ to 5	9
Back (entire)	5	18
Buttocks	5	18
Ears	½	5
Eye	½	4
Face	3	36
Foot	5	4
Groin and perineum	5	9
Hand	5	4
Scalp	5	9
Leg to knee	5	4
Neck	5	9
Thigh	5	4
Trunk (entire)	10	18
Trunk (upper)	10 (5)	9 (18)

sary thickness. Since the width of gauze varies with manufacturers, the length needed will have to be adjusted accordingly. Materials used for dressings should be free of lint and fillers that seem to irritate the skin and increase itching. In lieu of commercially available dressings, use of bleached muslin or linen has been suggested.

Powder beds The powder bed is used to keep powdered medications in contact with large areas of the body for a certain period of time. During this treatment, which is repeated three times daily and as necessary, the patient is virtually helpless, and the nurse must remember to provide for meeting his physiologic needs.

The nurse makes the foundation of the bed in the usual manner. However, rubber sheets and other protectors that contribute to warmth and perspiration are generally omitted, since the powder bed method of treatment is used to minimize moisture. The nurse places a full-sized sheet lengthwise over the foundation of the bed (Fig. 6-6, *A*) and distributes the prescribed powder evenly over the area on which the part of the body to be treated will be resting. In order to prevent caking and crusting, the amount of powder used should not be excessive. Sprinkling and patting the powder will aid in its even distribution (Fig. 6-6, *B*).

The patient lies on the powdered area, and the nurse treats intertriginous areas with powder, protecting them by double folds of soft gauze (Fig. 6-6, *C*). Areas that need to be protected

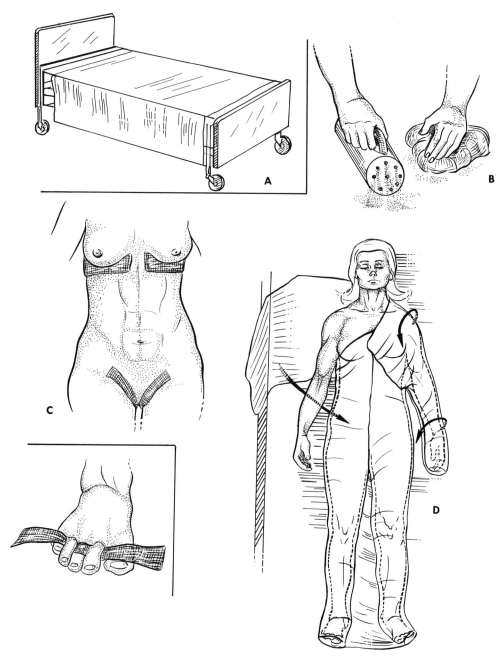

Fig. 6-6. Powder bed. **A,** A full-sized sheet placed lengthwise over the foundation of the bed. **B,** Application of powder to the sheet. **C,** Protection of intertriginous areas with gauze before the anterior surface of the body is powdered. **D,** A method of folding the sheet to keep powder in contact with the body.

from normal body moisture include the toes, groin, intergluteal folds, inframammary region, and axillas. After providing the necessary protection, the nurse powders the anterior part of the body. Soft gauze may be used to pat the powder onto the body. Lesions exuding moisture will require additional powder. The nurse then folds the sheet over the extremities and the trunk in a manner that will keep the powder in contact with the skin but will prevent contact between body surfaces (Fig. 6-6, *D*). Half sheets may be used for treatment of the legs or the trunk only, and pillowcases may be used for treatment of the arms.

Tub baths
Medicated tub bath

After the necessary medication, materials needed by the patient and materials needed to prepare the bath are assembled; the tub is scrubbed thoroughly with a suitable cleansing agent and rinsed completely. Then it is partially filled with water, and the medication is added.

Regardless of the medication ordered, the temperature of the prepared solution in the tub usually should be no less than 96° and no more than 100° F. Other temperatures for the bath solution may be prescribed. Stirring the solution with a bath thermometer will serve two functions: it will register the temperature of the solution and disperse the medication throughout the solution.

Most patients respond favorably to information and instructions regarding this form of therapy. However, it may be necessary for the nurse to reinforce explanations through positive actions. Most medicated baths are prescribed as half-hour treatments, but the duration may vary depending upon the needs of the patient as determined by the physician. The possibilities of the patient falling, fainting, or adding hot water should be anticipated and prevented whenever possible.

If the bath is being used to treat conditions of the skin, the nurse usually asks the patient simply to sit in the tub, relax, and permit the solution to bathe the lesions. In an effort to help the patient avoid further irritation of the skin, the nurse should instruct him not to rub or scrub during the bath. She should explain to him that, because its use may cause further irritation, a washcloth is not provided. Furthermore, he should be impressed with the importance of patting the skin dry with a towel rather than rubbing it, since any action that produces friction is likely to irritate the skin condition for which he is being treated.

In special instances, however, the physician may want the patient to scrub the skin. For example, he may leave orders that the patient with psoriasis be provided with soap and a washcloth and be asked to scrub thick, dry lesions with a hand brush. Any additional topical medications that are prescribed,

Table 6-2

Medications used in tub baths

Medication	Usual amount used*	Remarks
Potassium permanganate	6 Gm. (18 tablets, 5 gr., or 120 ml. of 5% solution	Tablets placed in waxed envelope may be pulverized with the aid of tongue blades; the drug is dissolved in pitcher of water, and the resulting solution is poured through several layers of gauze into bath water immediately prior to patient's entering the tub; straining of solution removes undissolved particles of drug, which will damage the skin chemically; a mixture of equal parts of vinegar and hydrogen peroxide will remove residual stains from tub.
Colloidal preparations (Aveeno, Soyaloid)	4 to 6 oz. or ½ to ¾ cup	Forcing cool water through the powder will place the colloid in solution; a large tea strainer permits rapid dispersion of colloid; since colloidal solutions are slippery, precautions should be used to prevent falling.
Corn starch, uncooked	½ lb.	If the physician wishes the starch solution to be cooked, a thick solution is made and heated until the mixture appears translucent.
Baking soda	¼ lb.	Stir until the soda is dissolved.
Sulfur	½ pt.	Avoid contact of eyes, mouth, and nose with this solution; remove the solution from normal skin with tap water.
Zinc sulfate	4 oz.	Dissolve the crystals in 2 L. of boiling water.
Entsufon (pHisoderm)	1 ½ oz.	Disperse the medication completely; other anionic surface agents may be prescribed.
Oil	1 ½ oz.	Cottonseed oil may be used.

*Amount listed is the amount of drug most frequently used for a conventional tub that is half filled with water. Twice the amount would be needed for larger tubs containing 30 gallons of water.

such as ointments, should be applied immediately following the bath.

The usual amounts of medication used in tub baths and remarks pertinent to their use are listed in Table 6-2.

Continuous tub bath   Occasionally, the physician prescribes a continuous tub bath in tepid water or medicated solution. The tub is cleansed as described for the medicated tub bath and filled with sufficient water to ensure immersion of the patient. To ensure a constant solution temperature of between 96° and 100° F. in a tub not equipped with thermostatic controls, a thermometer is placed in each end of the tub, and the temperature is adjusted as necessary every half hour. After the tub has been filled, a canvas hammock is secured over it (Fig. 6-7, *A*). Specially designed tubs contain extensions to which the hammock can be fastened. The hammock is covered with a clean sheet that extends over the rim of the tub (Fig. 6-7, *B*). The patient is permitted to wear a loin cloth, and a rubber ring or rubber pillow enclosed in a pillowcase is placed beneath his head and shoulders. He wears a harness around his chest to maintain his position and to provide for his safety when he sleeps (Fig. 6-7, *B* and *inset*). The ties of the harness are placed between the shoulder blades and are anchored to the end of the tub or to another immovable object. His chest is covered with a towel (Fig. 6-7, *C*) that has been saturated with the prescribed solution.

The nurse should place a board or tray table over the tub about 18 inches from the patient's face. She should cover them with a sheet to retain some heat, to ensure privacy, and to provide a surface on which may be placed items that the patient may need during this treatment, such as drinking water, a towel, and a handbell (Fig. 6-7, *C*). Contact with any electrical appliance is dangerous and must be prevented.

The nurse must observe the patient closely throughout the continuous tub bath. Any febrile reaction, a rapid, weak pulse, a feeling of faintness, or an increase in severity of symptoms, such as increased itching and burning, are indications to discontinue the treatment immediately and to notify the physician.

If the treatment is extended, the nurse should change the solution completely every 4 hours. She should change the linen at least twice daily and the hammock once daily.

Scalp medications   The application of medications to the scalp is usually preceded by a shampoo. In most instances the shampoo can be given with the patient seated near a sink. If the patient is confined to bed, the shampoo will be facilitated by positioning him so that his head is near the edge of the bed and by improvising a drainage trough to carry away the water. Such a trough can be

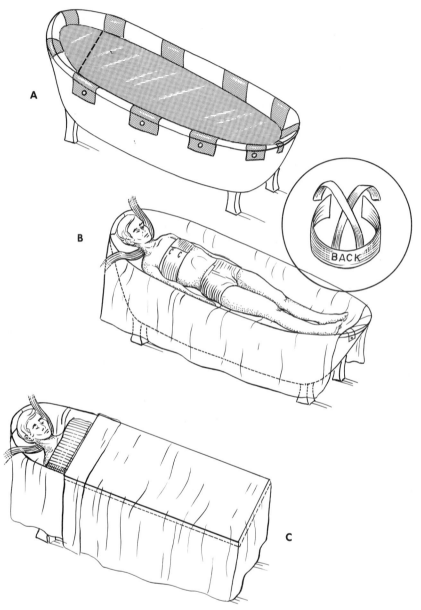

Fig. 6-7. Continuous tub bath. **A,** A canvas hammock is secured to the tub after the tub has been filled with the prescribed solution. **B,** The patient lying on the hammock that has been covered with a sheet. A waterproof pillow supports his head, and the harness around his chest is secured to the tub to maintain his position and to provide for his safety. **C,** The nurse covers the patient's chest with a towel saturated with prescribed solution. She places a board over the tub and covers it with a sheet to retain some heat, ensure the patient's privacy, and provide a surface on which materials he needs may be placed.

fashioned by rolling a rubber sheet toward both sides of the patient's head and placing the free end of the trough into a vessel that has been placed on a chair or the floor. This method is not necessary, of course, if special equipment for a bed shampoo is available.

The nurse should follow the physician's orders in regard to agents used for both washing and rinsing. She should suds the hair twice and rinse it 3 times following each application of suds. She should dry it with a towel and, if indicated, use a hair dryer. The nurse should be gentle, taking special precautions not to traumatize the scalp with her fingernails. The fingernails should be very short, and the nurse should make every effort to use only the fleshy portion of the fingertips.

The nurse combs the patient's hair and parts it in the middle. She applies the medication in the part and spreads it with the fingertips. Then she parts the hair at half-inch intervals and applies medication in each subsequent part until the entire scalp has been treated. The hair may then be parted and combed in the usual fashion.

When hot oil treatments to the scalp are ordered, the nurse applies the oil specified in the same way as medications. Then she wraps a Turkish towel, which has been saturated with very hot water and has had the excess removed by wringing, around the head. At stated intervals, the nurse removes the towel, remoistens it, and replaces it.

Questions for discussion and exploration

1. Why is it important psychologically that the nurse not wear gloves when applying a topical medication to a patient?
2. Under what circumstances would the nurse wear gloves to apply an ointment? What explanation should be given to the patient?
3. What does placing some ointment in the palms of the hands and spreading it on them accomplish in terms of patient care?
4. Describe the method of applying ointment and the underlying reasons for this method.
5. Plan the teaching that you should do when: (a) applying wet dressings, (b) applying ointments, (c) removing ointments, (d) applying lotions, and (e) preparing and giving therapeutic baths.
6. Why is it important that the technique used by all nurses administering treatments to a patient with a skin condition be consistent both in method and explanation? How can this be communicated to other nurses caring for this patient?
7. What merits might washed cotton pajamas have when worn as dressings over ointments as opposed to the merits of conventional dressings in relation to (a) mobility, (b) self-care, (c) independence, (d) inspection of the lesions, and (e) diversional activities?
8. Under what circumstances would a nurse decide that an additional application of ointment is indicated? What nursing observations are helpful in reaching such a decision? Of what might the patient complain that will suggest another application of ointment is indicated?
9. What is the most effective method of removing ointments from one's hands?
10. If the patient is able to stand during application of ointment or lotion to the lower extremities, how can you protect the floor and his feet?

11. Why should ointments be applied only in the direction in which hair grows?
12. For what reason is it recommended that cotton pajamas be washed before being worn as a dressing?
13. Why might a trial application of ointment be prescribed? What should this mean in terms of nursing responsibilities?
14. Why is it usually necessary to shake a lotion before applying it?
15. Discuss possible methods of applying lotions and the advantages and disadvantages of each.
16. If Mrs. J. has wet dressings over all body surfaces, what will happen to her body heat as moisture evaporates from the dressings? How can you prevent or reduce discomforts of which she is likely to complain unless anticipatory planning is done?
17. In what diversional activities can a patient who is in wet dressings participate? If the patient has ointment applied to the extremities? If lotion has been applied?
18. If you see a patient with a neurodermatologic condition scratching his arms, what are your nursing responsibilities to him and how will you fulfill them?
19. What is the purpose of occlusive dressings and when might you expect them to be prescribed?
20. What instructions would you expect a patient to need prior to a therapeutic bath? For what conditions might you expect the physician to ask that the patient scrub himself with a brush?
21. Why is it wise for the nurse working with patients who have lesions of the skin to keep her nails well trimmed? To remove finger rings?

Selected references   Bergersen, B. S., and Krug, E. E.: Pharmacology in nursing, ed. 11, St. Louis, 1969, The C. V. Mosby Co.

Brunner, L., Emerson, C., Ferguson, L., and Suddarth, D.: Medical-surgical nursing, ed. 2, Philadelphia, 1970, J. B. Lippincott Co.

Criep, L. H.: Dermatologic allergy: immunology, diagnosis, and management, Philadelphia, 1967, W. B. Saunders Co.

Leider, M.: Practical and pediatric dermatology, ed. 2, St. Louis, 1961, The C. V. Mosby Co.

Shafer, K. N., Sawyer, J. R., McCluskey, A. M., and Phipps, W. H.: Medical-surgical nursing, ed. 5, St. Louis, 1971, The C. V. Mosby Co.

Smith, D., Germain, C., and Gips, C.: Care of the adult patient, ed. 3, Philadelphia, 1971, J. B. Lippincott Co.

Stewart, W. D., Danto, J. L., and Maddin, S.: Synopsis of dermatology, ed. 2, St. Louis, 1970, The C. V. Mosby Co.

Tobias, N.: Essentials of dermatology, ed. 6, Philadelphia, 1963, J. B. Lippincott Co.

Wilkinson, D. S.: The management of skin diseases, New York, 1968, The Macmillan Co.

Chapter 7

Nutritional therapy

Opportunities to promote normal and therapeutic nutrition occur daily. The nurse's attitude toward and understanding of nutritional concepts and principles increase her effectiveness in carrying out this responsibility. Cultural, economic, religious, psychologic, and medical factors influencing acceptance of the diet must be considered if successful therapy is to be achieved. Patients and relatives may need practical and realistic guidance in applying principles of normal and therapeutic nutrition. These principles are discussed in basic nursing and nutrition textbooks.

Principles concerned with encouraging and assisting the patient and his relatives to accept diets requiring the use of gastric tubes are also discussed in basic textbooks. The patient who receives liquid feedings through a nasogastric tube or a gastrostomy should have the same attention given to his environment as does the patient who is able to eat normally. Such feedings are necessitated by certain surgical procedures, injuries, and illnesses. The environment should be conducive to digestion, and the patient and his relatives should be encouraged to conduct themselves as they would for a normal meal; the room should be tidy and free of odors and esthetically unpleasant materials. The conversation should be pleasant.

Prior to tube feeding, the nurse should give oral care to the patient as a means of helping to prevent nausea. If the nurse passes the tube just prior to the tube feeding, the patient should be allowed to rest before the feeding is begun. If the tube is withdrawn following feeding, oral care may do much to promote comfort. Unless doing so is contraindicated, the patient should be encouraged to assist in the plans for and in the execution of these techniques.

Gastric intubation   Gastric intubation is used to administer liquid feedings to patients who are unable to eat normally, and also to obtain specimens for laboratory studies, to irrigate or cleanse the stomach, or to decompress it (Chapter 9, pages 210 to 211). The physician, the nurse, or a skilled technician may do the intubation. The patient for whom intubation for therapeutic reasons is necessary following hospitalization is taught to do the intubation himself, or a member of his family is taught to do it for him. If recent surgical procedures or certain types of trauma have occurred, the physician will use his specialized knowledge to introduce the tube. In some hospitals, it is required that the physician intubate the patient the first time; in a few hospitals, the nurse is not allowed to intubate the patient at all.

A gastric tube may be passed into the stomach via the nose or the mouth. The nasogastric approach is generally preferred because the gag reflex seems to be stimulated less than when the oral approach is used. The nasogastric approach is usually used when the tube is to be left in place for an extended period of time. The oral route is used when deformities such as deviation of the nasal septum or absence of the hard palate exist, when intubation is planned for a relatively short period of time, when this route is preferred by the patient, or when the tube, such as the Ewald tube, is too large to be passed through the nares.

The size of the tube selected is influenced by the size of the patient and the purpose of the tube. A plastic or rubber tube, French size 12 to 18, is usually used for adult patients. The type of tube used varies with the supplies available and with the length of time the tube is to be left in place. Some of the newer tubes are radiopaque. One incorporates a sump type airway that partially suspends the tube and keeps it from direct contact with the mucosa (Fig. 11-5). The latter type prevents damage to the mucosa if suction is used and also facilitates collection of specimens since the tube does not become occluded as readily.

Rubber tubes must be chilled prior to insertion by placing them in a bowl of ice. This stiffens them, facilitating their passage, reducing friction, and lessening irritation of the mucosa. Plastic tubes are not chilled. They are naturally firm and slippery, qualities that facilitate intubation. Once the plastic tube is inserted into the upper gastrointestinal tract, the heat from the body makes it sufficiently pliable for conformance to the anatomy.

After explaining to the patient what must be done and why, the patient is placed in the desired position. A large bib, an apron, or a towel is placed over his chest to protect his clothing. Unless it is contraindicated, the patient is asked to assume a sitting position. The head of the bed may be elevated, or the patient is seated in a chair. A chair with a headrest may provide some comfort but is not essential.

The patient is encouraged to hold his head in a natural, upright position during the initial phase of intubation. If he is unable to sit up, he may lie on his back or on his right side. The latter position helps the tube to pass into the stomach. However, collection of specimens is easier if the patient is turned to his left side after the tube has been passed. Since this technique is not pleasant, it is important that the patient be positioned to promote optimum comfort.

The tube is advanced until it is placed well within the stomach. In the average-sized adult, this distance is about 45 cm. (18 inches) to 55 cm. (22 inches). If the tube is not premarked, the distance the tube must be passed to enter the stomach may be approximated by measuring the length of tubing needed to extend from the bridge of the nose to the tip of the xiphoid process (Fig. 7-1, *A*).

The tip of the tube is lubricated with normal saline, water, or a water-soluble lubricant. If the latter is used, only the very tip of the tube is lubricated; this is done by placing a small amount of the gel on a piece of gauze or tissue and rotating the tip of the tube in the gel to lubricate it. The tube must not be lubricated with water-soluble lubricants if samples are being obtained for cytology studies because the lubricant will interfere with visualization of cells. Oily materials such as mineral oil and petroleum jelly are not used because of the risk of lipid pneumonia developing if the tube or lubricant inadvertently enters the trachea.

Nasogastric intubation The person inserting the tube grasps it about three inches from its tip, lubricates it, and places it into the nostril, advancing it forward and downward (Fig. 7-1, *B*). During this stage of intubation the patient is encouraged not to wince, contort his face, or pull away since these acts make passage of the tube difficult. The patient's eyes will water during this phase. Whether eyeglasses or contact lenses are removed prior to intubation depends largely upon the desires of the patient and the preference of the person doing the intubation. When the person inserting the tube feels it pass into the pharynx, usually a distance of approximately 3 inches, the patient is instructed to flex his head until his chin rests on his chest (Fig. 7-1, *C*), to breathe shallowly, and to swallow repeatedly. Flexing the head forward helps

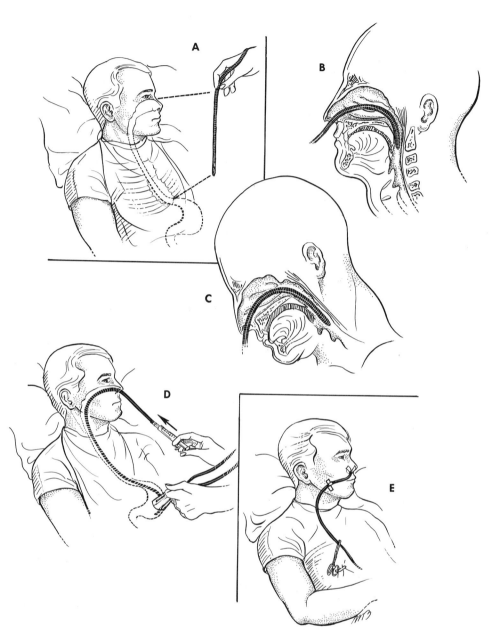

Fig. 7-1. Gastric intubation. **A,** The nurse approximates the depth of insertion by measuring the distance from the bridge of the nose to the tip of the xiphoid process. **B,** She encourages the patient to hold his head in a natural, upright position during the initial phase of intubation. Then she places the lubricated tip of the tube into the nostril, advancing it forward and downward. **C,** When the tube passes into the pharynx, the nurse instructs the patient to flex his head until his chin rests on his chest, to breathe shallowly, and to swallow repeatedly. **D,** The nurse checks placement of the tube by listening to the sound of air entering the stomach. She places the stethoscope distal to the xiphoid process. Other methods of checking the placement of the tube are described on page 176. **E,** The nurse tapes the tube to the nostril and clamps or connects it to suction.

the tube to enter the posterior pharynx rather than the mouth. If the patient is too ill to bend his head forward, an assistant may help, or pillows may be placed to help him assume and maintain this position. The tube is advanced as the patient swallows. This helps propel the tube into and down the esophagus by closing the epiglottis and increasing pharyngeal contraction and esophageal peristalsis. Swallowing interrupts inhalation temporarily, and shallow breathing minimizes the possibility of the tube being sucked into the trachea. The tube is advanced by feeding it forward with each swallow. If excessive gagging occurs, the advancement of the tube may be interrupted temporarily. The patient should be instructed to pant until this sensation passes. If resistance is met, the tube should not be advanced forcibly. The tube is withdrawn a short distance and carefully fed forward. If resistance is again encountered, a physician should be consulted.

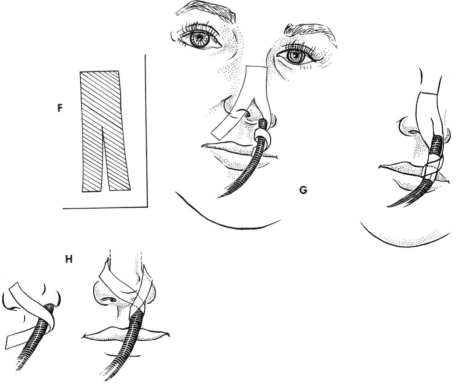

Fig. 7-1, cont'd. F, The nurse splits a length of adhesive tape for use in anchoring the tube to the nostril. **G,** She affixes the unsplit portion to the nose, wraps one of the split portions around the tube, and then wraps the other portion around the tube. **H,** A narrow strip of tape may be used to secure the tube.

Checking the placement of the tube

When the tube has been passed to the predetermined distance, its placement should be checked to be certain that it is in the stomach. The most accurate method of determining the exact placement of the radiopaque tube is with fluoroscopic visualization. In lieu of such equipment, other methods of checking placement, such as a syringe to aspirate gastric contents, are used. Failure to aspirate gastric contents, however, does not indicate conclusively that the tube is not in the stomach. It indicates only that the tube is not in contact with gastric contents. Changing the position of the patient or advancing the tube farther may bring the tube in contact with the contents of the stomach. A position useful for this purpose is a left side-lying one. However, in some cases effective use of the left side-lying position requires slight elevation of the head of the bed.

The left side-lying position helps the collecting end of the tube to gravitate toward the greater curvature where the contents pool when the patient is in this position. Another method of determining that the tube is in the stomach is to place the distal (free) end of the tube in a container of water and evaluate the rhythm of escaping air bubbles. Although some air may be released initially from the stomach, continued rhythmic escape of air bubbles coinciding with the respiratory rate of the patient probably means that the tube has entered the trachea. If the tube is passed through the larynx, the patient will be unable to speak or hum. If it has passed into the lower trachea, contact with the carina tracheae will induce violent coughing. Injection of 1 to 2 ml. of sterile normal saline will stimulate violent coughing if the tube is in the upper respiratory tract. Another method of testing placement in the stomach is injection of a small amount (approximately 5 mm.) of air through the tube. Then placement of the tube is checked by listening to the sound of air entering the stomach, with a stethoscope or one's ear placed over the stomach. A swooshing or popping sound is heard as the air enters the stomach (Fig. 7-1, *D*).

Securing the tube

After the tube is in place, it is secured with tape (Fig. 7-1, *E*). Either adhesive, masking, or nonallergenic tape may used. The method of securing the tube should not cause pressure on the tissues or obstruct vision. Pressure on the nose can cause necrosis if allowed to persist. One method of securing the nasogastric tube is to prepare a piece of tape, ½ inch wide and 2½ to 3 inches long, by splitting it lengthwise to its midpoint or a little farther (Fig. 7-1, *F*). The unsplit portion of the tape is affixed to the nose, and the divided lengths are wrapped around the portion of the tube proximal to the nose (Fig. 7-1, *G*). Another more simple method that seems to work quite well is to wrap a narrow strip of tape around the tube and attach the loose ends of the tape to the nose (Fig. 7-1, *H*).

Oral intubation When the tube is introduced through the mouth, the technique is essentially the same as described for nasogastric intubation, with a few exceptions. The tube is placed over the center and the back of the tongue (Fig. 7-2, A). The patient is instructed to suck on it as he might suck on a straw, and to swallow it as he might swallow a piece of spaghetti. When the tube has been

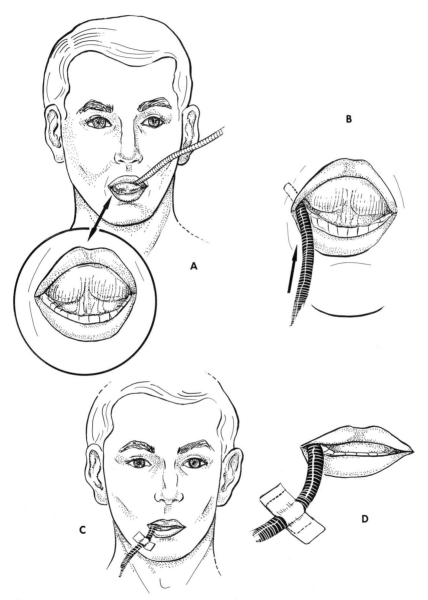

Fig. 7-2. Oral intubation. **A,** The nurse places the tube over the center and back of the tongue. **B,** When she has passed the tube about 6 inches, she places it in the left buccal area between the teeth and the cheek to reduce gagging. **C and D,** She anchors the tube to the chin with two pieces of tape, placing the first piece over the tube so that the two sides of the tape meet behind the tube and fixing the free ends of the tape to the chin. The second piece of tape is slightly longer than the first and is placed over the first to anchor it more securely.

passed about 6 inches, it is placed in the left buccal area, between the teeth and the cheek, to reduce gagging (Fig. 7-2, *B*). Then it is advanced as the patient swallows. Dentures that fit well need not be removed for intubation. They are helpful in maintaining the orally inserted tube between the teeth and the cheek. If excessive gagging occurs, the tube may be curling in the back of the throat. This is observed readily by looking into the patient's mouth. Anesthetic agents to relieve gagging should be used only with the physician's approval.

If the tube has been passed through the mouth, it is anchored to the chin with two pieces of tape. The first piece, about 1½ inches long, is placed over the tube so that the two sides of the tape meet behind the tube while the free ends of the tape are fixed to the chin. Another piece of tape, slightly longer than the first, is placed over the first piece to anchor it more securely (Fig. 7-2, *C* and *D*). The tube can then be clamped and its end covered and secured to the patient's clothing until a feeding is given. If the patient is ambulatory, he may prefer to drape the tube around his neck. If a sump tube is used, the end of the sump part can simply be placed over the connector, rather than clamping the tube (Fig. 11-5, *C*).

Irritation related to intubation   Permitting the patient to rest for a time after passing the tube allows him to adjust to its presence and to overcome feelings of gagging and nausea that may occur during intubation. The presence of the tube in the nasopharynx may cause irritation that can be eased with any of several methods. A physician's prescription is required for the use of drugs that are

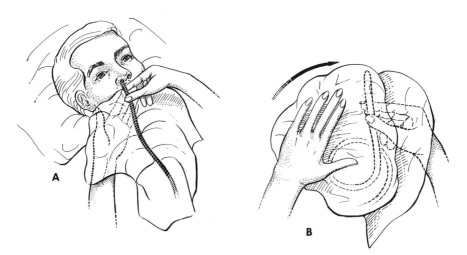

Fig. 7-3. Removal of the tube. **A,** The nurse draws the clamped tube through a towel held in a manner so that the tube is wiped of secretions as it is pulled through the towel. **B,** She wraps the tube in a towel or turns away from the patient momentarily and discards it.

applied locally or swallowed. Lozenges, a liquid antacid preparation, and anesthetic sprays or gels may be allowed. Antacids coat the mucosal lining of the pharynx, relieving irritation, while anesthetic agents relieve sensation in the area. Any of the nonsystemic antacid gels or creams seem to give some relief. Lidocaine (Xylocaine) spray, 2%, lidocaine viscous, and Cetacain are commonly used anesthetic agents.

While the tube is in place the patient tends to breathe through his mouth, thus drying the mucous membranes. In addition, the salivary glands are stimulated less than when one eats normally. Meticulous oral hygiene is indicated for the patient's comfort and to prevent complications such as parotitis. Lemon and glycerin mixtures coat the membranes as well as cleanse them. Allowing the patient to suck on sour candy stimulates salivation and helps to keep the ducts of the salivary glands patent. Occasional rinsing of the mouth with mouthwashes or water may be soothing; however, frequent rinsing seems to increase dryness and thirst.

Removal of tube To prevent liquid within the tube from escaping and being aspirated, the tube is clamped before it is removed (Fig. 7-3, A). If a sump type gastric tube is used, the end of the airway slipped securely over the end of the tube will serve this purpose. A mechanical clamp is preferable to pinching the tube or bending the tube over itself because this permits the person removing the tube to use both hands for this activity and to concentrate on encouraging the patient in cooperating. It also ensures that the tube will remain clamped during removal.

Any tape that was used to anchor the tube is removed, and a towel is placed beneath the tube. If the person removing the tube is right-handed, it is convenient to hold the towel by placing the left hand beneath it in such a manner that the tube will be wiped of secretions as it is pulled through the towel. The patient is instructed to take a deep breath and to exhale slowly; exhalation helps to prevent aspiration of liquids or even inhalation of the tube. During exhalation, the tube is pulled out with one continuous, rapid motion. The tip of the tube is caught with the towel, which is used to cover the tube (Fig. 7-3, B). If the person removing the tube wishes, he may place the tube within the towel or simply turn away from the patient momentarily while he discards the tube. Disposable tubes are discarded; tubes that are to be reused must be washed well, rinsed thoroughly, and sterilized.

Tube feeding The physician prescribes the amount, frequency, and kind of feeding that is to be administered through the tube. The formula for tube feeding can be prepared in advance and stored in the refrigerator. At feeding time, the nurse pours the specified amount of formula into a graduate measure and places it in a basin of warm water (Fig. 7-4, A). The temperature of the water should be such that the formula is warmed without producing coagulation. Warming the formula by letting it stand at room temperature for any length of time is a questionable

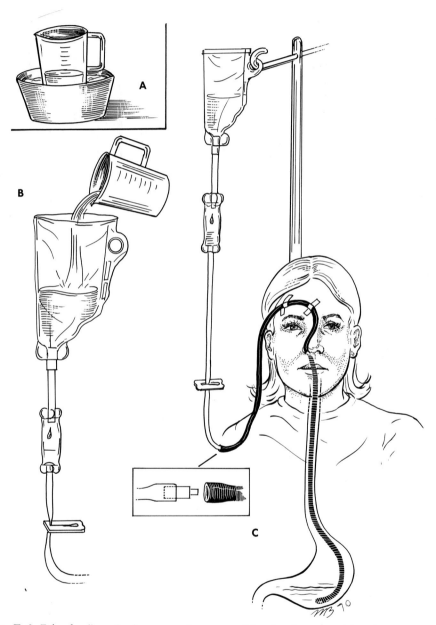

Fig. 7-4. Tube feeding. **A,** A measured amount of feeding is warmed in a basin of water. **B,** Formula is poured into the gavage container. **C,** After the tubing is freed of air, clamped, and connected to the gastric tube, the rate of flow is regulated. The inset shows one method of joining the tubes. (Courtesy Travenol Laboratories, Inc., Deerfield, Ill.)

practice because the ingredients and nature of most tube feeding formulas provide an excellent media for bacterial growth.

The nurse pours the formula into a gavage container suspended from an intravenous standard (Fig. 7-4, *B*). The tubing is freed of air, clamped, and connected to the gastric tube (Fig. 7-4, *C*). The patient should, of course, be in a sitting position. If this is not possible, he may be turned on his right side. Suction apparatus should be available if the patient being tube fed is unresponsive or unconscious.

The nurse regulates the rate of flow of the feeding by adjusting the clamp. The flow should be relatively slow in order to minimize unpleasant sensations that occur when formula passes rapidly through the nasopharyngeal portion of the tube. Ideally, 30 to 45 minutes are required to administer 200 to 300 ml. of liquid formula. Very rapid introduction of tube feedings, especially when the caloric content is high, is generally undesirable because of the increased incidence of diarrhea that seems to occur when this is done.

The formula is followed by a specific amount of water that rinses the tube and prevents coagulation of the formula within the tube. The volume of water used is unlikely to be greater than the volume of any given feeding. The occurrence of nausea or vomiting during feeding may indicate intolerance of the rate of administration, the volume, or the formula itself.

The nurse may administer drugs by pouring liquid medicine into the gavage container with the formula or water, or by pouring it directly into the tube through a funnel or the barrel of a large syringe that she has connected to the tube. If the form of medication ordered is not suitable for this method of administration, the physician should be consulted and the pharmacist should be requested to prepare a medication that can be administered safely and accurately through the gavage tube. When the feeding has been completed, the equipment used for gavage must be cleansed thoroughly or discarded.

Infant gavage differs from adult gavage in the volume of the feeding and in the specifications and preparation of the formula. Often a funnel or the barrel of a syringe is attached to the tube, the formula is poured into it, and its rate of flow is regulated by gravity. The rate of flow is therefore influenced by the distance between the tip of the tube and the tip of the funnel.

Funnel feeding   When mastication and movements of the lips are contraindicated, the nurse may administer liquids orally with the aid of a funnel to which a length of rubber tubing has been attached (Fig. 7-5, *A*). She places the tubing in the patient's mouth at a point distal to any surgical repair, usually at one

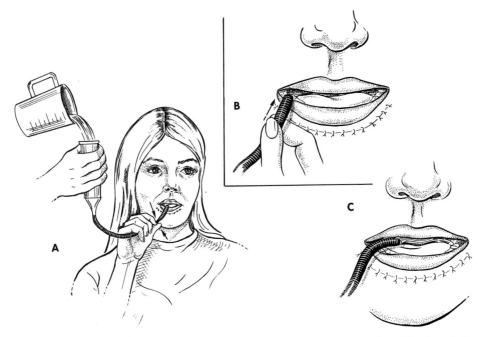

Fig. 7-5. Funnel feeding. **A,** After the tube is connected to the funnel and is placed, the patient regulates the flow of feeding with the fingers and tongue. **B,** The tube is inserted distal to surgical repair. **C,** The tube is directed so that the liquid is placed near the back of the patient's tongue.

corner of his mouth (Fig. 7-5, *B*), and directs it so that the liquid is placed near the back of the patient's tongue (Fig. 7-5, *C*). The. patient, even an infant, quickly learns to control the flow of liquid feeding with sucking actions and the position of his tongue. If this method is used to feed a very young or weak infant, a rubber bulb attached to the syringe may be necessary. The rubber bulb must be compressed gently, slowly, and continuously to control the rate of flow and prevent the introduction of air.

Infant feeders

Very tiny infants who do not have the strength to suck may be fed with the aid of an infant feeder. Such a feeder resembles a bulb syringe with an elongated nipple. Again, the pressure used to squeeze the bulb must be slow and gentle if the infant is to be kept from strangling.

Questions for discussion and exploration

1. If a patient who is intubated is found to be achlorhydric, what foods or drugs might be given to him to stimulate the secretion of hydrochloric acid?
2. What disease is ruled out if the patient secretes hydrochloric acid either with or without stimulation?
3. What are some of the factors (cultural, economic, religious, emotional, esthetic) that influence the acceptance of a diet or its components?
4. What are some of the causes and symptoms of nausea?
5. How do people react when nausea and vomiting occur? Why?

6. What are some of the nursing and medical measures used to relieve nausea and vomiting?
7. Under what circumstances is vomiting beneficial to the patient? How can vomiting be induced?
8. If the patient with a gastric tube gags easily and complains of a sore throat, what might you as a nurse do to lessen these problems?
9. When you walk into a room and find that the nasogastric tube in a patient has been looped back and up and taped to the nose and forehead, what should you look for? Why? What nursing action is indicated and why?
10. If you answer a patient's call and find him with a nasogastric tube in place and doing one of the following, think through the possible causes, methods of evaluating this situation, and appropriate nursing action for each:
    a. Patient is wretching
    b. Patient is vomiting
    c. Patient is coughing
    d. Patient seems to be choking and is pulling at the tube
    e. Tube is obviously slipping out of the nose
11. If the physician asks that a nasogastric tube be removed, how is this done? Discuss the rationale for the method you described.

Selected references

Bockus, H. L.: Gastroenterology, ed. 2, Philadelphia, 1963, W. B. Saunders Co., vol. 1.

Davenport, R. R.: Tube feeding for long-term patients, Amer. J. Nurs. **64:**121-123, 1964.

Davidsohn, I., and Henry, J., editors: Todd-Sanford clinical diagnosis by laboratory methods, ed. 14, Philadelphia, 1969, W. B. Saunders Co.

Davis, L., editor: Christopher's textbook of medicine, ed. 9, Philadelphia, 1969, W. B. Saunders Co.

Fason, M. F.: Controlling bacterial growth in tube feeding, Amer. J. Nurs. **67:**1246-1247, 1967.

Freidrich, H. N.: Oral feeding by food pump, Amer. J. Nurs. **62:**62-64, 1962.

Larson, C. B., and Gould, M.: Calderwood's orthopedic nursing, ed. 7, St. Louis, 1970, The C. V. Mosby Co.

Larson, D. L., Karzel, R., and Cameron, H.: Intestinal intubation with the aid of a magnetic tube, Surg. Gynec. Obstet. **115:**503-504, 1962.

Marlow, D. R., and Sellew, G.: Textbook of pediatric nursing, ed. 3, Philadelphia, 1969, W. B. Saunders Co.

Smith, A. V.: Nasogastric tube feedings, Amer. J. Nurs. **57:**1451-1452, 1957.

Williamson, P.: Office procedures, ed. 2, Philadelphia, 1962, W. B. Saunders Co.

Chapter 8

Intravenous fluid therapy

Selection of suitable equipment for venipuncture is guided by detailed information about the planned therapy. It is helpful to know the types of fluids that will be infused, whether the infusion is to be continuous or intermittent, the anticipated length of time over which therapy will extend, and the predicted need for blood transfusions. It is useful to know whether medications are to be administered and what the action of these drugs is upon the cardiovascular system. Knowledge that a drug is irritating to the vein or the heart will guide the selection of equipment and the rate of flow of solution.

Preparation for venipuncture   After obtaining the necessary equipment, the nurse selects and prepares the site of venipuncture. The site of choice is usually in the arm. For very short procedures such as a single-dose injection or withdrawal of a blood sample, the most conveniently located vein, frequently an antecubital vein, may be used. If therapy is to extend for a long period of time, it is preferable to choose a vein that is naturally splinted by long bones such as the ulna and the radius. The veins are distended by the application of pressure that permits arterial flow into the extremity but blocks the venous outflow. The use of a sphygmomanometer for this purpose is superior to the use of a tourniquet. The blood pressure cuff is applied as high on the upper arm as possible, in order to preserve accessibility of the antecubital veins. A pressure setting of 100 mm. of mercury should cause engorgement of the veins of most patients within 60 to 90 seconds (Fig. 8-1). When they are palpated, veins feel similar to flexible, hollow tubes.

If the venous pattern is not visible or palpable after a reasonable period of time, the nurse may apply hot packs. Hot packs applied to distend the veins should enclose the entire hand, the forearm, and extend well above the elbow for maximum effectiveness. (See Fig. 12-7.) The hot, moist pack is enclosed in plastic or another waterproof material to retain the heat and then is wrapped with a Turkish towel secured with bandage or safety pins. If a heating pad that can safely be placed in contact with moisture is available, it is placed directly over the hot, moist pack, wrapped securely around it, and covered with a towel to hold it in place. When a heating pad is used,

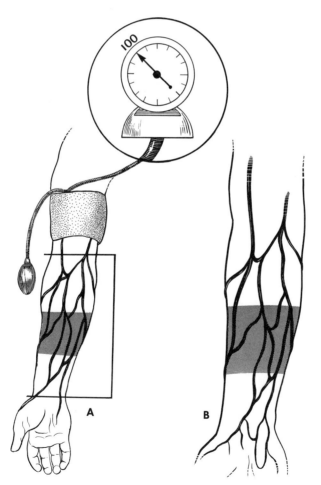

Fig. 8-1. Preparation for venipuncture. **A,** A sphygmomanometer is applied to the upper arm and inflated to distend the veins. **B,** An average pattern of superficial veins. The preferred area for fluid therapy is shaded.

pins are not used because of the dangers of puncturing the heating element. The hot, moist pack should be left in place for a minimum of 20 minutes and preferably for 30 minutes to ensure maximum distention of the veins. The skin must not be treated with oil before applying hot, moist packs to distend the veins because this increases the difficulty of venipuncture.

A right-handed person grasps the extremity with the left hand so that the thumb rests on the skin at a point approximately 2 inches distal to the selected site of venipuncture and exerts tension toward the hand. This tension minimizes the difficulty experienced when superficial veins retract or curl away from the

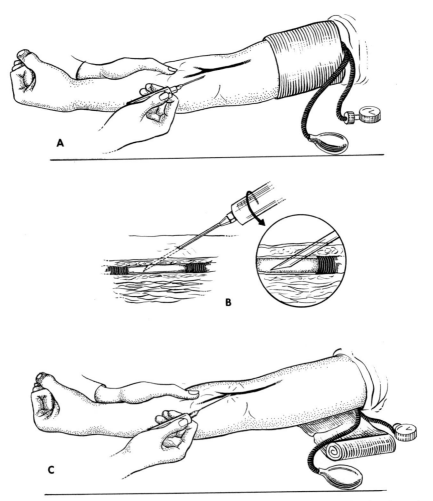

Fig. 8-2. Venipuncture with a steel needle. **A,** Tension of the thumb, distal to the site of venipuncture, stretches the skin and stabilizes the vein. The nurse inserts the needle, attached to a syringe, through the skin adjacent to the vein. **B,** She holds the needle at a little less than a 45° angle for penetration of the skin. When the needle enters the vein, the bevel is rotated to prevent puncture of the posterior wall of the vessel. **C,** The needle and syringe are lowered nearly parallel to the skin for advancement into the vein.

needle point and is helpful if it is maintained until the needle is in its final position within the vein (Figs. 8-2, *A* and *C* and 8-3, *A*, *B*, *D*, and *F*). Prior to puncturing the skin, the nurse cleanses the site with a suitable antiseptic such as 70% alcohol.

Venipuncture with a steel needle

To perform venipuncture with a steel needle, the nurse need seldom use a needle larger than 20 gauge. She attaches the needle to the syringe and inserts the needle through the skin adjacent to the vein (Fig. 8-2, *A*), holding the syringe at a little less than a 45° angle (Fig. 8-2, *B*). As soon as the needle has penetrated through the skin she lowers the syringe to a position almost parallel to the skin and advances the needle into the vein (Fig. 8-2, *C*). It is quite important that she keep direct contact with the patient's extremity while she manipulates the syringe, in order to avoid losing the vein or inadvertently puncturing the posterior wall of the vessel. As soon as the needle enters the vein, the nurse rotates the bevel to prevent puncture of the posterior wall (Fig. 8-2, *B*). She then advances the needle farther into the vein.

If the purpose of venipuncture is to obtain a sample of blood, the nurse does this before the pressure applied to the extremity by the blood pressure cuff is released. When the sample has been obtained, she releases the tourniquet, removes the needle, and applies pressure to the puncture site with a sterile compress until the bleeding subsides. When the purpose of venipuncture is to infuse a single bottle of fluid or blood, the nurse affixes the needle and tubing to the arm with adhesive tape, releases the tourniquet, and connects the tubing to the needle. The method of taping the steel needle to the arm is similar to that illustrated in Fig. 8-4, *B* and *C* for securing the plastic needle. A small piece of tape (Fig. 8-4, *B*, 3) is placed beneath the hub of the needle, and a longer piece of tape is placed over the top of the hub and applied to the skin on either side of the hub (Fig. 8-4, *C*). This stabilizes the needle.

Venipuncture with a plastic needle

The plastic needle is one of the various devices available for prolonged intravenous therapy. Some plastic needles are intended for single use only and are considered disposable. Others can be reassembled, sterilized, and reused. Plastic stylets to fit these needles are available and may be used when intermittent infusions are indicated. Each of the plastic needles encases a conventional steel needle that facilitates the introduction of the device. The tip of the steel needle extends a few millimeters beyond the tip of the plastic needle (Fig. 8-3, *C*).

The technique of introducing the plastic needle into the vein differs somewhat from the technique described for venipuncture with a steel needle. Although the demonstration of the vein and the preparation of the site are the same, the site should be selected carefully, because the plastic needle is used when prolonged infusion is desired. The introduction of the plastic needle is painful enough to make the use of a local anesthetic agent mandatory. A skin wheal that is approximately ½ inch in diam-

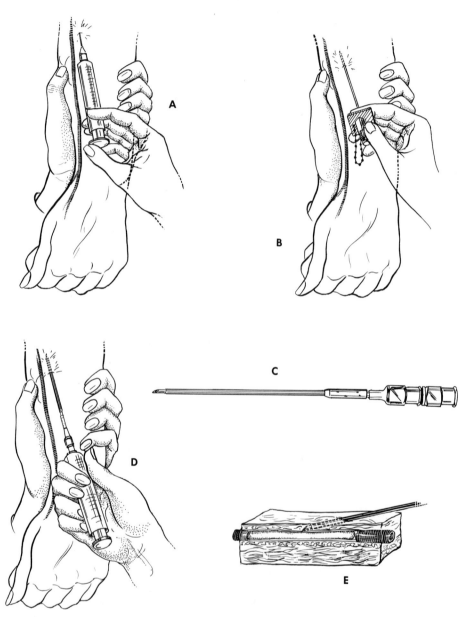

Fig. 8-3. Venipuncture with a plastic needle. **A,** Formation of a skin wheal with a local anesthetic agent. **B,** The nurse forms a pathway for the plastic needle by puncturing the skin with a large-bore steel needle. **C,** Plastic needle, Jelco I. V. catheter placement unit. **D,** The plastic needle with its metal insert is attached to a syringe for introduction through the preformed channel. **E,** Cross section showing a needle being introduced through the channel.

eter should be raised at the site selected for venipuncture (Fig. 8-3, *A*). Care to prevent the local anesthetic agent from entering the bloodstream should be exercised.

Introduction of the plastic needle is facilitated if a pathway for the plastic needle is provided by puncture of the skin with a

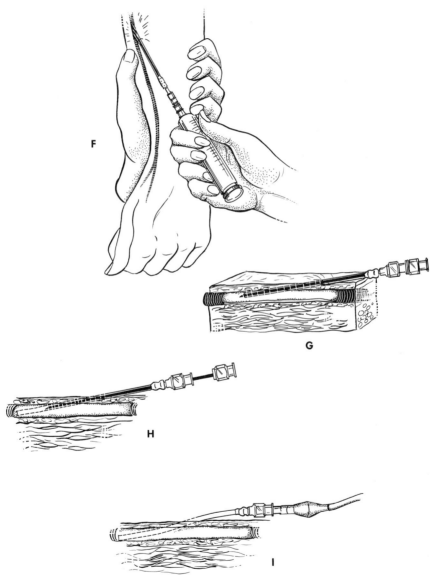

Fig. 8-3, cont'd. F, The nurse introduces the plastic needle into the vein. **G,** Cross section of a needle entering the vein. **H,** When the plastic part of the needle has entered the vein, the styletted steel needle is withdrawn about 0.5 cm. The needle is then advanced to its final position. **I,** After the plastic needle has been advanced to its final position, the styletted steel needle is withdrawn preparatory to administration of fluids. (Courtesy Jelco Laboratories, Raritan, N. J.)

large-bore steel needle such as a Lewisohn needle (Fig. 8-3, *B*). The diameter of the steel needle used to create the pathway should equal the diameter of the plastic needle that will be introduced. Care to avoid injury to the vein with this needle is necessary. Venipuncture with the plastic needle is performed by introducing the plastic needle through this preformed channel (Fig. 8-3, *D* and *E*). When the plastic needle has entered the vein (Fig. 8-3, *F* and *G*), the self-contained steel needle is withdrawn about 0.5 cm. (Fig. 8-3, *H*). The plastic needle is advanced as far as possible into the vein, and the self-contained steel needle is removed (Fig. 8-3, *I*).

Securing the plastic needle

A method of securing the plastic needle is shown in Fig. 8-4. Two narrow strips of tape circle the distal portion of the needle and are taped to the skin in a modified V pattern (Fig. 8-4, *A* and *B*). These tapes prevent slippage and loss of the plastic tube. Separation of the plastic tube from the hub occurs infrequently. The described method of anchoring the needle prevents loss of the plastic tube within the vein if such separation occurs. Two additional strips of tape are used to prevent the hub from

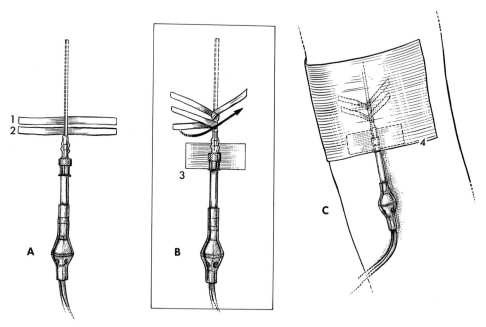

Fig. 8-4. Securing the plastic needle. **A,** Approximate placement of narrow strips of tape. The first tape is anchored before the second one is placed. The tape must adhere to the distal end of the plastic needle. **B,** Method of fastening tape to the needle and skin. Tape beneath the hub is placed with its adhesive side up. Its adherence to overlying tape prevents movement of the needle, which may contribute to separation and loss of the plastic tube. Tape should not interfere with injection into the needle. **C,** A large piece of tape completes stabilization of the needle. It is labeled to show the date of insertion and that a plastic needle is in place.

sliding sideways. The smaller strip of tape is placed under the hub (Fig. 8-4, *B*) so that it can adhere to the hub and to the larger strip of tape that is placed over it (Fig. 8-4, *C*). The tape will adhere better if excess hair is removed from the site beforehand. If the plastic tube becomes detached from the hub and floats in the vein, the person discovering this must prevent the tube from traveling through the circulatory system. A tourniquet, preferably a blood pressure cuff, will serve this purpose. The physician must be notified immediately so that he can remove the tube without delay. X-ray photographs are useful in locating the tube, which is radiopaque.

Use of veins in the hand

Occasionally, one may be tempted to use protruding veins of the hand for venipuncture. Results of the use of this site have not been too satisfactory. Often these veins are more brittle than veins of the lower arm, particularly in older people. Because an undue amount of motion of the hand is unavoidable, hematomas develop frequently; they are particularly painful in this area.

Application of splints

Splinting the arm can be avoided in many instances. If it is necessary because of the site of the venipuncture, the nurse should pad the arm board well and should apply it carefully. She should apply it to the back of the forearm and should extend it from the lower part of the upper arm to the back of the hand, immobilizing both the elbow and the wrist (Fig. 8-5).

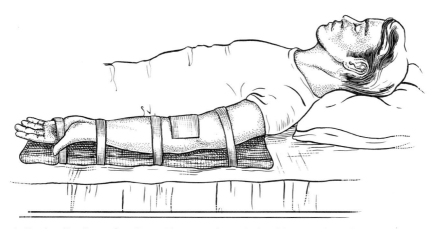

Fig. 8-5. Application of splints. The arm board should extend well beyond movable joints (elbow and wrist). Its use is necessary when the site of venipuncture is not splinted naturally by long bones. Bands used to secure the arm board should be snug, but not constricting.

Administration of solutions by intravenous infusion

To administer fluids intravenously, the nurse needs to obtain the designated solution and an appropriate length of tubing fitted with a drip chamber, needle adaptor, an adaptor to connect the tubing to the reservoir of solution, and a clamp to regulate the flow of solution. It is always advisable to administer fluids with a filter. Use of a filter is mandatory when whole blood is being administered. The filter used must be chosen according to the fluid being administered.

Disposable connecting tubing designed with all of these features is available from manufacturers of solutions for intravenous infusion. The nurse attaches the tubing to the reservoir of solution, suspends the solution several feet above the site of venipuncture, fills the drip chamber partially by squeezing it, frees the tubing and the filter, if one is incorporated into the administration tubing, of air by filling it with solution, interrupts the flow of solution with a clamp, and connects the tubing to the needle. In keeping with the physician's orders, she adjusts the rate of flow by regulating the clamp on the tubing, positioning the site of injection, and altering the height of the container of solution.

The method of connecting the tubing to the bottle varies with the equipment. If the container is fitted with a threaded cap, the cap is removed and replaced with a threaded dispensing cap attached to tubing. If the container of solution is fitted with a rubber stopper sealed with a thin rubber covering, it is important that the covering diaphragm be removed before the tubing adaptor is inserted into the stopper. The adaptor is placed securely into the larger of the openings, not the smaller airway opening. If the container of solution incorporates an entry port into its design, the spike adaptor of the intravenous administration tubing is inserted into the entry port until it penetrates the seal. The adaptor is then twisted until it is securely in place. Asepsis should be maintained throughout this technique (Figs. 8-6 to 8-8).

The rate of flow of the solution can be determined by using the following formula:

$$\frac{\text{Number of milliliters of solution} \times \text{number of drops per milliliter}}{\text{Number of hours over which solution is to be administered} \times 60 \text{ (minutes)}}$$
$$= \text{drops per minute}$$

The number of drops per milliliter delivered varies with the manufacturer and the equipment used. The labels should be consulted to learn the approximate number of drops per milliliter delivered by a particular system. Direct observation of the rate of flow is necessary because of the number of factors that may cause the flow rate to vary.

Attaching a second container of solution

A second container of solution can be attached to the primary container of solution. Although the bottles of solution may be attached in a series with a short length of tubing, it is preferable to attach two bottles with a Y connector that permits the two solutions to be administered either simultaneously or intermittently. The method of attachment is similar regardless of the equipment available. Sterile Y tubing complete with adaptors to fit the containers of solution is available from the manufacturer. An adaptor is attached to each bottle of solution in the manner described previously. Both bottles of solution are suspended, and air is removed from the tubing. The two solutions will tend to mix, depending upon the position of the clamps on the tubing and the specific gravities of the solutions. Mixing can be prevented by closing the clamp on one extension of the Y tubing (Figs. 8-6, *E* and 8-8, *H*).

Addition of medications and attachment of tubing

Medications may be administered simultaneously as a part of the intravenous infusion solution or separately through the needle that has been placed in a vein. Before administering any drug intravenously, the nurse must make certain that the preparation available is suitable for intravenous administration. For example, preparations that are unsterile or have an oil base are not suitable. If the preparation is to be administered by intravenous drip, the nurse must ascertain that the medication is compatible with the intravenous solution and any other drugs that are to be added to the same solution. For this information, the nurse must consult reliable sources of information. The pharmacist is consulted whenever necessary.

To administer the medication separately, the nurse cleanses the rubber inset of the tubing near the needle with an antiseptic, interrupts the flow of solution, and injects the drug by piercing the rubber inset with a small needle, frequently 25 gauge, attached to the drug-filled syringe. It is important that she observe for the presence of air bubbles in the tubing and for solution leaking from the tubing. If the rubber inset in the tubing does not seal itself, air can be pulled into the tubing by the flow of solution and result in air embolus. The use of large-bore needles is undesirable; these tend to remove a core of rubber tubing and cause leakage to occur. Various mechanical devices facilitating injection of drugs are available as a part of different brands of tubing.

The method of adding drugs to the solution will vary with the type of equipment used and the time at which the drug is added to the solution. If the container of solution is fitted with a threaded cap, the drug can be poured or injected directly into the open bottle of solution before the dispensing cap is attached to the container (Fig. 8-6, *B*). If the

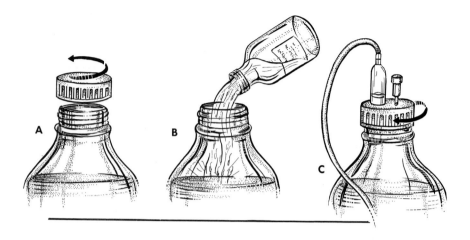

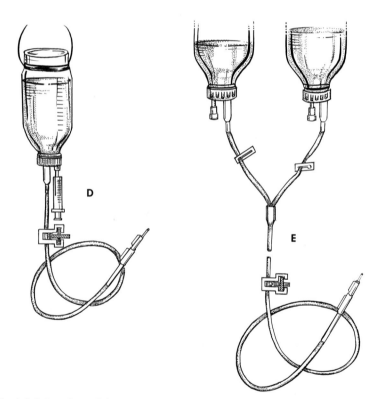

Fig. 8-6. Administration of fluids with threaded cap type of covering. **A,** After the metal seal is removed, the cap is removed. **B,** Medication is added. **C,** Infusion tubing is attached by applying the adaptor to the bottle. **D,** The bottle of solution is suspended, and the tubing is freed of air and attached to the needle. Medication can be injected with a syringe; the air filter is removed and the syringe inserted into the opening. **E,** Fluids may be attached with a Y tube for simultaneous or intermittent administration. (Courtesy Abbott Laboratories, North Chicago, Ill.)

bottle is fitted with a rubber stopper sealed with a thin sheet of rubber, the drug can be injected through the rubber diaphragm into the opening intended for the insertion of the tubing adaptor (Fig. 8-7, *C*). Fig. 8-6, *C* shows infusion tubing attached by applying the adaptor to the bottle. The bottle of tubing is suspended, and the tubing is freed of air and attached to the needle (Fig. 8-6, *D*). Fluids may be attached with a Y tube for simultaneous or intermittent administration (Fig. 8-6, *E*).

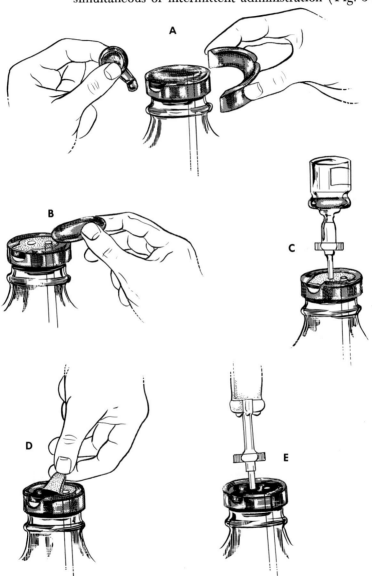

Fig. 8-7. Administration of intravenous fluids with the metal seal type of covering. **A,** The nurse removes the metal seal covering the bottle. She removes the metal cover, **B,** and adds medication through the rubber seal, using a special medication vial, **C.** Injection must not be placed in the airway. The nurse removes the rubber seal, **D,** and inserts the adaptor on the intravenous tubing, **E.**

Continued.

Fig. 8-7 shows administration of intravenous fluids with the metal seal type of covering. After the metal seal covering the bottle and the metal cover are removed, medication is added through the rubber seal, using a special medication vial (Fig. 8-7, *A* to *C*). This special medication vial can also be used for the administration of fluids supplied in plastic containers

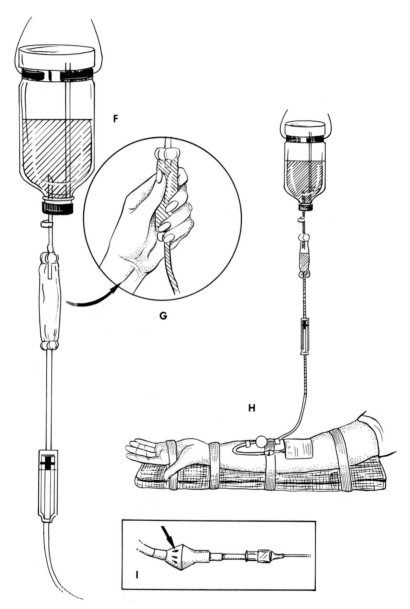

Fig. 8-7, cont'd. F, The bottle of solution is suspended, and the tubing remains clamped until the adaptor for the needle is uncovered. **G,** The nurse frees the tubing of air by permitting fluid to fill it completely. She squeezes and releases the drip chamber to partially fill it. **H,** The tubing is attached to the needle. **I,** The arrow points to self-sealing sites for injection into the flashbulb. (Courtesy Baxter Laboratories, Inc., Morton Grove, Ill.)

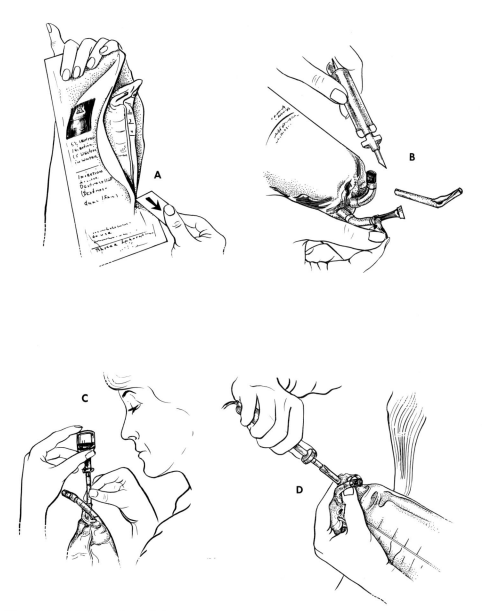

Fig. 8-8. Administration of intravenous solution in plastic containers (Viaflex solution packs). **A,** The nurse removes the container of solution from its protective covering by tearing the wrapper along a premarked line. **B,** She removes the protective coverings from the adaptor spike and the port into which it will be inserted. These parts must be kept sterile. **C,** She may add medication contained in vials to the solution before the adaptor spike of the intravenous tubing is uncovered and inserted into the port. Some vials are pumped with a device that is built into the vial to force the medication into the intravenous solution; others require that the bag of solution be compressed and released alternately to draw the medication into the bag. When no medication is to be added, this step is omitted. **D,** After adding the medication, the nurse inserts the adaptor spike of the intravenous tubing into the port of the plastic solution pack.

Continued.

shown in Fig. 8-8, *C.* The medication vial is equipped with a special adaptor to fit the opening in the bottle's stopper. As a precaution against overdosage and contamination, it is left in place until the rubber seal is removed. Addition of the drug must be made with the aid of a syringe after breaking the rubber seal. It is important with this type of bottle that the drug be introduced through the correct opening, since functioning of the reservoir is dependent upon patency of the airway. The airway will be blocked or dislodged if the drug is inserted through it. If the container is fitted with an air filter, the filter can be removed, even after the container has been suspended, and a syringe filled

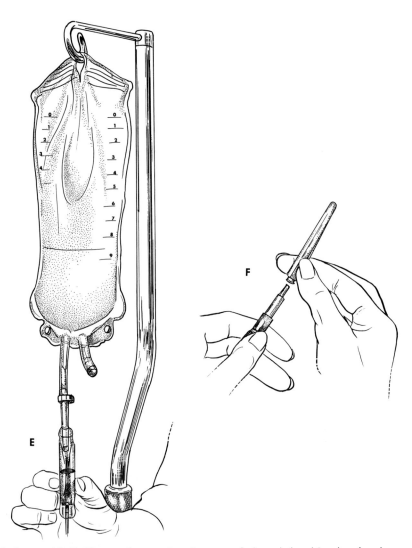

Fig. 8-8, cont'd. E, The pastic container is suspended, and the drip chamber is squeezed and released to partially fill it. **F,** The nurse removes the covering from the adaptor that connects the tubing to the needle, and, following this, clears the tubing of air by filling it with fluid.

with medication can be inserted into this opening (Fig. 8-6, *D*). The syringe is not fitted with a needle. After the drug has been injected, the syringe is removed and the air filter is replaced; the solution should be swirled to ensure complete mixing of the drug with the solution.

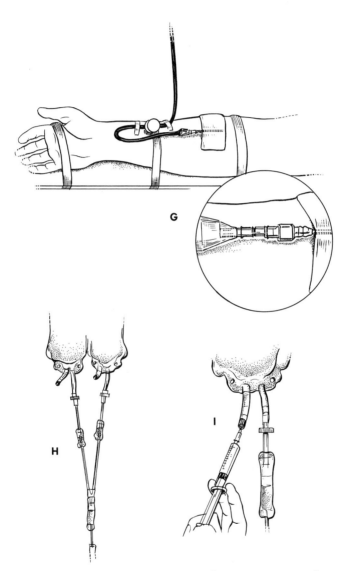

Fig. 8-8, cont'd. G, The tubing is connected to the intravenous needle or catheter. **H,** A Y tubing may be used to connect two containers of solution. These may be administered alternately or simultaneously by regulating the flow of solution with the clamps on the tubings above the drip chamber. Solutions that are to be administered simultaneously must be compatible with each other. **I,** Medication may be injected into the solution before or after the container has been suspended. The covering over the port through which the medication is injected must be cleansed with a suitable antiseptic before the sterile needle is inserted. (Courtesy Baxter Laboratories, Inc., Morton Grove, Ill.)

After adding medication to intravenous fluid supplied with a metal seal type of covering, the rubber seal is removed, the adaptor on the intravenous tubing is inserted, and the bottle of solution is suspended. The tubing is freed of air by permitting fluid to fill it completely, squeezing the drip chamber and releasing it to partially fill it. The tubing is attached to the needle (Fig. 8-7, *D* to *H*). Fig. 8-7, *I* illustrates the arrow pointing to self-sealing sites for injection into the flashbulb.

Fig. 8-8 shows administration of intravenous solution in plastic containers. The nurse removes the container of solution from its protective covering by tearing the wrapper along a premarked line. She then removes the protective covering from the adaptor spike and the port into which it will be inserted, seeing to it that these parts are kept sterile (Fig. 8-8, *A* and *B*). If the container of solution is equipped with an entry port and a port for administering medication, either of two methods may be used. The spike of preparations that come equipped with it may be inserted into the entry port and the bag of solution squeezed to force air into the medication vial, then released to allow the medication to flow into the bag of solution (Fig. 8-8, *C*). Some vials incorporate a pumping device that can be used to force the solution into the bag (Fig. 8-7, *C*).

After adding the medication, the nurse inserts the adaptor spike of the intravenous tubing into the port of the plastic solution pack and suspends the plastic container, squeezing and releasing the drip chamber to partially fill it (Fig. 8-8, *D* and *E*). The nurse removes the covering from the adaptor that connects the tubing to the needle, after which the tubing is cleared of air by filling it with fluid (Fig. 8-8, *F*). The tubing is connected to the intravenous needle or catheter, as shown in Fig. 8-8, *G*. A Y tubing may be used to connect the two containers of solution, and they may be administered alternately or simultaneously by regulating the flow of solution with the clamps on the tubings above the drip chamber (Fig. 8-8, *H*). The nurse must see to it that any solutions administered simultaneously are compatible with each other.

Medication can be added to the solution through the medication port with a needle and syringe either before or after the bag of solution has been suspended (Fig. 8-8, *I*). The surface of the medication port should, of course, be cleansed with an antiseptic solution such as 70% alcohol to preserve asepsis. To determine the amount of solution remaining in the bag, grasp the sides of the bag and pull gently in opposite directions. The upper, empty part of the bag will collapse, and a fairly accurate reading can be obtained. Flow rate can be maintained during ambulation or transport by exerting gentle, steady pressure on the bag instead of suspending the bag.

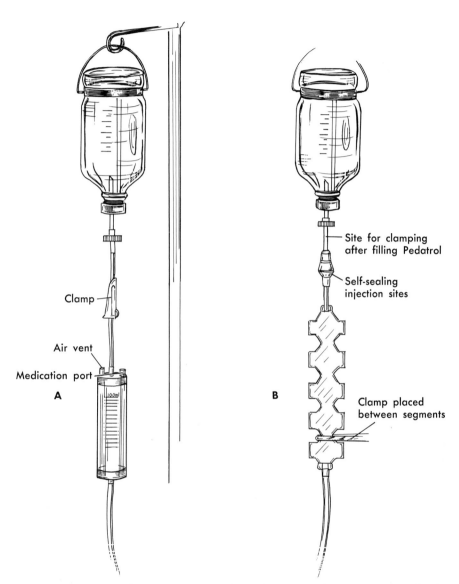

Clamp

Air vent

Medication port

A

Site for clamping
after filling Pedatrol

Self-sealing
injection sites

B

Clamp placed
between segments

Fig. 8-9. In-line devices for administration of small amounts of solution and medications. **A,** In-line burette (Buretrol) for intravenous administration of measured amounts of fluid or medication. Clamp above burette is used to regulate flow of solution from the bottle to the burette. Medication may be injected through the medication port after cleansing it with a suitable antiseptic. **B,** The Pedatrol may be used to control the amount of fluid administered. When filled, each section contains approximately 10 ml. of solution. A clamp may be placed above any section to ensure that no more than the amount of solution below the clamp will be administered in a given period of time. Segments below the level of the clamp will collapse at the same rate that the solution leaves them. Medication can be injected into the solution through the self-sealing injection sites provided in the flashball. The site must be cleansed with a suitable antiseptic before the medication is introduced. (Courtesy Travenol Laboratories, Inc., Deerfield, Ill.)

In-line devices

In-line devices are used to deliver small amounts of solution and medication.

In-line burette. The nurse may place a burette in the line between the container of solution and the intravenous administration tubing, as illustrated in Fig. 8-9, *A*. The clamp above the burette regulates the flow of solution into the burette, and the nurse may close it when the burette is being used to administer medication diluted with a small amount of solution. When the burette is used, the administration tubing must be freed of air, as described previously. The nurse can inject medication into the burette through the self-sealing rubber covering the medication port. She must cleanse it with a suitable antiseptic agent prior to inserting the needle. A size 20 or 22 gauge needle is recommended because a larger needle may prevent the rubber from sealing itself and may lead to contamination. The rate of flow of solution is regulated by the clamp on the administration tubing leading from the burette to the needle used for intravenous infusion.

Pedatrol. A Pedatrol is placed in the line between the container of solution and the administration tubing (Fig. 8-9, *B*). Again, the administration tubing must be freed of air. The Pedatrol is used to deliver a controlled volume of solution. Each segment of the Pedatrol will hold approximately 10 ml. of solution, and the entire Pedatrol will hold 50 ml. of solution. The amount of solution permitted to leave the Pedatrol is controlled by placing a clamp between the desired segments on the tubing between the Pedatrol and the flashball, or just above the flashball. Medication can be added through the self-sealing injection sites in the flashball. For this purpose the tubing above the flashball may be clamped. This is used primarily in pediatric nursing when the amount of solution administered must be carefully controlled.

Changing intravenous administration tubing

It is sometimes necessary to change intravenous administration tubing if it has been used too long, if the filter becomes obstructed, or if the tubing becomes contaminated. Some institutions have established policies that require the tubing to be changed on a regular basis. This is easiest to do if two persons work together and if the changing of the tubing can be planned to coincide with the addition of a new container of solution. The new container of solution is prepared as described previously; depending upon its design, the administration tubing is connected to it and freed of air. During this time, the other person loosens the tubing from the needle. When the new container and solution are ready, the person who is removing the adaptor of the old tubing from the needle clamps the tubing and maintains a gentle pressure at the end of the indwelling needle. This prevents blood from flowing out of the needle when the tubing is changed. The old tubing is removed, and the adaptor of the new tubing is placed in the needle. The actual changing of the tubing at the point of connection to the needle should be done rather quickly, and asepsis must be preserved. It is somewhat more difficult for one person to change tubing for the administration of intravenous infusions.

Possible mechanical difficulties

At frequent intervals, the nurse should determine that the intravenous infusion is functioning properly. If the needle has been properly positioned within the vein and has been well secured, it is unlikely that infiltration will occur. However, the flow of solution may be slowed or stopped by mechanical difficulties as well as by infiltration of solution into the tissues due to puncture of the vessel wall by the needle. Mechanical difficulties most frequently encountered include obstruction of the tubing, obstruction of the filter, obstruction of the airway leading into the reservoir of fluid, and obstruction of the needle. Kinking of the tubing is readily located by observation and inspection and is easily corrected. If the container has an air filter, it may need to be removed and inspected. Tubing containing an in-line filter should be changed when enough particulate matter has been filtered out to slow the flow appreciably. Flow of the solution may be obstructed if the bevel of the needle is occluded by the wall of the vein. Rotation of the needle will correct this.

The nurse can prevent clogging of the needle by flushing solution through the needle at half-hour intervals. If the solution flows freely, the needle is probably in the vein. If the nurse can feel the entire length of the needle within the vein, infiltration has not occurred. Fluid infiltrating the interstitial space tends to obscure palpation of the needle.

Another method of checking the placement of the needle is to clamp the administration tubing, detach it from the needle, and observe blood flow. If blood flows back, the needle is in the vein. If no blood flows back, the needle is either outside the vein or the vein is collapsed. In the latter case, outflow of blood will be produced if the needle is in the vein with a blood pressure cuff applied to the upper part of the arm and inflated to approximately 70 mm. of mercury. Other methods such as lowering the bottle below the venipuncture site in hopes of obtaining return of blood into the tubing are not dependable. It is extremely difficult to aspirate blood with a plastic syringe because this must be done very slowly and gently; more rapid aspiration tends to pull the walls of the vein over the end of the needle. This occludes the lumen of the needle even though the needle may be placed properly.

However, if a glass syringe is used, the force of the blood will move the plunger back. To be effective, the inside of the barrel and the outside of the plunger must be wet with sterile solution.

Termination of
an infusion

The nurse begins termination of an infusion by clamping the tubing through which the solution is flowing. She loosens the tape fixing the needle and tubing to the skin (Fig. 8-10, *A*). She must hold the needle firmly while she removes the tape, in order to prevent unnecessary trauma to the vein and surrounding tissues. With one hand the nurse holds a sterile cotton pledget over the site of insertion, and with the other hand she slowly withdraws the needle, using care to keep the hub of the needle flush with the skin. As soon as she has completely removed the needle, she applies pressure to the wound with the sterile pledget for the period of time necessary to stop

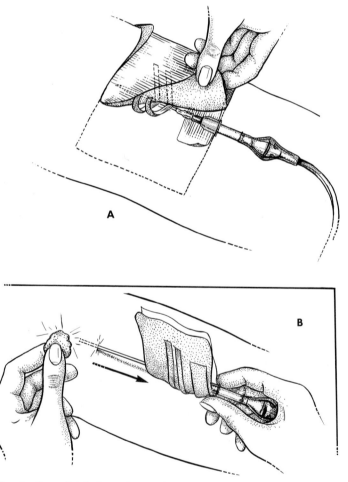

Fig. 8-10. Termination of infusion. **A,** To discontinue an intravenous infusion, the nurse loosens tape adhering to the skin but does not remove tape from the needle. **B,** She withdraws the needle and applies direct pressure to the site with a sterile pledget until bleeding stops.

bleeding from the wound. The pledget can be secured with a strip of adhesive tape if desired (Fig. 8-10, *B*), or a Band-Aid may be applied to the puncture site.

Measurement of central venous pressure

Central venous pressure may be measured at frequent intervals for varying periods of time with the aid of an indwelling plastic catheter or needle and a simple venous pressure set. This set is basically an intravenous set with a calibrated open-end sidearm that is used as the pressure manometer. The physician positions the needle or catheter within the vein and sets the level of the manometer scale and tubing on the intravenous stand. When a needle is used, the physician places it in the external jugular vein. It is preferable to insert a small catheter into the antecubital vein and advance it about 24 inches so that the tip of the catheter is placed close to the right atrium.

The nurse may assist the physician with this technique. The venous pressure set is attached to the container of solution in the manner described for connecting tubing for intravenous infusion. The stopcock on the venous pressure set is closed, the solution is suspended, and the drip chamber is squeezed and released to partially fill it with solution. The manometer scale, marked in centimeters, is taped to the intravenous stand in such a way that the zero mark on the scale is at the level of the right atrium of the patient's heart. This level is half the distance from the sternum to the skin of the back when the patient is in a recumbent position. The sidearm tube should be taut, and an intravenous stand attached to the bed should be used to keep the level of the scale constant if the height of the entire bed is changed (Fig. 8-11, *A*). Accurate readings can be obtained only if the zero mark on the manometer scale is level with the patient's right atrium. The patient must be in a recumbent position (Fig. 8-11, *A*).

To fill the intravenous tubing with fluid, the nurse turns the stopcock so that the extensions from the stopcock, which are across from each other, are aligned with the intravenous tubing. The third projection points downward and away from the manometer (Fig. 8-11, *B*). This position permits fluid to flow through the intravenous tubing only and prevents fluid from entering the manometer. Filling the intravenous tubing before attempting to fill the manometer prevents air bubbles from getting into the solution in the manometer. Next, the sidearm manometer is filled to a level of 10 to 15 cm. by turning the stopcock so that its adjacent projections align with the tubing leading from the reservoir of solution and with the manometer (Fig. 8-11, *C*). Because central venous pressure is measured in relation to atmospheric pressure, solution

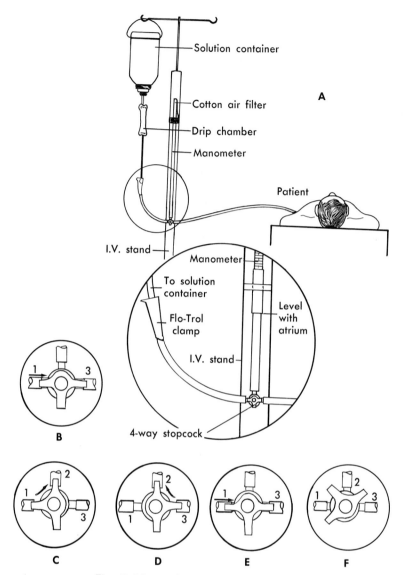

Solution container

Cotton air filter

Drip chamber

Manometer

A

Patient

I.V. stand

Manometer

To solution container

Flo-Trol clamp

Level with atrium

I.V. stand

4-way stopcock

B

1 3

C

1 2 3

D

2 1 3

E

1 3

F

2 1 3

Fig. 8-11. For legend see opposite page.

should not be permitted to contact the air filter at the top of the manometer if one is incorporated into the design. It is advisable to retain at least an inch of space between the column of solution and the filter. Next, the protective covering over the needle adaptor on the intravenous tubing is removed and the adaptor is inserted into the indwelling catheter or needle. The rate of flow of the solution should be sufficient to maintain patency of the indwelling catheter or needle and may, therefore, be quite slow.

To measure central venous pressure, the nurse turns the stopcock so that one extension is aligned with the tubing

Fig. 8-11. Measurement of venous pressure. **A,** Venous pressure set in use. Fluid flows from the container to the patient when venous pressure is not being measured. The calibrated scale on the sidearm manometer is used to read venous pressure. For the reading, the patient must be in a recumbent position with the zero mark on the manometer scale level with the patient's right atrium. **B,** To fill the intravenous tubing, the four-way stopcock is turned so that the extensions from the stopcock are aligned with the intravenous tubing only (1 and 3). The extensions on the stopcock may be thought of as pointing the direction of flow. The tubing is then attached to the indwelling catheter or needle. **C,** To fill the manometer, the stopcock is turned so that one extension is aligned with the tubing leading from the container of intravenous solution, 1, and the other extension is aligned with the tubing leading to the manometer, 2. **D,** To read venous pressure, the stopcock is turned so that one extension is aligned with the tubing leading to the manometer, 2, and the other extension is aligned with the tubing leading from the patient, 3. The level of solution in the manometer is pushed down by air pressure on the column of fluid in opposition to the venous pressure from the patient. The level of solution in the manometer settles and pulsates at the level of venous pressure. The venous pressure reading is taken, recorded, evaluated, and used to alter the nursing care of the patient. **E,** To maintain patency of the intravenous needle or catheter, the stopcock is turned so that the two extensions are aligned with the tubing leading from the bottle, 1, to the patient, 3. **F,** The flow of solution is stopped in all directions when the stopcock is positioned so that the extensions are not aligned with the tubing or the manometer. (Courtesy Baxter Laboratories, Inc., Morton Grove, Ill.; Travenol Laboratories, Inc., Deerfield, Ill.)

leading to the manometer, and the other extension is aligned with the tubing leading from the patient (Fig. 8-11, *D*). The level of the solution in the manometer tube will settle and pulsate at the level of the central venous pressure. The nurse turns the stopcock so that the two extensions are aligned with the tubing leading from the bottle to the patient to maintain patency of the intravenous needle or catheter (Fig. 8-11, *E*). To continue intravenous infusion between readings, the nurse repositions the stopcock. The flow of solution is stopped when the extensions from the stopcock are not aligned with the tubing or the manometer (Fig. 8-11, *F*).

Central venous pressure readings are recorded on the patient's chart. The physician should be informed of significant changes or trends in venous pressure. Unless the physician specifies otherwise, it is assumed that a venous pressure reading between 5 and 20 cm. of water is reasonably safe.

The physician utilizes venous pressure in the diagnosis and treatment of inadequate circulation. High venous pressure in the presence of hypotension suggests myocardial insufficiency, which may be treated with cardiotonic drugs. Low venous pressure suggests low circulating blood volume or peripheral vasodilatation, conditions treated by increasing the blood volume. Intelligent observation can prevent the venous pressure from rising above the desired reading and avoid infusion of excessive amounts of blood or fluids.

Questions for
discussion and
exploration

1. What factors determine the choice of needles or catheters used for intravenous infusion?
2. What sites can be used for venipuncture? What factors influence the selection of a particular site?
3. What are the advantages of using a sphygmomanometer instead of a narrow tourniquet?
4. What is the importance of applying manual traction distal to the site of venipuncture?
5. Contact with the extremity is emphasized in the text. What is the value of maintaining contact with the extremity during venipuncture?
6. Why is the tourniquet not released until a blood sample is obtained and why must it be released before infusion is begun?
7. If you notice that an intravenous infusion is leaking and upon palpation discover that the plastic part of the needle has come apart from the hub and is felt a few inches away from the site of venipuncture, what nursing action is indicated?
8. What is the purpose of a splint, when should it be used, and how must it be applied to serve its purpose?
9. Calculate the rate of flow in drops per minute when 800 ml. of solution is to be administered in 6½ hours and the manufacturer's information states that the solution provides approximately 10 drops per minute.
10. As you enter Mrs. G.'s room, you notice that her intravenous solution is not running. She complains that her arm hurts. What information do you need and what will you do to determine if the intravenous needle is in place, why it is not working, and to make Mrs. G. comfortable?
11. Jack E. is upset about having intravenous infusions for several days. He complains bitterly and threatens to discontinue the intravenous infusion himself. You know that he has been bleeding in the gastro-intestinal tract and that the "needle" is really an intravenous catheter. What approach might you use with him?
12. When the physician orders a penicillin preparation to be added to an intravenous solution, how will you learn if the preparation ordered is compatible with the solution being administered? If it is not compatible, what is your nursing responsibility?
13. Jane R., aged 17, is admitted in a poor nutritional state. When the physician orders hyperalimentation solution to be given intravenously, what are the nurse's responsibilities?
14. When assisting Mr. D., a postoperative patient, to ambulate, you notice that the intravenous solution is running poorly and blood is visible in the tubing proximal to the needle. What nursing action is indicated?
15. When blood transfusions are given, nursing care and patient activity may be limited to essential care only. Why? What are the signs and symptoms of an adverse reaction to a transfusion and what nursing action is indicated for each?
16. By what methods can you check the placement of a needle in the vein?
17. Of what value are central venous pressure readings to the physician?
18. What errors in technique can cause erroneous readings of central venous pressure?

Selected references

Adriani, J.: Techniques and procedures of anesthesia, ed. 3, Springfield, Ill., 1969, Charles C Thomas, Publisher.

Adriani, J.: Venipuncture, Amer. J. Nurs. 62:66-70, 1962.

Betson, C., and Use, L.: Central venous pressure, Amer. J. Nurs. 69: 1466-1468, 1969.

Chow, R.: Innovations in IV equipment, Amer. J. Nurs. 62:80-81, 1962.

Crouch, M. L., and Gibson, S. T.: Blood therapy, Amer. J. Nurs. 62:71-76, 1962.

Donn, R.: Intravenous admixture incompatibility, Amer. J. Nurs. **71**:325, 1971.

Grant, J. N., Moir, E., and Fago, M.: Parenteral hyperalimentation, Amer. J. Nurs. **69**:2392-2395, 1969.

Haselman, J.: Teaching principles of intravenous therapy, J. Nurs. Educ. **2**:21-23, 34-42, 1963.

Imperiale, M., and Krebs, T.: The intravenous therapy nurses, Amer. J. Nurs. **61**:53-54, 1961.

Massa, D. J., Lundy, J. S., Faulconer, A., Jr., and Ridley, R. W.: A plastic needle, Proc. Mayo Clin. **25**:413-415, 1950.

Metheny, N., and Snively, W. D.: Nurse's handbook of fluid therapy, Philadelphia, 1967, J. B. Lippincott Co.

Michel, F.: The vexing core, Amer. J. Nurs. **71**:768, 1971.

Moffitt, E. A., and Sessler, A. D.: The circulation in anaesthesia, Canad. Anaesth. Soc. J. **11**:173-181, 1964.

Programmed instruction: Intravenous infusion of vasopressors, Amer. J. Nurs. **65**:129-152, 1965.

Russell, M. W., and Maier, W. P.: The ABC's of C.V.P. measurement, RN **69**:34-35; 68-69, 1969.

Shanck, A. H.: The nurse in an intravenous therapy program, Amer. J. Nurs. **57**:1012-1013, 1957.

Voda, A.: Body water dynamics, Amer. J. Nurs. **70**:2594-2601, 1970.

Chapter 9

Elimination

Assistance, instruction, encouragement, and preliminary explanation of the planned care must accompany techniques used to promote elimination. The nurse must assure the patient by her words, actions, attitude, and facial expression that elimination of waste material is a normal, healthy process. Provision of privacy encourages elimination.

Intestinal decompression When peristalsis is lacking or intestinal obstruction occurs, the physician may insert a gastrointestinal tube to remove gaseous and liquid materials. This treatment, called decompression therapy, is used to relieve abdominal distress.

When such therapy is planned, it should be recognized that swallowing a tube is unpleasant under the best conditions. Preparation of the patient and the tube is likely to be similar to that described for gastric intubation in Chapter 7, pages 172 to 175. In addition, the balloon should be tested for capacity and leaks and should be freed of excess air. Frequently the physician passes the tube through the nostril into the intestinal tract and gives the nurse instructions concerning positioning of the patient and advancing and irrigating the tube.

After the tube has passed through the pylorus, the nurse may be requested to position the patient on his right side without a pillow and with the foot of the bed elevated about 12 inches for 2 hours. At the end of this time, the physician will determine whether the tube is in the duodenum; if it is, he will give instructions to advance the tube. The rate of advancement may be as much as 6 inches every half hour.

To anchor the tube during the intervening time, the nurse can place a piece of split rubber tubing about 1½ inches long around the tube and tape it to the patient's forehead. She can pull the tube through the split rubber tubing to provide necessary slack for its advancement. Prior to advancement of the tube, the nurse tells the patient what is to be done and why. She places him in a high Fowler's or a sitting position unless this is contraindicated. Prior to each succeeding advancement of the tube, she should lubricate the nostrils and the portion of the tube that is to be advanced. The nurse asks the patient to swallow small amounts of water and advances the tube at the exact time swallowing occurs. Some patients find it helpful to hold a small amount of ice in their mouth, swallowing the liquid as the ice melts. This limits the intake when obstruction or fluid and electrolyte balance is a problem.

If the patient is unable to swallow, the nurse should stroke the area from the upper end of the sternum to the chin in an upward direction, and the tube should be advanced when the larynx rises. Once the tube has been advanced to the desired position, the nurse should tape it securely. Otherwise, peristalsis will continue to propel the tube.

Application of suction is discussed in Chapter 10, and irrigation of the tube is discussed in Chapter 11.

Enemas   Preparation varies with the type of enema prescribed. When disposable enemas are used, the manufacturer provides directions for preparation and administration. For one type, the nurse places the patient in a left lateral position unless the knee-chest position has been specified (Fig. 9-1, *A*). She removes from the rectal tube the protective cover containing a lubricant for its lubrication, inserts the rectal tube into the rectum, and compresses the plastic container for injection of the solution (Fig. 9-1, *B* to *D*).

Another type of disposable enema is illustrated in Fig. 9-2. For its use, the nurse places the patient in a left lateral position (Fig. 9-2, *A*). She exerts pressure on the tube proximal to the bead, expelling orange bead from the tube into the bag. Dislodgment of the bead permits the solution to flow through the tube, and this dislodgment can be done either before or after the rectal tube has been inserted (Fig. 9-2, *B*). The nurse removes the Measur-Gard protector cover from the tip of the container with a rotating motion, distributing lubricant in the container onto the tip of the rectal tube (Fig. 9-2, *C*). She may move the guard to a position on the tube representing the dis-

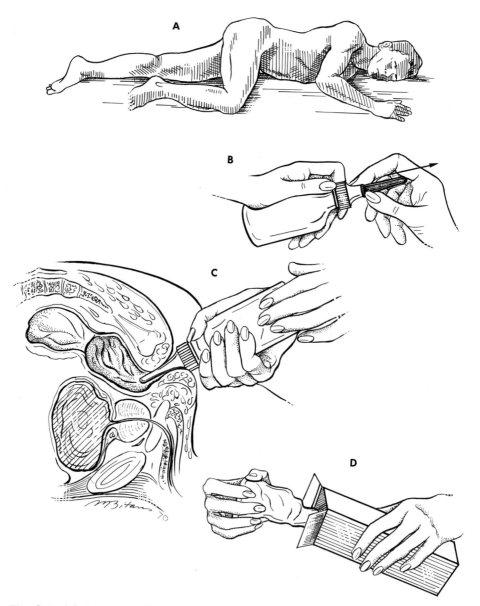

Fig. 9-1. Administration of a disposable enema (Fleet enema). **A,** The nurse places the patient in a left lateral position unless the knee-chest position has been specified. **B,** She removes the protective covering from the rectal tube and lubricates the tube with a lubricant contained in this cover. **C,** Then she inserts the lubricated rectal tube into the rectum and injects the solution by compressing the plastic container. **D,** The used container may be replaced in its original container for its disposal. (Courtesy C. B. Fleet Co., Inc., Lynchburg, Va.)

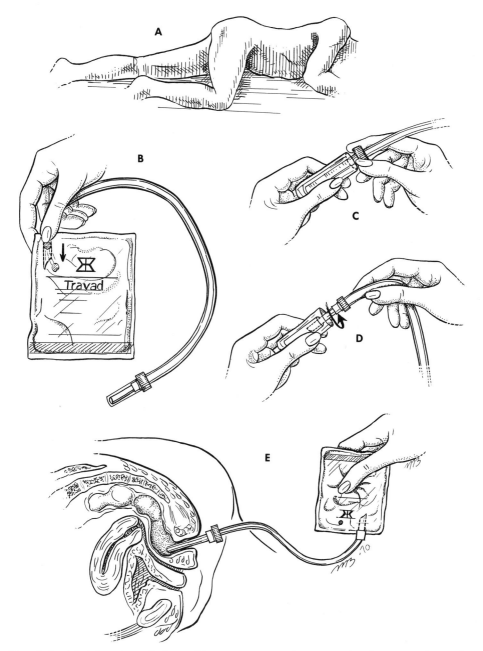

Fig. 9-2. Administration of disposable enema (Travad enema). **A,** The nurse places the patient in a left lateral position. **B,** The nurse should expel orange bead from the tube into the bag by exerting pressure on the tube proximal to the bead. This can be done either before or after the rectal tube has been inserted. Dislodgment of the bead permits the solution to flow through the tube. **C,** The nurse removes the Measur-Gard protector cover from the tip of the container with a rotating motion. This distributes lubricant in the container onto the tip of the rectal tube. **D,** She may move the guard to a position on the tube that represents the distance the rectal tube is to be inserted. **E,** After the tube has been inserted, the nurse squeezes the bag until the desired amount of fluid has been administered. The used equipment may be replaced in its original package for disposal. (Courtesy Travenol Laboratories, Inc., Deerfield, Ill.)

tance the tube is to be inserted (Fig. 9-2, *D*). After insertion of the tube, the nurse squeezes the bag until the desired amount of fluid has been administered (Fig. 9-2, *E*). Then she places the used equipment in its original package for disposal.

Equipment and solution

If disposable enemas are not used, the nurse prepares equipment and solution in a service area and takes them to the nursing care center where she administers the enema. She connects a 1-foot to 2-foot length of rubber tubing with an adaptor to a size 18 to 20 French catheter. She places a shutoff clamp or pinchcock on the tubing attached to the irrigating container and coils the tubing and catheter loosely around the container. Then she places all three on a tray that contains lubricant, tissue, and protective pads and prepares the prescribed amount and kind of solution, placing them in the container. Temperature of the solution is tested with a thermometer and should not exceed 110° F.; more commonly 105° F. or less is used. If the water is too warm, the intestinal mucosa may be injured; if it is too cold, unnecessary cramping may occur. Table 9-1 lists the ingredients and proportions for enema solutions.

Positioning the patient

The nurse assists the patient in assuming the desired position and protects his bed with disposable pads or waterproof material covered with a cloth. Choice of position is influenced by the condition of the patient and the results desired. A left lateral position may be used to cleanse the rectum.

If a small amount of solution is used, the nurse may attach the catheter directly to a funnel. She places the prepared solution in a graduated measure and pours it into the funnel.

A flat, back-lying position with the legs flexed is useful if the patient is unable to control the anal sphincter. In this situation, the nurse inserts the catheter after placing the bedpan and uses a rubber glove to protect the hand holding the catheter in place during administration of the solution. Support of the lumbar region with pillows or a folded bath blanket adds some comfort to this position.

The knee-chest position, prescribed occasionally, must be used cautiously if the patient is weak, debilitated, or elderly. Unless the mattress is completely protected and the bed can be lowered, it may be desirable to place a large foam rubber mat covered with a cloth on the floor of the bathroom, asking the patient to assume the knee-chest position on this mat. It is imperative that the nurse provide complete privacy and ensure the patient's safety when this position is used.

If the 3-maneuver enema is used to eliminate or reduce the need for several cleansing enemas, the nurse places the patient in a right lateral position for administration of the solution (Fig.

Table 9-1

Enema solutions*

Name of enema	Type	Ingredients	Additional information
Alum	Astringent	Alum, 2 Gm. (30 gr.) Water, 500 ml. (1 pt.)	If not expelled after 30 minutes, siphon solution from colon with rectal tube
Glycerin and water	Carminative	Glycerin, 30 to 90 ml. (1 to 3 oz.) Water, 500 ml. (1 pt.) or Glycerin, 30 ml. (1 oz.) Water, 90 ml. (3 oz.)	Sometimes referred to as G and W enema Referred to as "cup" enema
Milk and molasses	Carminative	Equal amounts of milk and molasses: 90-250 ml. (3-8 oz.) of each	Warm milk to 110° F.; add molasses, followed by a cleansing enema
1-2-3	Carminative	Magnesium sulfate, 30 Gm. (1 oz.) or 50% solution (1 oz.) Glycerin, 60 ml. (2 oz.) Water, 90 ml. (3 oz.)	Dissolve magnesium sulfate in boiling water; add glycerin and cool to 105° F.
Peroxide	Cleansing	Hydrogen peroxide, 15 ml. (½ oz.) Water, 500 ml. (1 pt.)	Insert rectal tube after 10 minutes
Oil retention	Softening	Mineral, cottonseed, or olive oil, 120-240 ml. (4-8 oz.)	To be retained indefinitely; may be followed by cleansing enema
Saline, physiologic	Cleansing	Salt, 4 Gm. (1 tsp.) Water, 500 ml. (1 pt.)	
Soapsuds	Cleansing	Soap solution, 30 ml. (1 oz.) or Powdered soap, 1 tbsp. Water, 1,000 ml.	
Soda	Cleansing	Sodium bicarbonate, 20 Gm. (5 tsp.) Water, 1,000 ml.	
Starch	Emollient, vehicle for medications	Starch, 4 Gm. (1 tsp.) Water, 8 oz.	Mix starch with 2 oz. cold water; slowly add 6 oz. boiling water; add prescribed medication; administer slowly with a small catheter (12-14 French), retained
Tap water	Cleansing	Water, 1,000 ml.	
Turpentine	Carminative	Turpentine, 4 ml. Soap solution, 30 ml. Water, 500 ml.	Stir well; turpentine is irritating to mucous membranes; follow with cleansing enema

*Temperature of the solution on administration should be 105° F. The total amount of solution may be increased or decreased as necessary, if the proportions of the contents remain the same.

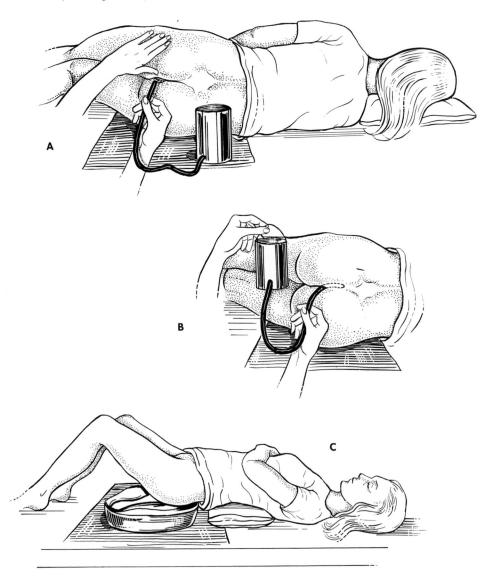

Fig. 9-3. Three-maneuver enema. **A,** The nurse places the patient in right lateral position for administration of the solution. **B,** She administers the solution. **C,** The hips are elevated as the patient is turned; evacuation occurs with the hips at a higher level than the chest, shoulders, and head. The lumbar area is supported with a pillow or lumbar pad.

9-3, *A* and *B*). Then she elevates the hips of the patient as he is rolled onto his back. Evacuation occurs with the hips at a higher level than the chest, shoulders, and head (Fig. 9-3, *C*). A pillow under the back and a small pillow beneath the head may promote comfort in this position.

Administering the   The nurse expels air in the tubing by releasing the clamp
solution   until the catheter is completely filled with solution. She then

reapplies the clamp and lubricates the tip of the catheter. Asking the patient to bear down to relax the sphincter, she inserts the catheter and advances it gently.

The nurse may insert the catheter 4 to 6 inches for cleansing the rectum and 6 to 8 inches for retention enemas. Inserting the catheter beyond this distance or forcing its advancement can produce injury to the wall of the colon. If advancement seems impaired, it may be due to a fecal mass or to folds of tissue. The nurse may withdraw the catheter slightly and then ease it forward. Introducing the solution very slowly may permit it either to flow around the mass of fecal material or to distend the colon, removing obstruction caused by the folds of tissue.

Generally, the nurse administers the solution slowly by elevating the container of solution 18 to 24 inches above the level of the hips. More rapid administration stimulates peristalsis, causing intestinal cramping and reducing ability to retain the solution. Cramping is relieved by interrupting the flow of solution temporarily, by lowering the container to slow the rate of flow, or by lowering the container below the level of the hips to permit gas to escape from the colon.

After the nurse administers the solution, she withdraws the catheter and applies pressure to the anal area to minimize spasms of the sphincter. Depending upon the purpose of the enema, the nurse may encourage the patient to retain the solution for a period of 10 minutes or more. Unless doing so is contraindicated, the patient may be permitted to expel the enema in the bathroom. If the enema solution is not expelled within a reasonable length of time, the physician may ask the nurse to administer another enema in the hope that additional solution will stimulate peristalsis, or he may ask her to remove or siphon the solution already administered. This procedure is described in the next section.

Rectal tube When discomfort is related to flatus or liquids in the rectum that the patient is unable to expel voluntarily, the physician may order a rectal tube. Frequently, the rectal tube is used in conjunction with drugs such as glycerin suppositories. A physician's order is required because certain pathologic problems and surgical procedures contraindicate the use of a rectal tube.

The nurse lubricates and inserts the tube as described for enemas. Usually she leaves it in place 20 minutes. A longer period of time tends to produce spasms of the anal sphincter, which ultimately may produce relaxation of the sphincter. Infrequently it may be necessary to tape the tube to the buttocks to anchor it. Provision for drainage is essential.

Disposable units, consisting of a rectal tube connected to a flatus bag, are available (Fig. 9-4, *A*). The lubricated tip of the

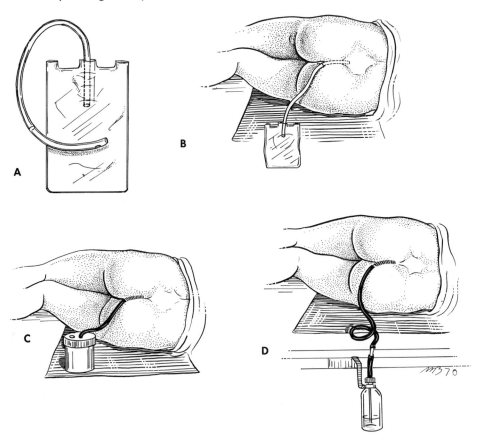

Fig. 9-4. Rectal tube. **A,** Kenwood flatus bag. Projections on either side of rectal tube are air vents. **B,** Lubricated tip of flatus bag is inserted and flatus bag rests on the bed. (Courtesy Will Ross, Inc., Milwaukee, Wis.) **C,** The rectal tube drains into a vented container. **D,** The rectal tube drains into a vented bottle suspended from the bed. Escaping gas causes water to bubble.

flatus bag is inserted, and the flatus bag rests on the bed (Fig. 9-4, *B*). The rectal tube drains into a vented drainage container (Fig. 9-4, *C*). If the container is suspended from the bed, placing a measured amount of water in it will cause "bubbling" when flatus escapes (Fig. 9-4, *D*), thus giving some indication of the effectiveness of this measure. When a tube is inserted into a colostomy for similar reasons, the length of time it is allowed to remain in place may be longer because the stoma has no sphincter. Attention should be given to control of odor, and a section in this chapter is entitled "Control of Odor."

Fecal impaction   The nurse should make every effort to prevent the occurrence of fecal impaction. Preventive measures, including adequate fluid intake, exercise, diet, laxatives, and cleansing enemas, are especially important for elderly persons and for those patients receiving drugs known to be constipating. Thus, laxatives and enemas are often prescribed following the use of barium sulfate.

If contents harden within the colon, obstruction of varying degrees results. Then, diarrhea, which characteristically has a foul odor, may pass around the fecal mass and cause fecal incontinence. It can occur within a 24-hour period. In addition to diarrhea, the patient may complain of rectal pain and inability to defecate. Ignoring symptoms at this stage can result in serious imbalance of fluids and electrolytes.

Early treatment of fecal impaction includes administration of medicated suppositories, oil retention enemas, or both. This treatment should be followed by a cleansing enema, and subsequent cleansing enemas may be ordered as necessary.

Late treatment of fecal impaction involves digital manipulation to break and remove the obstructing mass. For this procedure, the nurse places protective pads beneath the patient, who assumes a Sims' position. A bedpan is convenient for receiving the fecal material as it is removed. The nurse or the physician wears a clean rubber glove, lubricates the forefinger well, and uses it to break up and remove the obstructing fecal mass. Following removal of the impaction, the area should be cleansed and the patient allowed to rest, for this procedure causes considerable discomfort.

Abdominal stoma Rehabilitation of the patient with an abdominal stoma is dependent upon his acceptance of this method of elimination and upon the development of a basic but satisfactory self-care program. To promote such rehabilitation, it is necessary for the nurse to develop a positive approach that combines acceptance, compassion, firmness, knowledge, and skill.

By the time the patient is dismissed from the hospital, he should be able to demonstrate that he knows how to care for his stoma. He should also be aware of agencies available to help him. Information concerning "ostomy" clubs and surgical supply houses is useful.

Generally, the patient who has learned to care for his stoma adapts the procedure to meet his own needs. This, as well as his participation in planning his care, should be encouraged.

Skin care Fig. 9-5, *A* shows the anatomic location of a stoma. Discharge from an abdominal stoma contains material irritating to the skin. Efforts to keep the surrounding skin and adjacent incision clean, dry, and protected are important in preventing odor, irritation, excoriation, and infection (Fig. 9-5, *B*). Intensity of care and selection of techniques are influenced by the fluid state and the nature of the discharge. Thus, provision for drainage and methods of skin care will be similar for ileostomies, drain-

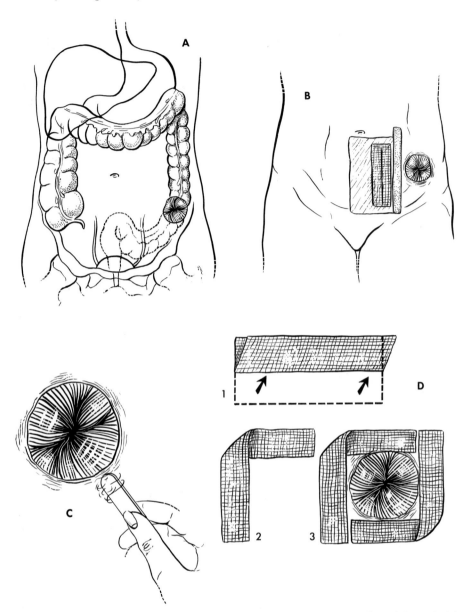

Fig. 9-5. Colostomy dressings. **A,** Anatomic location of a stoma. **B,** The adjacent incision is protected from contamination with a "dam" made of waterproof material. A strip of waterproof tape seals the material to the skin. **C,** After cleansing and drying of the area around the stoma, the prescribed ointment is applied. **D,** Gauze strips are folded and placed around the stoma.

ing fistulas, transplants of the ureters to the abdominal wall, and liquid drainage from a colostomy.

The skin can remain healthy only if it is kept clean and dry. The nurse usually uses mild soap and water to sponge the skin until it is clean; then she rinses it thoroughly and blots it dry. If the skin becomes irritated or infected, other cleansing agents and protective ointments may be used. If heavy ointments are

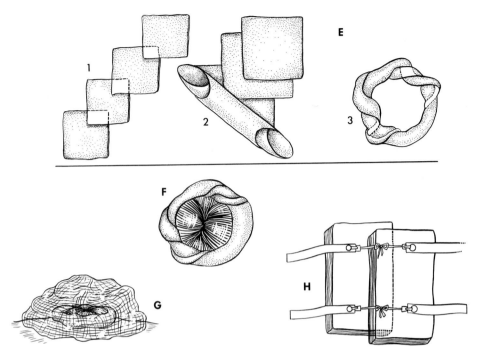

Fig. 9-5, cont'd. E, Layers of Cellucotton are used to form a circular dressing, popularly called a doughnut dressing. After the material is formed into a roll, the ends are interlocked with a twisting motion. **F,** The circular dressing is placed around the stoma. **G,** The stoma is covered with layers of gauze, then with fluffed Cellucotton. **H,** Dressing is completed with large abdominal dressing pads held in place with Montgomery straps.

used, an organic solvent such as oil will remove them. Prior to further treatment, old medications must be removed completely.

Colostomy care

Colostomy dressings. If discharges are semiliquid, the nurse may place dressings around and over the stoma to receive its discharges. During the initial period of stomal activity, dressings are necessarily large and absorbent. Later, stomal activity is regulated with diet and periodic irrigation. If a dressing is necessary, a small one may provide adequate protection. It may consist of only a folded tissue covered with a small sheet of waterproof material held in place with colostomy belt, girdle, wide athletic support, or undergarments made of stretchable material.

The skin around the stoma is protected with petroleum jelly or prescribed ointments and gauze dressings (Fig. 9-5, *C* and *D*). If the stoma protrudes from the abdominal wall, absorbent pads, available with a precut, centered opening for the stoma, may be used to prevent pressure on it. During the immediate postoperative period, the immature stoma will protrude and may be protected with a doughnut dressing (Fig. 9-5, *E* and *F*) fashioned from absorbent material. The stoma is covered with layers of gauze, then with fluffed Cellucotton. The dressing is completed with large abdominal dressing pads held in place with Montgomery straps (Fig. 9-5, *G* and *H*). The dressings should be somewhat fluffy in order to increase absorbency. The materials used vary. Cellucotton pads are available with or without a moisture-resistant backing.

Colostomy irrigations. Colostomy irrigations should be planned for a time that will be compatible with the individual's pattern of daily activity. Ideally, they are given at the same time every day. Some consider prebreakfast irrigation ideal, while others prefer evening irrigation. Frequency of irrigation varies; satisfactory results have been obtained from biweekly irrigation, from irrigation on alternate days, and from daily irrigations.

The size of the catheter used for colostomy irrigation may vary with the size of the stoma. To irrigate the stoma of an adult patient, a size 24 to 26 French catheter is usually suitable. This size is of some value in dilating the stoma. Tap water or physiologic saline solution is prepared and injected in amounts needed for satisfactory results. Variations from 500 ml. to more than 2,000 ml. have been reported. Commonly, 1,000 ml. of normal saline or tap water is prepared at a temperature of 105° F. Occasionally, a mild soapsuds enema or a medicated solution such as 2% neomycin may be prescribed.

If the patient has a temporary loop colostomy, also called a double-barreled colostomy, the nurse or the physician should tell him which stoma or opening leads to the proximal end of the colon and which leads to the distal end. If the colostomy is located in the ascending colon, the lower stoma or opening usually enters the proximal loop. When the stomas or openings are located beside each other, the one on the patient's left enters the proximal loop; if one opening is placed above the other in the sigmoid, the upper stoma enters the proximal loop. If the colostomy involves the transverse colon, the stoma or opening leading to the proximal loop is usually located on the patient's right side. If the stoma or opening involves the descending colon, the upper stoma usually enters the proximal loop and the lower stoma or opening usually enters the distal loop.

When doing a 3-way irrigation, the nurse usually irrigates each stoma and the rectum until clear returns are obtained. The following sequence is suggested: (1) proximal loop, (2) distal loop, and (3) rectum. Irrigation of the rectum is like an enema, but solution may escape from the distal stoma. This sequence is followed because drainage from irrigation of the proximal loop may enter the distal loop, and drainage from the distal loop may enter the rectum.

If excessive backflow of the irrigating solution occurs, advancing the enema catheter farther into the colon will usually correct the problem. The nurse must never advance the catheter forcibly. Any resistance that is encountered is treated as described on page 217. After the catheter is in place, the nurse releases the clamp, and the solution flows by gravity from a distance of 1½ to 2 feet above the stoma. The nurse guides the patient by suggesting that the irrigation container should be at the level of the shoulder.

Commonly, the nurse teaches the patient to seat himself on the toilet or on a chair facing the toilet during irrigation. This position permits the irrigation return to flow directly into the toilet. Occasionally a patient may prefer to stand and lean over the toilet. If he is confined to bed, the patient may lie on his side, near the edge of the bed. In this case the bed should be well protected. Receptacles for collecting the returns must be available, because it is difficult to leave the bedside once the irrigation is begun.

Various types of irrigating appliances are available. In some, the nurse introduces the catheter through an opening in the appliance that can be occluded after the solution is introduced and the catheter is removed (Fig. 9-6, *A* to *C*). In others, to allow introduction of the catheter, the nurse pulls away from the stoma the ring or dome to which the drainage tubing is attached (Fig. 9-6, *D*). If an irrigating device is not used, a pad of cloth or sponge rubber held over the stoma helps to control leakage while the solution is introduced. A large basin can be held tightly against the abdomen to collect the returns if an irrigating device is not used, or a trough can be fashioned from waterproof material and taped to the abdomen.

If the patient is unsure that the returns are complete, the end of the drainage sleeve can be closed and the appliance can be worn for a period of time. During this interval, the patient may resume other activities. Often, the returns are complete within an hour. The abdomen is washed and dried, and a dressing is applied to the stoma. The equipment is washed, dried, and aired in preparation for subsequent irrigations.

Instead of a catheter or a rectal tube, the nurse may use an irrigating tip such as the Laird tip, manufactured by John F. Greer Company. Irrigating tips are available in several sizes. Size is selected so that only a small portion of the tip protrudes from the stoma when the tip is inserted. A tip that is too small will slip completely into the colon; one that is too large will protrude some distance. The tip is used to limit penetration of the colon, dilate the stoma, and fill the colon with irrigating solution. It is thought to be of considerable value in preventing perforation, particularly when the tissue is diseased and friable. If the stoma protrudes for some distance outside the abdominal wall, use of the tip may be unsatisfactory because the

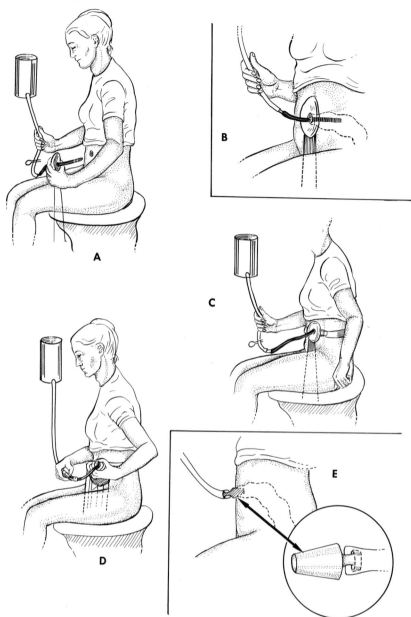

Fig. 9-6. Colostomy irrigation with a catheter, **A** to **D**, or with the Laird tip, **E. A,** The catheter is introduced through an opening in the irrigating appliance. After the desired amount of solution has been introduced, the opening through which the catheter was introduced is sealed. **B,** Cross section shows the catheter inserted and the irrigation appliance in use. **C,** The container of irrigating solution is placed at shoulder level or approximately 1½ to 2 feet above the stoma. **D,** The catheter may be introduced through the open top of the appliance. **E,** The Laird tip may be used to irrigate a colostomy without using an irrigating appliance. The size of the tip is individually selected and should fit into the stoma so that it acts like a cork. A properly fitted tip extends about ¼ inch on the outside of the stoma and must never be so small that it could slip into the colon. After the irrigation is complete, the tip is removed and the returns flow through a drainage sleeve or into a receptacle held beneath the stoma. The inset shows an enlarged view of the Laird tip attached to tubing. (Courtesy John F. Greer Co., Oakland, Calif.).

lumen inside the abdominal wall is likely to be smaller than the lumen outside the abdominal wall (Fig. 9-6, *E*).

Drainage bags. Some physicians prefer that a bag not be applied to a colostomy except for brief periods following irrigation and during episodes of diarrhea. However, a temporary drainage bag or a permanent appliance is fitted to a stoma that discharges fluids.

A measuring guide can be used to determine the most desirable size of opening in the drainage bag or appliance (Fig. 9-7, *A*). The guide is basically a premeasured series of rings or cutout circles and is available from surgical supply houses (Fig. 9-7, *A, inset*). It may be used to mark the temporary drainage bag (Fig. 9-7, *B*) for accurate enlargement of its opening (Fig. 9-7, *C*). The ideal size of opening provides a space of ⅛ inch between the aperture of the bag and the exterior aspect of the stoma. Complications such as fistulas may develop if the appliance is fitted too close to the stoma.

The nurse must see to it that the skin is clean and thoroughly dry preparatory to application of the drainage bag. Placing cotton balls or other absorbent material over the stoma when drainage tends to be continuous helps to keep the area dry. This material acts as a wick and is replaced as it becomes saturated. A double-faced adhesive disc (stoma seal) may be used to seal the drainage bag to the skin. Double-faced adhesive discs are convenient and easy to apply and remove. Neither cementing agents nor solvents are needed; this reduces skin reactions and irritations. Some persons prefer that a protective substance such as tincture of benzoin or a commercial cement be used to seal the bag to the skin. After the first coat of either is applied in a thin layer and allowed to dry, a second thin coat is applied to increase adherence.

After the adhesive surface is exposed and a stoma seal applied (Fig. 9-7, *D*), the nurse applies the temporary drainage bag carefully so that a complete seal is obtained. Pressure is first used to seal the part of the bag that is proximal to the opening; then the remaining part is sealed smoothly to the abdominal wall (Fig. 9-7, *E*). This is done to prevent drainage from seeping beneath the bag, destroying the seal. Air is removed from the bag, which is then pleated, closed, and fastened securely at the distal end (Fig. 9-7, *F*).

Periodically, drainage is emptied by opening the distal end of the bag (Fig. 9-7, *G*). If the bag is collecting urinary drainage or material from a fistula, any cleansing must be done very carefully. If the drainage is from an intestinal stoma, the nurse may rinse the bag with cool water while it is cemented to the skin. She rinses the bag applied over the colonic stoma with warm water (Fig. 9-7, *H*), dries the lower part of the bag, and reseals it (Fig. 9-7, *I* and *J*).

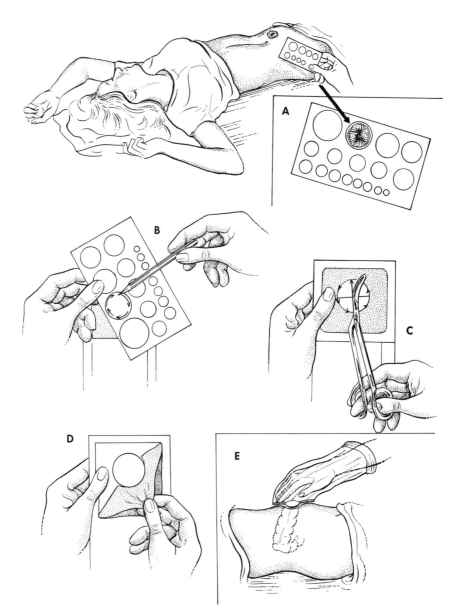

Fig. 9-7. Temporary drainage bags. **A,** A measuring guide is used to determine the size of the opening in the drainage bag. A safety margin of $\frac{1}{8}$ inch around the stoma is allowed. **B,** The measuring guide is used to mark the desired size of opening. **C,** The opening is enlarged by first cutting diagonally. The opening is completed by cutting along the marked circle. **D,** The adhesive surface is exposed by removing the backing. A stoma seal may be applied. **E,** The adhesive surface of the bag is applied.

A variety of permanent appliances is available. Choice of the appliance depends upon the individual's needs. Some are fastened to the abdominal wall with double-faced adhesive discs or cementing agents; others are held in place with an elastic belt. The nurse must adjust the latter to fit properly, without leakage or pressure on the stoma. Further adjustment is necessary when

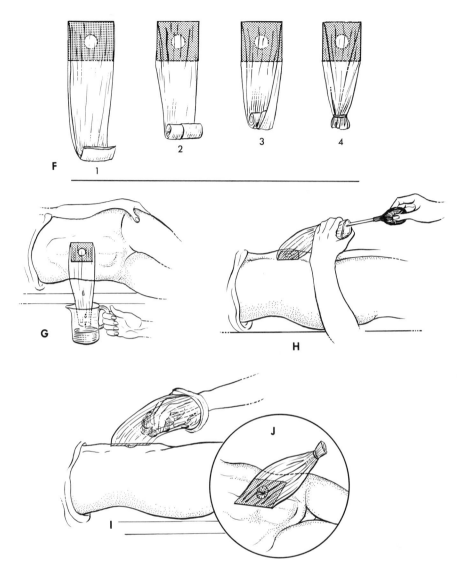

Fig. 9-7, cont'd. F, Air is removed from the bag, which is closed by folding it up at least twice, then toward the center. The seal is secured with a rubber band. **G,** The bag is emptied whenever necessary. **H,** The bag applied over the colonic stoma is rinsed with warm water. **I,** The lower part of the bag is dried. **J,** The bag is resealed.

the patient lies down because position changes the contour of the abdomen somewhat. The bag itself may be disposable or reusable. Reusable bags should be replaced with a second bag while being washed, dried, and aired. Rubber or very heavy plastic appliances are usually powdered lightly.

Treatment of skin irritation. Irritation of the skin may be treated with karaya gum powder sprinkled on the skin. This powder has adhesive ability also. If digestive agents are responsible for the irritation, the karaya gum powder can be mixed with concentrated aluminum hydroxide or other antacid preparations, or a paste of antacid may be used.

Allowing a bottle of antacid to stand for several weeks and then pouring off the top liquid is one method of obtaining an antacid paste. A commercial preparation of karaya and aluminum hydroxide gel, Neo-Karaya, is available. Healing of excoriated areas can be promoted with exposure to air and lights. This can be done by placing the patient on a Foster reversible orthopedic bed, Stryker turning frame, or CircOlectric bed and turning him face downward, permitting drainage to drop from the stoma without contacting the skin. (See Chapter 3, pages 59 to 64.) The nurse should place a basin beneath the stoma to collect drainage. If this equipment is not available, the nurse can place the patient in a side-lying position and fold a piece of rather heavy plastic under the lower edge of the stoma to funnel drainage into a basin. The latter method is more difficult to use, but satisfactory results have been reported.

Control of odor. Cleanliness is essential in controlling odor. Each time the nurse empties an ileostomy or colostomy bag, she should rinse it thoroughly with cool water. Hot water coagulates protein, making cleansing difficult; if used in rubber bags it increases the permeability of the rubber to odor. The nurse may rinse the bag with a deodorant solution if the patient wishes. Patients report good results from placing one of the following in the bottom of the stoma bag: commercially available deodorant tablets, a piece of cotton saturated with rubbing alcohol or mouthwash, bicarbonate of soda (baking soda), a chlorine tablet (gr. 4.6), aspirin (two tablets, 5 gr. each), charcoal tablets, charcoal obtained by crushing a charcoal barbecue briquette, vinegar, sodium benzoate, and ordinary room deodorant. Substances such as alcohol and certain mouthwashes must be used cautiously because they are irritating to the mucous membrane. Contact of irritating agents with the stoma should be avoided.

The physician may prescribe an oral deodorant that acts internally. A common prescription is for bismuth subgallate or bismuth subcarbonate, ½ tsp. three times daily. Because any oral medication may produce undesirable reactions, these medications should be used only with the physician's approval and direction.

Various methods are used to control odor in the room. Modern air conditioning is helpful. Aerosol sprays may be used, if tolerated by the patient. Some of these destroy odor; others mask it. Persons with allergies may be adversely affected by sprays. Methyl salicylate in which a wick has been placed may be helpful in controlling severe odors that occur with fecal fistulas and grossly infected wounds. Preference for commercial room deodorizers is an individual matter.

Some patients find it helpful to avoid or restrict the eating of certain foods, particularly those that cause formation of gas. Others tolerate most foods.

Questions for discussion and exploration

1. If the physician plans to start intestinal decompression, what supplies should you have at the bedside?
2. What are your responsibilities in preparing the patient for insertion of a gastrointestinal tube? In advancing it? In preventing or relieving irritation of the nostril?
3. What responsibilities does the nurse have in preventing fecal impaction from occurring?
4. How does an enema ordered to cleanse the rectum differ from an enema used to cleanse the colon, that is: (a) distance tube is inserted, (b) amount of solution used, and (c) position of the patient?
5. Discuss the nurse's role in helping the patient being prepared for reentry into normal living following (a) colostomy, (b) ileostomy, and (c) ileal bladder (ileal conduit).
6. Mr. Y. has been told that a stoma is necessary. What information should be given to him in order to help him accept his diagnosis, need for intervention, and prevent postoperative discouragement?
7. Prepare a teaching plan for a patient who is admitted to the hospital for surgery that will result in colostomy.
8. In order to help Mr. A., a patient with chronic ulcerative colitis who is facing an ileostomy, you might decide to ask a person with an ileostomy to visit him. List criteria you would use to select the visitor so that this would be a positive experience. How would this differ if the patient were a young mother?
9. What is the nurse's role in helping the patient with a stoma maintain family relationships?
10. In what way might a busy executive with a stoma need to modify his living patterns? How might a homemaker modify her patterns of living? How could a college freshman modify his patterns?
11. What are some methods that a patient might use to control odor?
12. Mr. Z. asks how soon he'll be permitted to return to work following a colostomy. What facts must you know in order to answer his question honestly?
13. What information do you need to obtain in order to teach a patient colostomy care? Why?
14. Why is gentleness in cleansing and dressing a stoma emphasized?
15. How would you adapt a hospital procedure for irrigating a colostomy to the patient on complete bedrest? To a bathroom in the patient's home?
16. Mr. K. complains of his stoma being "inappropriately noisy." What ways might he deal with this problem and still remain active in society?
17. While bathing Mrs. J., she states that she always takes an enema daily if she has not had a bowel movement before 10 A.M. How can you use yourself therapeutically in reference to this statement?

Selected references

American Cancer Society: Care of your colostomy, a sourcebook of information, New York, 1964.

Barnes, M. R.: Clean colons without enemas, Amer. J. Nurs. **69:**2128-2129, 1969.

Dericks, V. C.: Rehabilitation of patients with ileostomy, Amer. J. Nurs. **61:**48-51, 1961.

Dubois, E. C.: Hints on the management of a colostomy, Amer. J. Nurs. **55:**71-72, 1955.

Goligher, J. C., deDomal, F. T., Watts, J. McK., Watkinson, G., and Morson, B. C.: Ulcerative colitis, Baltimore, 1968, The Williams & Wilkins Co.

Hammer, L. G., Sawyer, J. G., Sister Monica, and McKnight, J.: The three-maneuver enema, Amer. J. Nurs. **62:**72-73, 1962.

Happenie, S. D.: Colostomy, a second chance, Springfield, Ill., 1968, Charles C Thomas, Publisher.

Horowicz, M.: Profiles in OPD: a rectal and colon service, Amer. J. Nurs. **71:**114-116, 1971.

Ingles, T., and Campbell, E.: The patient with a colostomy, Amer. J. Nurs. **58:**1544-1546, 1958.

Katona, E. A.: A patient-centered, living-oriented approach to the patient with an artificial anus or bladder, Nurs. Clin. N. Amer., pp. 623-634, December, 1967.

Katona, E. A.: Learning colostomy care, Amer. J. Nurs. **67:**534-541, 1967.

Lindner, J.: Inexpensive colostomy irrigation equipment, Amer. J. Nurs. **58:**844, 1958.

QT Boston: Manual for ileostomy patients, ed. 5, Boston, Mass., 1965, QT Inc.

McKittrick, J. B., and Shotkin, J. M.: Ulcerative colitis, Amer. J. Nurs. **62:**60-64, 1962.

Mayo, C. W.: A handbook of operative surgery: surgery of the small intestine and large intestine, ed. 2, Chicago, 1962, Year Book Medical Publishers, Inc.

Saxon, J.: Techniques for bowel and bladder training, Amer. J. Nurs. **62:**69-71, 1962.

Secor, S. M.: Colostomy care—1964, Amer. J. Nurs. **64:**127, 1964.

Secor, S. M.: Colostomy rehabilitation, Amer. J. Nurs. **70:**2400-2401, 1970.

Shaw, B. L.: Current concepts of stomal care, RN **32:**52-57, 1969.

Sill, A. R.: Bulb-syringe technique for colonic stoma irrigation, Amer. J. Nurs. **70:**536-537, 1970.

Stafford, N. H.: Bowel hygiene of aged patients, Amer. J. Nurs. **63:**102-103, 1963.

Steigmann, F.: Are laxatives necessary? Amer. J. Nurs. **62:**90-93, 1962.

Tillery, B., and Bates, B.: Enemas, Amer. J. Nurs. **66:**534-537, 1966.

United States Department of Health, Education, and Welfare: Public Health Publication No. 1304, Health Information Series, No. 124, 1965.

Chapter 10

Drainage and suction

Drains may be placed in various anatomic locations to remove fluids or air. The purpose and location of the drain determine whether its placement is a medical or nursing function. Therefore, when an incision is necessary, the surgeon places the drain. If the drain is inserted through a normal orifice, the nurse may be permitted to introduce the drain. Often, the nurse shares with the physician responsibility for the placement and care of drains. For example, by positioning the patient and advancing the tube as ordered, the nurse may assist the physician who introduces a Miller-Abbott tube into the intestinal tract. However, a nurse does not insert a drain without a physician's order.

Knowledge of whether insertion of the drain requires aseptic technique is essential. Sterile technique is used if the area is normally sterile. Clean technique may be permitted if the area is not normally sterile. Strict aseptic technique is used for urethral catheterization, but clean technique is usually permitted for gastrointestinal decompression.

After a drain is in place, care to ensure its patency and to keep it free of tension is essential. The drain is anchored to prevent dislodgment and provide comfort. Flow of drainage depends upon gravity, pressure, capillary attraction, or suction. The purpose and location of the drain, the kind, amount, and viscosity of drainage, the pathology and anatomic location, and the preferences of the attending physician influence the methods used to promote the flow of drainage.

The nurse should observe all drainage systems periodically to determine that factors influencing satisfactory function are present. She should develop a habit of observation that ensures the proper functioning of all aspects of the drainage system whenever she sees one in use. A commonly encountered problem, loose connections between drainage tubes, can be corrected by tightening connections or by replacing parts; applying a water-soluble lubricant to the connection point provides a temporary seal. Other problems include disconnection of suction machines from the source of electricity or lack of patency in the drains.

Drainage of the urinary bladder   Voluntary micturition should be promoted when indicated. With the permission of the physician, the nurse helps the patient to assume the normal position for voiding. Not infrequently, the female patient needs to be guided in leaning forward slightly to relax the urethral sphincter. Micturition is further promoted by ensuring privacy, utilizing a positive approach, and using comfort measures such as warming the bedpan. It is desirable to permit the patient to use bathroom facilities whenever possible. A collecting basin placed in the bowl of the toilet is used whenever a record of output is necessary. Other measures such as the sound of running water may help some patients void.

Frequently, responsibilities for and judgments concerning urethral catheterization are delegated to the nurse who performs catheterization of the female patient. Commonly, a male nurse, a urology technician, or the physician catheterizes the male patient. Ureteral catheterization is performed by the physician.

Catheterization is indicated in the presence of obstruction or paralysis, in the absence of voluntary micturition, after surgery or trauma involving contiguous pelvic organs, and as an aid to clinical evaluation. Careful observation and evaluation in light of the physician's order, of the individual's fluid intake and output, bladder distention, and discomfort are imperative.

Traumatic catheterization predisposes the urinary tract to infection. If difficulty is encountered in passing the catheter, the physician should be consulted.

Anomalies and certain surgical procedures may obscure the female urethra. Normally, the meatus is located between the clitoris and the vagina. It must be exposed and identified. If the orifice is not in the usual anatomic location, it may be found lateral to the usual location. Following gynecologic procedures, edema and swelling may obscure the orifice. Following radical vulvectomy, identification of the meatus can be exceedingly difficult because it may be located beneath a fold of tissue. The nurse may need to consult the surgeon in order to learn its location.

Urethral catheterization of the male and female patient

utilizes the same principles and similar equipment. However, the method of packaging equipment and supplies modifies the technique.

The indications for urethral catheterization, the need for intermittent or continuous drainage of the bladder, and the size and condition of the urethra influence the selection of the catheter. For catheterization of the male, a coudé catheter or a finely woven silk catheter may be used. Special skill is needed to introduce metal or glass catheters. The introduction of retention cathe-

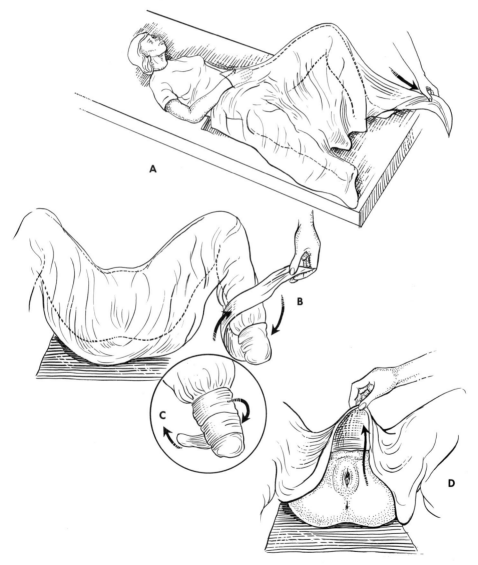

Fig. 10-1. Draping the perineal area. **A,** A sheet, placed diagonally over the patient, is arranged to cover the legs and feet. The corner of the sheet is straightened preparatory to wrapping the foot. **B,** Wrapping the foot. **C,** The foot rests on a corner of the drape, anchoring it. **D,** The perineal area is exposed by lifting the corner of the drape.

ters necessitating the use of a stylet is a physician's responsibility. If the catheter is to be retained, one with an inflatable bag is likely to be selected. Sediment is less likely to collect around catheters treated with silicone; patency of these catheters is maintained longer than patency of latex catheters. A straight catheter, French size 12 to 16, is usually selected, if the purpose of catheterization is to relieve distention, obtain a sterile specimen, or instill medication.

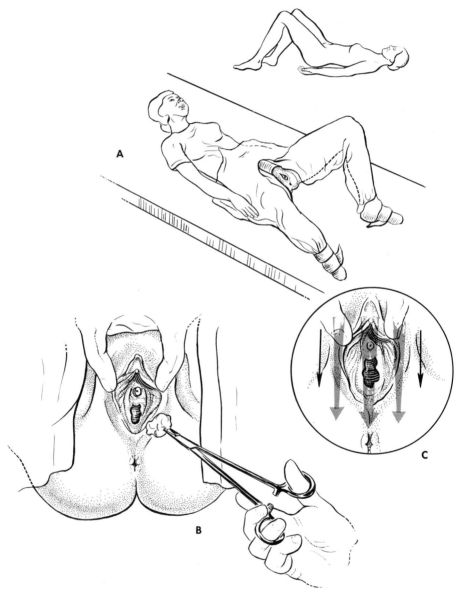

Fig. 10-2. Catheterization of the female patient. **A,** The nurse positions and drapes the patient. **B,** She separates the labia minora with the left thumb and forefinger and begins cleansing. **C,** Cleansing proceeds downward and outward.

Female catheterization Prior to positioning the patient, the nurse must provide privacy and explain the purpose of the technique. The patient who trusts the nurse performing the technique and who understands that the catheter is inserted into the bladder to remove urine for a designated purpose is more able to cooperate. Referring to the catheter as a small tube and telling the patient that the catheter will be in the bladder temporarily often relieve undue apprehension. In addition, assuring privacy through adequate draping

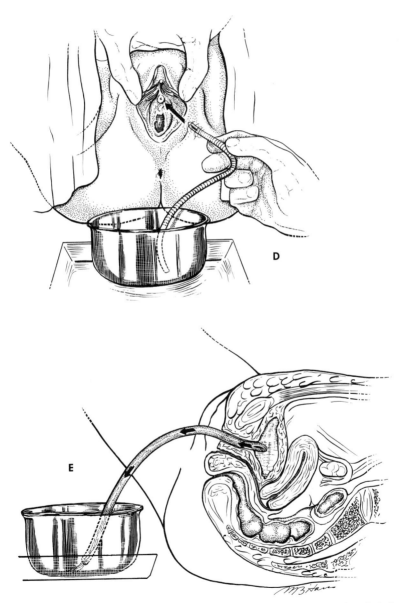

Fig. 10-2, cont'd. D, The lubricated catheter, held in the right gloved hand, is inserted. The free end of the catheter rests in a sterile receptacle. **E,** The catheter, inserted through the urethra into the bladder, drains into a sterile receptacle.

and screening avoids discomfort and anxiety due to unnecessary exposure. Explaining that passing the catheter does not produce pain but may cause some temporary discomfort may also be helpful.

After placing a protector beneath the patient's buttocks, the nurse drapes the perineal area as described in Fig. 10-1, directs additional light toward the meatus, and assembles the previously sterilized equipment in a convenient location.

Ideally, the nurse positions the patient on a gynecology table. If this is not done, she positions the patient in a back-lying position with her knees flexed and legs abducted (Fig. 10-2, *A*). This locates the bladder above the level of the meatus, permitting urine to escape through the catheter by gravitation.

Next, the nurse washes her hands well with soap and water and puts on sterile rubber gloves, as shown in Figs. 2-1 and 2-5. Using her thumb and forefinger to separate the labia minora, she retracts the tissue slightly upward in order to expose the meatus (Fig. 10-2, *B*). She cleanses the meatus and the surrounding area with a suitable solution. A solution of benzalconium chloride, pHisoHex, or green soap, followed by sterile normal saline or water, might be used. The nurse applies the solution by saturating cotton sponges or pledgets held with sterile forceps. Preceding this, she may irrigate the area externally. The downward direction of cleansing must proceed from the anterior to the posterior, thereby preventing contamination of the perineal area with organisms normally found in the anal area. Cleansing proceeds outward (Fig. 10-2, *C*). A fresh sponge is used for each cleansing stroke. During cleansing, the meatus may separate slightly, aiding in its identification.

After cleansing the area, the nurse must keep the labia separated. She places a sterile collecting basin near the area. With her other hand she picks up the catheter, lubricates its tip 1 to 1½ inches, and moves it to the work area, where she drops the distal end of the catheter into the sterile collecting basin. She inserts the lubricated tip through the meatus and urethra into the bladder (Fig. 10-2, *D*), at which time urine will flow through the catheter into the basin (Fig. 10-2, *E*). The fact that the female urethra is approximately 1½ to 2½ inches long and that the opening in the straight catheter is about ½ inch from the tip of the catheter indicates that a straight catheter will be inserted a total distance of approximately 2 to 3 inches.

The nurse holds the catheter throughout the drainage period. When urine ceases to flow, she withdraws it slowly to permit complete drainage of the bladder. Immediately after she removes the catheter, she uses a sterile sponge to apply gentle pressure to the meatus and to remove lubricant from the area. After the area has been dried, the patient is made as comfortable as possible. Notation of the amount, color, odor, and other important characteristics of the urine should be made. The used equipment is washed and sterilized unless disposable equipment is used.

Retention catheter When continuous or intermittent bladder drainage is necessary, a catheter with an inflatable bag may be used. The previously described technique is used to cleanse the area and insert the catheter. The nurse inserts the catheter beyond the distal portion of the uninflated balloon, approximately 3 to 4 inches (Fig. 10-3, *A*). When the bladder has been drained, the bag is inflated.

Catheters are available with inflatable bags of varying sizes; the size of the bag determines the amount of solution or air needed for its inflation. The amount needed is usually imprinted on the distal extension from the catheter used to inflate the balloon.

Four basic types of bag catheters are available, each requiring a somewhat different method of inflation (Fig. 10-3, *B*). In one type, the nurse injects through an open sidearm sterile solution or air used to inflate the bag, which is then folded over itself and fastened with a clamp, rubber band, or fishline. A similar catheter is inflated by penetrating a seal in the end of the sidearm with a needle or the tip of a syringe and injecting the solution through it. A third type inflates itself when a prepositioned clamp is loosened. In a fourth type, a metal clamp may be used to compress the catheter.

After the bag is inflated, the nurse connects the catheter to sterile drainage tubing that extends into a sterile drainage container (Fig. 10-3, *C*). She tapes the catheter itself to the patient's thigh, lessening tension on it and thereby preventing discomfort (Fig. 10-3, *D*). She secures the drainage tubing to the foundation of the bed in such a way as to ensure drainage. The container may be hung on the side of the bed (Fig. 10-3, *E*). Teaching the patient to adjust the drainage tubing increases his mobility. If he is ambulatory, the nurse should help him to manage the drainage tubing and container so that he may achieve increased independence. Helping him to understand the principles of drainage by gravity will assist him to realize the importance of keeping the drainage tubing and bottle lower than the bladder.

Generally, the nurse does not disconnect, clamp, or irrigate the indwelling catheter without the permission of the attending physician. Sitz baths may be given without contamination if the catheter remains connected. Irrigation of catheters is discussed in Chapter 11, pages 259 to 261. If the catheter is to be disconnected from the drainage tubing, it is first clamped; then it is disconnected, and a sterile plastic catheter plug is placed into the end of the catheter. A sterile drainage tube protector is placed over the connection on the drainage tube, or each end is

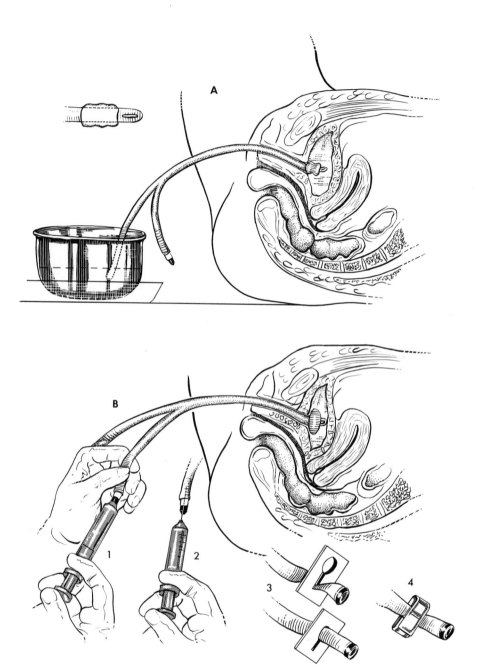

Fig. 10-3. Insertion of a retention catheter with an inflatable bag. **A,** The catheter with an inflatable bag is inserted. The enlarged view shows the relationship of the deflated bag to the eye of the catheter. **B,** Methods of inflating the bag: **1,** the tip of the filled syringe is placed directly into the sidearm extension, the solution is injected, and the sidearm is folded over itself and clamped; **2,** solution is injected through a needle or the tip of a syringe that pierces the self-sealing end of the sidearm; **3,** the prepositioned clamp is released from the sidearm of a self-inflating type of catheter; **4,** a metal clamp may be used to compress the catheter.

covered with sterile gauze sponges held in place with a sterile rubber band. Previously sterilized packages containing gauze sponges, rubber bands, and a clamp are convenient for this purpose.

In an attempt to reduce infection, the point of juncture between the catheter and the meatus may be cleansed daily for

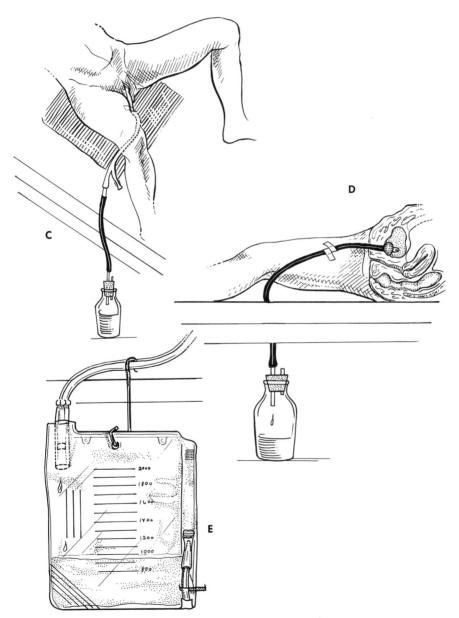

Fig. 10-3, cont'd. C, The catheter is connected to sterile tubing that extends into a sterile container, providing straight drainage. **D,** The catheter is taped to the inner aspect of the thigh. **E,** The drainage container may be suspended from the side of the bed. **(E,** Courtesy Baxter Laboratories, Inc., Morton Grove, Ill.; Travenol Laboratories, Inc., Deerfield, Ill.)

male patients and twice daily for female patients. Gentle hygienic cleansing is almost never contraindicated, and it is particularly important to cleanse the area well when the patient is unable to do so. As well as cleansing the points of juncture routinely, the nurse may do so prior to disconnecting or reassembling the connection.

Collection of urine specimens

Clean voided specimens (midstream, clean-catch urine specimens). Increased use of clean voided specimens for laboratory studies has reduced the frequency of catheterization. Before the specimen is collected, the patient's bladder should contain a fair amount of urine, and factors contributing to contamination should be reduced to a minimum. For this reason, the nurse should direct the patient to insert a tampon if a vaginal discharge is present, should cleanse the meatus and adjacent tissues, and should direct the patient to pass at least an ounce of urine to cleanse the urethra before the specimen is collected.

If a special table is available, the nurse positions the patient on it. The back of the table is raised so that the patient is in a sitting position with her feet in stirrups and her legs abducted. If such a table is not available, cleansing is done while the patient is seated on the toilet with her legs well apart. Throughout the entire cleansing and until the specimen has been collected, the labia must be held apart. Cleansing is done as for catheterization. A solution of 1:3 pHisoHex and water or another suitable agent is used. Each cleansing stroke begins above the meatus and proceeds toward the anal area. Opinions vary on whether cleansing should begin at the midline and proceed outward or whether it should begin at the inner aspect of the labia majora and proceed to the midline. A single sterile sponge is used for each cleansing stroke. Following this, the area is cleansed again with sterile sponges and sterile normal saline or sterile water. After the specimen is collected, the area is dried with sterile sponges in single-directional strokes.

The nurse instructs the patient to void forcefully without permitting the labia to close. After the patient has passed an ounce or more of urine, the nurse collects the specimen by catching the stream of urine in a sterile collecting container. During the catch, it is important that the flow be sufficient to force the stream away from the tissues and directly into the bottle. Gentle retraction of the tissues may be helpful in directing the stream. As soon as the nurse has collected the specimen, she caps it, using sterile precautions, labels it, and places it in the refrigerator or has it cultured immediately. If the patient wishes, she may finish voiding as soon as the specimen has been collected.

Collection of a midstream specimen from the male patient is based on similar principles. Many patients can be taught to carry out this technique satisfactorily; otherwise, a urology technologist or the physician assists the patient.

The area is cleansed with a circular motion, beginning at the meatus and working away from it. Sufficient urine, at least 2 ounces, is passed to cleanse the urethra, and the stream is stopped momentarily and directed into the container. As soon as the specimen has been collected, urination should be stopped. Complete emptying of the male bladder is accompanied by possible contamination of the specimen with prostatic fluid; therefore, it is important that the bladder contain a fair amount of urine before the specimen is collected. Following collection of the specimen, the bladder can, of course, be emptied completely.

Catheterized specimens. If the purpose of catheterization is to obtain a sterile specimen for culture, the patient's bladder should contain a fair amount of urine. Ideally, he should void an amount sufficient to cleanse the urethra immediately prior to the cleansing of the surrounding area and insertion of the catheter. It is desirable that the female patient pass an ounce or more of urine; the male patient should pass at least 2 ounces.

Continuous irrigation and drainage

Continuous irrigation and drainage of the bladder is used in selected cases. Sterile irrigating solution flows into the bladder at a specified rate, often 30 to 60 drops per minute. The height of the siphon tube regulates the amount of intravesical pressure. If straight drainage is used to empty the bladder continuously, the drain leading from the catheter must be below the level of the bladder and must be arranged so that drainage by gravity is possible (Fig. 10-4, *A*). Increased intravesical pressure is produced when the drainage tube is arched (Fig. 10-4, *B*). This produces a modified type of tidal drainage that should not be used without direction from the physician. If straight drainage apparatus is used for this purpose, the physician determines the height of the siphon tube.

Tidal drainage

Following certain types of trauma to the bladder, tidal drainage may be used to empty it periodically. This mechanically controlled method of bladder drainage is used to promote bladder function. It is used to increase muscle tone and to reduce hypertonicity of the bladder that would cause it to empty frequently.

In addition to equipment used to catheterize with a 3-way retention catheter, the nurse needs a sterile tidal drainage set, sterile solution, and an intravenous standard from which the solution is suspended. After inserting and inflating the retention catheter, she places its distal end in a sterile basin or connects it to straight drainage until the tidal drainage apparatus is assembled.

The nurse assists the physician as necessary. She places the intravenous standard beside the bed or attaches it to the bed.

The collecting receptacle may be hung from the bed; if a bottle is used, it may be placed on the floor. Strict aseptic technique is used in assembling the apparatus. All parts of the apparatus except the upper end of the manometer, when one is used, are connected. During assembly of the equipment, open ends of tubes may be covered with sterile gauze or sealed with a sterile catheter plug and drainage tube protector to prevent their con-

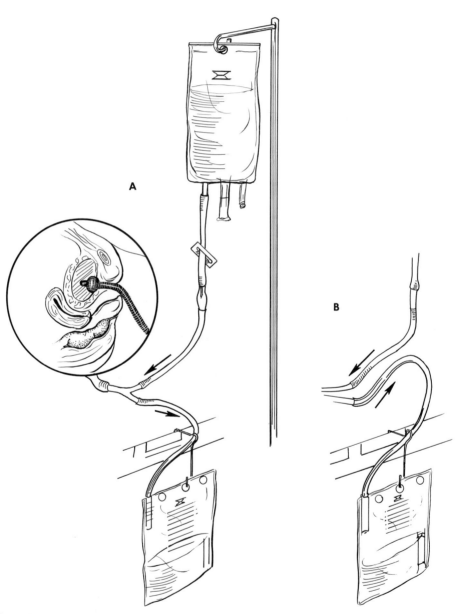

Fig. 10-4. Irrigation and drainage. **A,** Solution flows into and drains out of the bladder continuously. **B,** Modified tidal drainage results when the tube draining the bladder is elevated. This tube must not be arched without instructions from the physician. (Courtesy Baxter Laboratories, Inc., Morton Grove, Ill.; Travenol Laboratories, Inc., Deerfield, Ill.)

tamination. Disposable tubing sealed with temporary coverings that ensure sterility is available. The siphon tube is clamped, and the prescribed solution is used to expel air from the drainage set. The siphon loop must be filled with solution to prime it. When the tube that leads to the catheter is filled with solution and therefore free of air, flow is interrupted, and the tube is connected to the catheter. The rate of flow is regulated according to the physician's orders, often at 30 to 50 drops per minute. The height of the siphon tube is selected by the physician and will need adjusting when the bed is raised or lowered unless the loop is attached to a pole incorporated into the design of the bed.

Throughout this treatment, the nurse must be certain that all tubing is kept patent and free of kinks and pressure. Adequate fluid intake must be ensured, and as much as 3,000 ml. of solution may be given in a 24-hour period unless doing so is contraindicated. It is imperative that the nurse observe for distention of the bladder and that she observe and note the length of the cycle. Usually the bladder is expected to empty every 2 to 3 hours. The nurse adds additional irrigating fluid when necessary.

When tidal drainage is interrupted for purposes such as ambulation, the nurse connects the catheter to straight drainage or clamps it in accordance with the physician's orders. If the catheter is to be disconnected, an equipment set containing a basin, a clamp, gauze sponges or catheter plug and drainage tube protector, and a sterile towel are needed. The nurse disconnects the catheter and connecting tubing and holds them over the basin to drain; then she places them on the sterile towel until the catheter is clamped. The ends of the catheter and the tubing are covered with gauze sponges and secured with rubber bands or sealed with a stirle catheter plug and drainage tube protector.

Intravesical pressure can be measured if the tidal drainage apparatus incorporates a manometer and scale. The nurse or physician fastens the calibrated scale to the intravenous standard with the zero mark parallel to the level of the bladder. She clamps the siphon tube leading from the bladder, allows a predetermined amount of solution to enter the bladder, and measures the resulting pressure by reading the mark on the scale that parallels the level of fluid in the manometer. She then records the pressure and unclamps the siphon tube (Fig. 10-5).

Biliary drainage   If the common bile duct is entered surgically, the surgeon inserts a T tube to splint the duct and maintain its patency. The tube should be kept sterile, and a drainage system should be provided. A simple method of providing for straight drainage that permits independent activity consists of attaching a disposable but sterile collecting bag to the T tube. Bags containing a valve that prevents drainage from reentering the drainage tube are available.

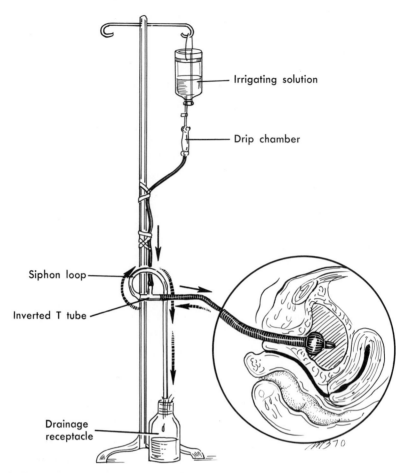

Fig. 10-5. Tidal drainage. After the tubing is connected to the irrigating solution and filled with solution to clear it of air, it is connected to the indwelling urinary catheter. The siphon loop must be filled with solution to prime it. The inverted T tube is level with the symphysis pubis, and the height of the siphon loop, often about 10 cm., is set by the physician. When intravesical pressure is equal to that in the siphon loop, siphon action begins and will continue until the contents in the bladder have emptied into the drainage receptacle. The rate of flow of the irrigating solution is prescribed by the physician. When periodic determination of pH of the urine is used to determine the rate at which the irrigating fluid should flow, the sample for testing should be obtained directly from the catheter.

The bag may be folded and secured to the patient's binder or to the uppermost layer of dressings by safety pins passed through slits incorporated into the design of the bag for this purpose (Fig. 10-6, *A*). The bile bag can be secured with adjustable latex belts and special buttons supplied with the bag. It may be folded as shown in Fig. 10-6, *A* or unfolded as shown in Fig. 10-6, *B*. Preparatory to emptying the bag into a graduated measure, the distal end of the bag is elevated to prevent escape of drainage, and the cap is removed (Fig. 10-6, *C* and *D*). After the bag is emptied, the cap is replaced; the bag is again secured in a position that

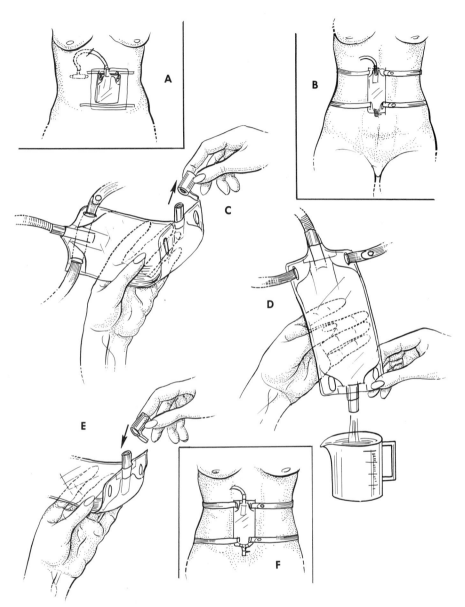

Fig. 10-6. Biliary drainage (Bardic bile bag). **A,** The nurse can fold and secure the bile bag to the patient's binder or to the uppermost layer of dressings with safety pins passed through the slits incorporated into the design of the bag. **B,** She can secure the bile bag with adjustable latex belts and special buttons supplied with the bag. It may be folded as shown in A or unfolded as shown. **C,** Preparatory to emptying the bag, the nurse elevates its distal end to prevent escape of drainage, and removes the cap. **D,** She drains the contents of the bag into a graduated measure. The hand beneath the bag supports it and positions it to aid in draining the contents from the bag. **E,** After the bag is emptied, the cap is replaced. **F,** The bag is again secured in a position that prevents tension on the T tube and facilitates gravity drainage. (Courtesy C. R. Bard, Inc., Murray Hill, N. J.)

prevents tension on the T tube and facilitates gravity drainage (Fig. 10-6, *E* and *F*). The amount, color, and odor of the bile are observed and recorded. Occasionally it is necessary to empty the bag more frequently than every 3 to 4 hours. This depends on the amount of bile escaping into the bag and the size of the bag used.

Chest drainage   Following surgery, it is extremely important that air not enter the drainage tube leading from the chest cavity, that patency of the drains be maintained, and that an acceptable method of drainage be used. Orders aimed at maintaining patency of the drain may include periodic stripping (Fig. 10-7, *B*) and milking (Fig. 10-7, *C*) of the chest catheter.

Precautionary measures such as taping the tubing to the chest wall, sealing all connection points, and fastening the electric plug of the suction machine to the outlet with waterproof adhesive tape help to prevent accidental interruption of the system. In addition, a pair of clamps should be readily available, for if the system is interrupted for any reason, the nurse must clamp the chest catheters immediately. The nurse should place the clamp on the catheter close to its point of entry through the chest wall. A second clamp placed distal to the first is used as a precautionary measure. Straight forceps are used because they can be applied quickly. The inside surface of the blades should be free of sharp points or teeth that could damage the tubing. When the chest drainage system is functioning well, some fluctuation of drainage in the drainage tube can be observed with each respiration; a wide fluctuation of drainage in the tube may indicate leakage.

If the fluctuation of drainage or the amount of suction becomes less or greater than the prescribed range, the physician will wish to be notified at once. Often, more than a borderline fluctuation outside the prescribed range is considered an indication for clamping the chest tubes immediately. If the gauge consists of a sidearm manometer, the area directly behind the permissible range of fluctuation can be shaded or colored to facilitate visualization. Any material of contrasting color may be applied; however, it must not interfere in any way with the reading of the manometer.

If the chest tube is dislodged accidentally, the nurse must seal immediately the site through which the tube entered the chest. This can be done by forming an airtight seal with the hand, a piece of adhesive tape, or several layers of petroleum jelly gauze placed over the site and held with gentle pressure. Although these methods carry some risk of contamination, failure to seal the drain site immediately will permit air to enter the pleural cavity, causing pneumothorax.

Water-sealed drainage Water-sealed drainage consists of a bottle fitted with a 2-hole stopper through which tightly fitted tubes extend. One tube is short and acts as an escape route for air in the bottle (Fig. 10-7, *A*). The other tube, which is connected to the drain, extends 1 to 2 inches below the surface of water previously placed in the bottle. Possibility of ascending infection is lessened by using sterile equipment and water. The water acts as a seal or valve,

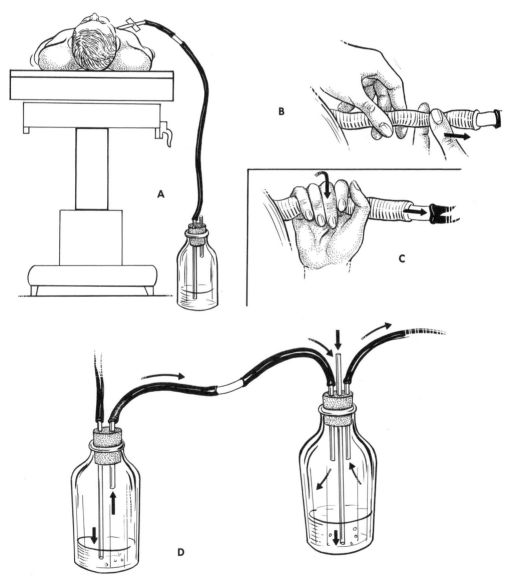

Fig. 10-7. Chest drainage. **A,** Water-sealed drainage. **B,** Stripping a drain. **C,** Milking a drain. **D,** Regulated suction.

Continued.

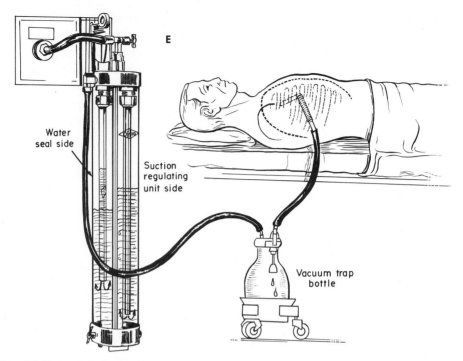

Water
seal side

E

Suction
regulating
unit side

Vacuum trap
bottle

Fig. 10-7, cont'd. E, Combination water manometer and underwater seal used for water-sealed drainage only or combined with suction. (Courtesy Ohio Chemical & Surgical Equipment Co., Madison, Wis.)

permitting air or fluid to escape into the bottle and preventing its reentry into the chest cavity. The bottle is placed on a level lower than the cavity being drained, often on or near the floor, permitting gravity to drain fluid into the bottle.

In order to maintain effective water-sealed drainage, the drain must be placed carefully, the water seal and air escape must be maintained, and the tubing must be arranged so that straight drainage is possible. When the bottle is changed, the chest tube must be clamped.

Regulated suction   Sometimes suction is reduced by connecting a water-sealed drainage bottle between the patient's drain and the suction apparatus. The number of bottles connected in a series will determine the degree to which suction will be reduced (Fig. 10-7, *D*). This is referred to as regulated, cut-down, or bubble suction.

Machines that   Machines that incorporate water-sealed drainage and principles
incorporate   of electric suction are available. In some, an electrically driven
principles of   motor heats the air within the system to a preset level, expand-
water-sealed   ing it and forcing it into the atmosphere. At prescribed intervals
drainage and   the cycle is interrupted and the air remaining cools, producing
electric suction   a partial vacuum that results in mild suction. As suction is

created, the level of the liquid in the manometer rises, indicating the amount of suction. The weight of the liquid used in the manometer influences the amount of suction possible. Thus, use of mercury permits more suction than does use of an equal amount of water.

A combination water manometer and underwater seal that can be used for water-sealed drainage only or be combined with suction is available (Fig. 10-7, *E*). The drainage bottle containing a vacuum trap is placed on the floor, and the combination manometer and underwater seal is mounted on the wall near the source of suction. This arrangement facilitates observations and eliminates problems encountered when all equipment is placed on the floor. After the equipment is prepared and checked for proper functioning, the nurse connects it to the chest catheter. She then opens the clamp on the catheter slowly and observes the rate of bubbling at the lower end of the manometer, adjusting it as necessary. Directions of the manufacturer should be consulted for details concerning the operation and repair of this equipment.

Electric suction pumps

Several electrically operated suction machines are available. Among these are the Gomco thermotic drainage pump and the Emerson suction machine. Satisfactory operation of these machines depends upon establishing and maintaining airtight connections between the drains and the drainage bottle, connecting the machine to a source of electricity, and maintaining patency of the drainage system.

Questions for discussion and exploration

1. When Mr. T. is returned to his room from surgery, you are the only nurse present to help the nonprofessional personnel transfer him from the surgical cart to his bed. Before this is done, you have a responsibility to make certain that any drains inserted into him will not be displaced. How will you determine this (a) if his chart is not available? (b) if his chart is available?
2. If in the preceding situation, an orderly insists that speed is urgent because he must return to the surgical suite, what is your obligation to the patient? How might you tactfully handle this situation?
3. If drains are in place, what are your responsibilities in relation to each of the following and why?
   a. Urinary catheter intended for straight drainage
   b. Urinary catheter intended for tidal drainage
   c. Gastrointestinal tube
   d. Penrose and cigarette drains
   e. Biliary drainage
   f. Chest drains
   g. Straight drain placed in the hepatic duct
   h. T tube placed in remaining stump of duodenum for decompression purposes
4. Mrs. K. has not voided for 12 hours. How can you systematically determine whether her bladder is distended?
5. What can you do to assist Mrs. K. to void voluntarily?
6. Mr. Q. states that he feels like he must urinate but cannot do so while lying on his back. What factors will determine whether or not he will

be allowed to stand by his bedside or walk to the bathroom? If he has recently returned from surgery and is too weak to stand by himself, how could you handle this situation?

7. If the physician orders "up to void" for a surgical patient who has chest tubes in place, think through the steps you would follow if the patient is (a) a 15-year-old boy weighing 180 pounds, (b) a 35-year-old man weighing 165 pounds, (c) a 60-year-old priest weighing 165 pounds, (d) an 80-year-old lady weighing 98 pounds.

8. What observations should you make routinely in relation to the drains listed in question 3?

9. Write out a plan of teaching and action for situations in which you are asked to obtain a clean-catch specimen from a female patient?

10. How would you alter the preceding plan for (a) a child or (b) an adult male patient?

11. When you pass a room in which a patient who has drains resides and observe the following, what action should you take and why?
    a. Drainage in the receptacle on the floor is red
    b. Drainage in the reservoir is about to overflow
    c. Suction machine is not functioning
    d. Patient is manipulating drain

12. What systematic observations should you make routinely related to a patient who has drainage of any type?

Selected references

Delehanty, L., and Stravino, U.: Achieving bladder control, Amer. J. Nurs. **70:**312-316, 1970.

Dittbrenner, Sister Marilynn, and Herbert, W. M.: Regimen for a thoracotomy patient, Amer. J. Nurs. **67:**2072-2075, 1967.

Drummond, E. E., and Anderson, M. L.: Gastrointestinal suction, Amer. J. Nurs. **63:**109-113, 1963.

Fordham, M. E.: Cardiovascular surgical nursing, New York, 1962, The Macmillan Co.

Fuerst, E. V., and Wolff, L. V.: Fundamentals of nursing, ed. 4, Philadelphia, 1969, J. B. Lippincott Co.

Hunt, E. L., and Magee, M. J.: Collecting urine specimens, Amer. J. Nurs. **57:**1323-1324, 1957.

Linden, R., and Keane, A. J.: The catheter team, Amer. J. Nurs. **64:**128-132, 1964.

Mackinnon, H. A.: Urinary drainage: the problem of asepsis, Amer. J. Nurs. **65:**112, 1965.

McGrath, D., and Kruger, B. K.: Chest suction using mercury instead of water, Amer. J. Nurs. **62:**72-73, 1962.

Revolution in chest drainage, RN **68:**50-51, March, 1968.

Sagath, E. E.: Using a pleural pump postoperatively, Amer. J. Nurs. **62:** 102-103, 1962.

Santora, D.: Preventing hospital-acquired urinary infection, Amer. J. Nurs. **66:**790-794, 1966.

Saxon, J.: Techniques for bowel and bladder training, Amer. J. Nurs. **62:** 69-71, 1962.

Tudor, L.: Bladder and bowel retraining, Amer. J. Nurs. **70:**2391-2393, 1970.

Williams, T. J., and Julian, C. G.: Tidal drainage in the postoperative bladder, Amer. J. Obstet. Gynec. **83:**1313-1317, 1962.

Winter, C. C., and Roehm, M. M.: Sawyer's nursing care of patients with urologic diseases, ed. 2, St. Louis, 1968, The C. V. Mosby Co.

Chapter 11

Irrigations

Irrigation may be used to maintain patency of drains or to cleanse, soothe, and medicate wounds, body areas, channels, and cavities. A physician's order is necessary for most irrigations. If the purpose of the irrigation is to be achieved, the following information should be known: (1) the reason for the irrigation, (2) the specific area or drain to be irrigated and its size, (3) the need for clean or sterile technique, (4) the kind, strength, and amount of solution, (5) the amount and kind of pressure to be used for introducing the solution, (6) the method of removing the solution following irrigation, (7) frequency of irrigation, and (8) equipment needed.

As a guide, clean technique is usually permitted if the area being irrigated is normally contacted by air or food. Sterile technique is used when solution enters an area normally considered to be sterile. With either technique, care must be exercised to prevent the introduction of contaminants.

The solution prescribed is usually quite dilute. Often, a physiologic strength is prescribed. The amount used varies with the nature and purpose of the irrigation.

As a general rule, only gentle pressure is used to introduce solutions internally. The height of the irrigating solution above the area being irrigated determines the force of gravity. This height can be used to control the amount of pressure used. The force and rapidity with which it is applied to the bulb or the plunger of a syringe will influence the amount of pressure and rate at which the solution will be introduced. The amount of pressure used is directly related to the pathophysiology of the tissues involved and their relationship to other anatomic structures. The main indication for forceful pressure occurs when irrigation is used to cleanse an infected wound of accumulated secretions, enabling it to heal by granulation.

If undue pressure is necessary to introduce the solution or its instillation produces discomfort, the nurse should interrupt the irrigation and consult the physician.

The method of removing the solution varies with the nature of the irrigation. When fluid and electrolyte balance is precarious, the physician may ask that the solution be aspirated with a syringe immediately following instillation. The nurse must do this gently in order to avoid trauma to the tissues. In other instances, she may remove the solution by reestablishing suction or gravity drainage. In either case, it is important to observe whether the solution returns. If solution does not return, the drain may be blocked by a mucous plug. Measures to dislodge it, such as milking or stripping the drain, may be necessary, or the drain may need to be changed. The nurse must ask the physician for permission to do this; some drains are placed only by the physician. With some irrigations, the solution is allowed to return by itself. The rate is influenced by the force of gravity and deviations in pressure.

Irrigation of the eye

Irrigation of the eyelids and conjunctival sac serves to cleanse and soothe the tissues. Its need is indicated by the presence of discharges, inflammation, infection, or superficial irritation. Prior to irrigation, the nurse should protect the bed beneath the patient's head from drainage. She may remove accumulated secretions gently with moistened pledgets.

The nurse should pour the irrigating solution over the area from a distance no greater than 4 inches. She may use an undine irrigating bottle, soft-bulb syringe, or eyedropper. The nurse positions the patient with his head turned in the direction of the eye that is to be irrigated (Fig. 11-1, *A*). This can be accomplished whether he is lying in bed or seated in a chair. This position and seeing to it that the solution flows from the inner canthus to the outer canthus of the eye prevent contamination of the opposite eye (Fig. 11-1, *B* and *C*).

Knowledge that the eye is sensitive to touch and temperature guides the nurse in this technique. Unless contraindicated, the prescribed solution should be lukewarm, that is, between 95° and 100° F. The nurse holds the eyelids apart, without exerting pressure on the eye itself, and asks the patient to look toward

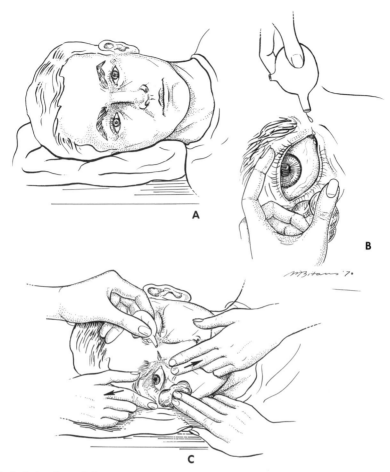

Fig. 11-1. Irrigation of the eye. **A,** The nurse turns the patient's head toward the eye that is to be irrigated. **B,** Solution flows from the inner canthus to the outer canthus of the eye. The irrigator is held less than 4 inches away from the eye. **C,** The patient may assist by retracting the lower eyelid and collecting irrigating solution with absorbent material.

the top of his head. This prevents the solution from flowing onto the sensitive cornea, which not only causes discomfort but also squinting, an activity that can be very damaging to the eye that has been treated surgically. The hand separating the lids may be rested on the underlying skeletal structures surrounding the eye (Fig. 11-1, *B*). The patient is permitted to assist by holding the pledgets or the basin used to collect the irrigating return and by retracting the lower eyelid to expose the conjunctival sac (Fig. 11-1, *C*).

Irrigation of the ear   Irrigations with water, 2% to 4% boric acid solution, 0.8% bicarbonate of soda (1 tsp. to 500 ml.), or normal saline are used to cleanse the external auditory canal.

Although the patient may lie down for this technique, it is preferable to seat him and protect the area to which solution might escape with a suitable drape. The nurse assists the patient in tilting his head slightly in the direction of the ear that is to be irrigated. The patient is permitted to hold the basin into which returning solution flows (Fig. 11-2, *A*).

To expose the auditory canal, the nurse must pull the earlobe of an adult downward and backward (Fig. 11-2, *A* and *B*) and that of a child upward and backward (Fig. 11-2, *C* and *D*). If desired, she may manipulate the auricle of the ear rather than the lobe, but in the same direction.

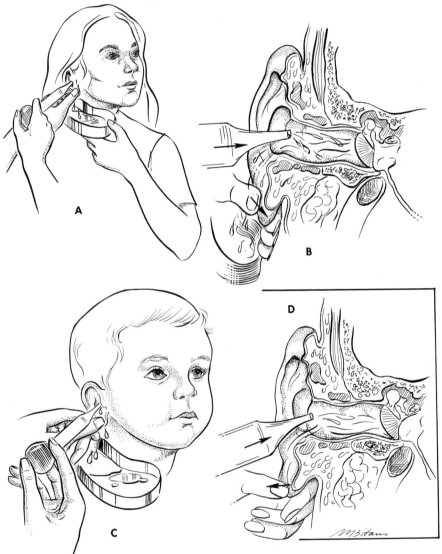

Fig. 11-2. Irrigation of the ear. **A,** The method of exposing the external ear canal in an adult. The nurse tilts the patient's head toward the ear being treated. The patient holds the basin for collecting solution as it returns. **B,** Front view showing retraction of external ear and direction of solution against the side of the canal. **C,** Exposure of the external ear canal in a child. **D,** Front view showing retraction of child's ear and direction of solution against the side of the canal.

Because the injection of cool solutions produces discomfort, the temperature of the prescribed solution should be 105° to 108° F. The nurse directs the flow of solution toward the side of the canal (Fig. 11-2, *B* and *D*). She should not inject it forcefully or direct it toward the eardrum, because doing so causes discomfort and can, in some instances, create additional problems. If pain or dizziness results, the nurse should interrupt the irrigation until further instructions can be obtained.

Irrigation of the mouth and throat

Occasionally, irrigation is used to remove secretions and relieve inflammation in the throat or to cleanse an oral wound. The nurse prepares the kind and strength of solution prescribed. The permissible temperature ranges between 100° and 120° F. and is altered according to the patient's tolerance to heat.

The nurse can position the patient in a sitting position with his head tilted forward over a collecting basin or sink. She can achieve the desired rate of flow by holding the irrigating solution just slightly above his mouth (Fig. 11-3, *A*). A rapid rate of

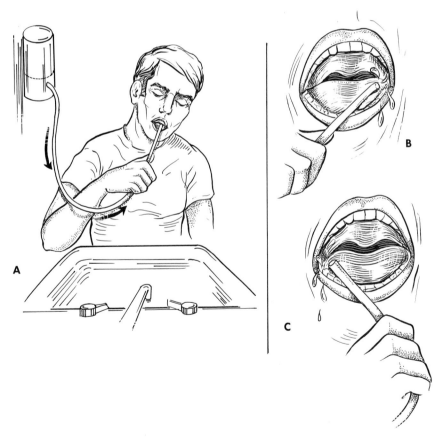

Fig. 11-3. Irrigation of the mouth and throat. **A,** The patient's head is held forward, over a sink. Solution flows from a height slightly above the level of the mouth. The patient is permitted to direct the flow of solution. **B,** Solution is directed toward the area being treated. **C,** Solution is not directed at the uvula or the base of the tongue.

flow may stimulate the gag reflex or may produce discomfort due to irritation.

The patient may direct the irrigating solution against the affected part. He will be more comfortable if the solution is not directed toward his uvula or the base of his tongue. Breathing through his nose will also facilitate this irrigation. Deep breathing should be discouraged because it can cause aspiration of solution. If necessary, the nurse or the patient can clamp the tubing intermittently for his comfort. Having the patient tilt his head first to one side and then to the other during this procedure will increase irrigation results (Fig. 11-3, *B* and *C*).

Drainage tubes
Irrigation of
gastrointestinal
tubes

When the irrigation of a nasogastric or gastrointestinal tube such as the Levin or Miller-Abbott tube is ordered, the frequency is likely to extend from 1-hour to 8-hour intervals. Knowledge that irrigation is sometimes undesirable emphasizes the importance of obtaining a physician's order. Although other dilute solutions are sometimes ordered, it is common to use 20 to 60 ml. of normal saline solution for each irrigation. This solution is used in an attempt to replace chloride ions that are removed with irrigation and suction. It can be made by dissolving 4 Gm. (1 tsp.) of sodium choride in 500 ml. of water. Clean technique is usually permitted.

The nurse fills an Asepto syringe or a calibrated syringe fitted with an adaptor with the designated amount and kind of solution and then frees it of air. If a T connector is placed between the gastrointestinal tube and the tube leading to suction (Fig. 11-4, *A*), the nurse inserts the tip of the syringe into the short length of tubing that extends from the T connector. She directs the syringe slightly downward and rests it in the palm of her hand. She uses the thumb and forefinger of the same hand to occlude the extension tube (Fig. 11-4, *B*). With the other hand she transfers the clamp from the extension tube to the tubing that leads to the suction apparatus. The clamp is placed relatively close to the connector, for the solution will flow to this point. The thumb and forefinger that have been pinching the extension tubing are now free to secure this tubing over the tip of the syringe (Fig. 11-4, *C*). The solution is instilled slowly and gently; semirotation of the plunger may be helpful in controlling this rate. The patient is likely to feel the solution flow through the nasopharyngeal portion of the tube. If ordered, the nurse aspirates the solution immediately by slowly drawing back on the plunger. To reestablish suction, she occludes the extension tubing with her thumb and index finger, removes the syringe (Fig. 11-4, *D*), and transfers the clamp back to the extension tube (Fig. 11-4, *E*).

If a straight connector is in place, the nurse must separate

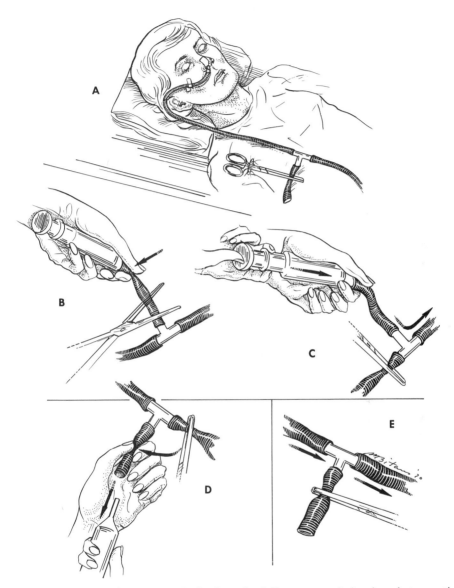

Fig. 11-4. Irrigation of gastrointestinal tubes. **A,** A T connector is in place between the gastrointestinal tube and the tube leading to suction. The short length of tubing extending from the T connector is clamped. **B,** A syringe filled with the designated solution is inserted into the extension tubing and rested in the palm of the hand while the thumb and forefinger occlude the extension tube during transfer of the forceps. **C,** The forceps is placed on the tubing leading to suction. The thumb and forefinger are used to secure the extension tubing over the tip of the syringe. Solution is injected into the gastrointestinal tube. **D,** The extension tubing is occluded with thumb and forefinger for removal of the syringe and transfer of the clamp. **E,** The clamp is reapplied to the extension tubing, reestablishing suction.

the tube from the connector and insert the syringe into the free end of the gastrointestinal tube. If the tube leading to suction is clamped before the tubing is separated, air will not be pulled into the suction apparatus. When a motor-driven suction machine is used, clamping the tube prevents air from rushing into the vacuum and creating a noise that may startle or annoy the patient. With certain types of suction, such as the 3-bottle suction, this may save considerable time, for once the siphonage mechanism is interrupted, it must be recreated.

When a balloon type of gastrointestinal tube is used, care must be exercised so that irrigating fluid is not introduced into the balloon. This is a matter of becoming familiar with the various types of tubes and the markings used to indicate which extension leads to the balloon.

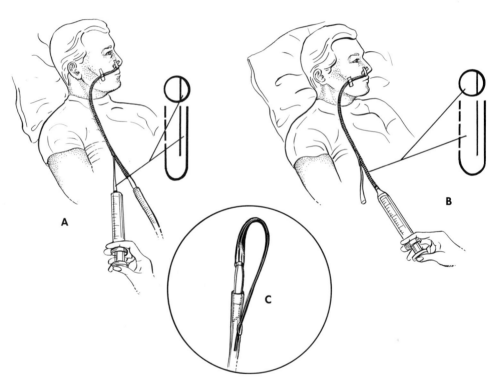

Fig. 11-5. Irrigation of the Salem sump tube. **A,** The tube may be irrigated through the funnel end of the air vent lumen without disconnecting the tube from suction. Cross section shows the part of the tube that is being irrigated. **B,** The stomach may be irrigated by introducing the irrigant through the main part of the tube after it has been disconnected from suction. Cross section shows the part of the tube through which the solution enters the stomach. **C,** The funnel end of the air vent lumen can be placed over the connector placed in the distal end of the tube, when suction is to be interrupted for a time. This eliminates the need for clamps. During ambulation, the tube can be draped around the back of the patient's neck or secured to his gown. (Courtesy Sherwood Medical Industries, Inc., St. Louis, Mo.)

The Salem sump tube may be irrigated through the funnel end of the air vent lumen without disconnecting the tube from suction. The part of the tube being irrigated is shown in the cross section in Fig. 11-5, *A*. The stomach may be irrigated by introducing the irrigant through the main part of the tube after it has been disconnected from suction, and Fig. 11-5, *B* shows in the cross section the part of the tube through which the solution enters the stomach. When suction is to be interrupted for a time, the funnel end of the air vent lumen can be placed over the connector placed in the distal end of the tube, thus eliminating the need for clamps. The tube can be draped around the back of the patient's neck or secured to his gown during ambulation (Fig. 11-5, *C*).

Irrigation of urethral catheters

The closed system of irrigating retention catheters is described in Chapter 10, pages 241 and 242. This method may be applied continually or intermittently. For example, the surgeon may ask that continuous drainage and irrigation be used in the immediate postoperative period following transurethral resection. If an anterior-posterior repair has been done, tidal drainage may be used on a fairly continuous basis, but the physician may allow the nurse to interrupt it when the patient is ambulating. (See Chapter 10, pages 241 to 244.)

Internal irrigation of the catheter, achieved with adequate intake, is preferable to manual irrigation, which involves separating the catheter from the drainage tube and is accompanied by risk of introducing contaminants. However, when patency is questionable, irrigation with sterile solution and equipment may be ordered. If the urine is quite clear, it is not usually necessary to irrigate retention catheters more than once or twice daily. Catheters left in place for long periods of time are changed at regular intervals, often every week. Use of silicone-coated catheters seems to reduce the problem of sediment collecting around the catheter and blocking the flow of urine. Presence of large amounts of macroscopic materials, such as shreds of mucus or purulent material, indicates the need to irrigate more frequently or even continuously. Physiologic saline, 2% boric acid, or other dilute solutions are used. Either a syringe or a funnel may be used to introduce the solution into the catheter.

The nurse places the irrigation set on a sterile field between the patient's thighs. If the equipment is packaged individually, the inside of the wrapper provides a sterile area. After the nurse carefully disconnects the catheter, she places its free end in the sterile basin and places the open end of the drainage tube within the sterile wrapper (Fig. 11-6, *A*), thus minimizing the possibility of contamination. The solution may be poured into a sterile funnel attached to the catheter (Fig. 11-6, *B*). Air pres-

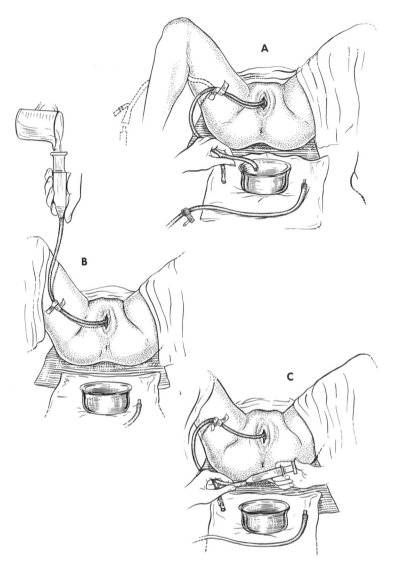

Fig. 11-6. Irrigation of a urethral catheter. **A,** The catheter is disconnected from the drainage apparatus. The drainage tubing lies on the sterile field, and the catheter drains into a sterile basin. **B,** Instillation of sterile solution utilizing a funnel through which solution is poured. **C,** Instillation of irrigating solution with a syringe.

sure and gravity cause the solution to flow into the bladder. If the nurse uses a syringe to introduce the solution, she fills it and inserts it into the catheter, injecting the solution slowly (Fig. 11-6, *C*). Approximately 30 to 60 ml. of solution is introduced. The nurse drains the solution from the bladder by disconnecting the syringe or funnel and permitting the solution to flow into the basin. The irrigation is usually repeated until the return is clear. The nurse in charge should be notified if the solution does not return. This may indicate that the eye of the catheter is blocked. Sometimes the nurse can correct catheter blockage by milking the catheter to dislodge mucus; she may need to change the catheter.

Surgically inserted drains

Irrigation of surgically inserted drains requires skillful technique, together with special knowledge of the exact anatomic location of the drain and of the condition of the surrounding tissues. Often, when such an irrigation is indicated, a doctor assumes this responsibility. Needed supplies will probably include a sterile solution of normal saline, a sterile 10-ml. syringe, and sterile gloves.

Wounds

Nursing responsibility for wound irrigation varies. In general, nurses are permitted to irrigate wounds known to be infected or contaminated. Because of the problems involved, a wound that enters the peritoneal cavity is usually irrigated by the physician.

The nature of the wound is evaluated by the physician, who decides if a catheter is to be inserted, the direction and depth of its insertion, the solution to be used, its strength, and the frequency of irrigation. This information should be a part of the nursing care plan and should be altered as the condition of the wound changes.

Solutions prescribed, which are usually very dilute, include 2% hydrogen peroxide, 0.5% sodium hypochlorite (modified Dakin's solution), physiologic saline, antibiotic solutions, and proteolytic enzyme solutions. The amount of solution used varies with the size of the wound and the amount and kind of drainage present. Commonly, the wound is irrigated until the return flow appears to be clear. Thus, the amount of solution used may vary. An amount of 120 to 200 ml. or more is often needed to irrigate an abdominal wound.

It is more comfortable for the patient if the solution is at room temperature or warmer. The temperature of the solution must not exceed 39° to 40° C. (103° to 105° F.), and *heating is contraindicated if increased temperature destroys or releases the active ingredients*. Reliable sources should be consulted for information related to the properties of specific solutions.

Anterior wound irrigation

For anterior wound irrigation, the nurse needs the prescribed solution, some type of bed protector, and a sterile irrigation tray (Fig. 11-7, *A*) containing a graduated measure, a catheter, a kidney basin, a syringe, and forceps or rubber gloves.

After the dressing is removed and placed in a waxed bag or wrapped in several layers of newspaper, the nurse assists the patient in assuming a side-lying position. The side to which she turns the patient depends upon the presence of other wounds and drain sites and upon his physical comfort (Fig. 11-7, *B*).

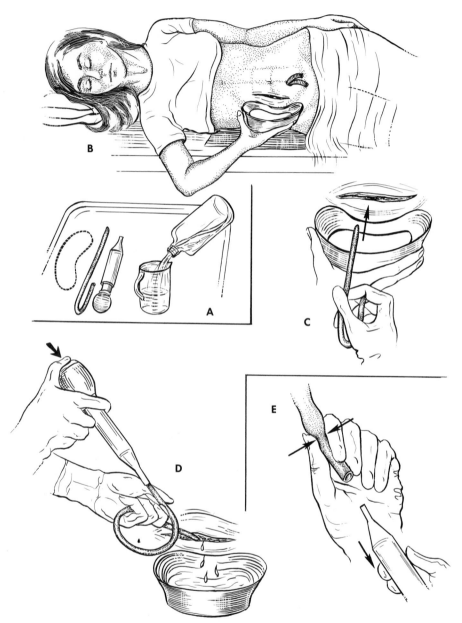

Fig. 11-7. Anterior wound irrigation. **A,** Solution is poured into a graduated measure. **B,** The patient, in side-lying position, holds a collecting basin beneath the wound. Proper positioning prevents contamination of the drain site above the wound. **C,** The gloved hand directs the catheter into the wound. **D,** The wound is irrigated by instilling solution with a syringe. **E,** The catheter is occluded while the syringe is detached from it for refilling. This prevents aspiration of contaminated solution.

Immediately prior to opening the tray, the nurse must wash her hands thoroughly. If she is working alone she first pours the prescribed solution into the graduated measure (Fig. 11-7, *A*), gauging the amount needed by the appearance of the wound. Unless the solution has been warmed previously, she may place the graduated measure containing the solution in a basin of warm water. The kidney basin is removed from the tray and held snugly against the abdomen, below the wound. This can be done by the patient, if he is able, or by an assistant (Fig. 11-7, *B*).

The nurse may handle the catheter with sterile forceps or gloves. She guides it gently into the wound until it reaches the desired depth (Fig. 11-7, *C*). If resistance is encountered, she does not advance the catheter forcefully but withdraws it slightly and redirects it. She attaches the filled syringe to the catheter and instills the solution (Fig. 11-7, *D*). Unless forceful instillation is desirable, irrigation should be gentle. When the syringe is empty, the nurse pinches the catheter to prevent accidental aspiration of the irrigation return while the syringe is being disconnected (Fig. 11-7, *E*). These steps are repeated until the return is clear. If a catheter is not to be inserted, the nurse sprays solution directly onto the wound until it appears clean.

At the completion of the irrigation, the nurse, beginning at the incision and proceeding outward, dries the area with sterile sponges. After she has done this, she applies abdominal lights or dry, sterile dressings. When finished, she should make notations concerning the amount of solution used, the nature of the irrigation returns, and other pertinent observations.

Posterior wound irrigation

Similar equipment, technique, and positioning can be used to irrigate wounds following posterior resection. If the wound is close to the perineal area, folded Cellucotton or gauze will prevent drainage from flowing over the perineal area (Fig. 11-8, *A*). A catheter is not usually needed, but the syringe may be fitted with a short length of rubber tubing (Fig. 11-8, *B*). The gluteal tissues may be retracted by the patient or taped to maintain exposure of the wound.

The nurse should report any evidence of adhesion formation and, if instructed, interrupt this process by wiping these areas with a sterile cotton applicator.

Anal sprays

Following rectal procedures such as hemorrhoidectomy, the physician may order anal sprays for cleansing and comfort. The nurse positions the patient in a side-lying or Sims' position and instructs him to retract the upper buttock with his hand so that adequate exposure is obtained (Fig. 11-9, *A*). When the patient does the retracting himself, little if any discomfort occurs. The

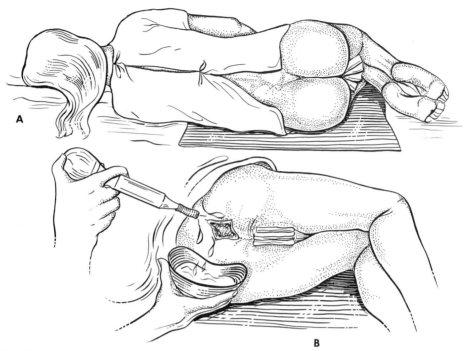

Fig. 11-8. Posterior wound irrigation. **A,** A patient prepared for posterior wound irrigation. Folded material is used to prevent solution from flowing over the perineal area. **B,** A syringe fitted with a short length of rubber tubing is used to irrigate the wound. A basin collects solution as it returns.

presence of a cotton wick, medications, or dressings in or over the anal area indicates that further orders are necessary before proceeding with the irrigation.

A 60-ml. syringe is filled with warmed solution. This is sprayed gently against the wound and absorbed by several layers of Cellucotton held gently against the tissues distal to the wound (Fig. 11-9, *B*).

Anal irrigations   Following certain rectal procedures, particularly hemorrhoidectomy, the physician may prescribe anal irrigation. This can be carried out by the patient if the nurse instructs and assists him as necessary. Most patients prefer to do this technique themselves and are able to do so with coaching.

One method requires an irrigating container, tubing, connector, clamp, and a No. 18 French catheter. These are assembled in the same way as is equipment used for enemas. Approximately 400 ml. of tap water is placed in the irrigating container. Temperature of the water should not be greater than 105° F.

Anal irrigation is carried out in the bathroom with the patient seated on the toilet. Therefore, this treatment is not done until the patient is ambulatory. The nurse suspends the irrigat-

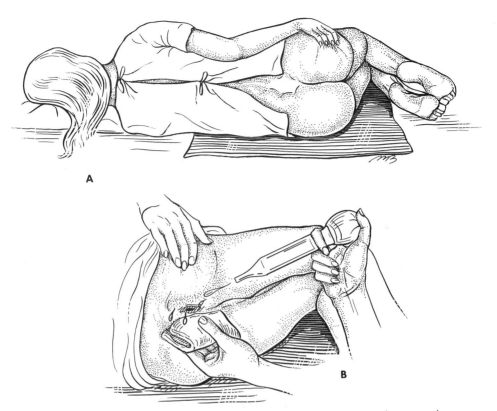

Fig. 11-9. Anal spray. **A,** The patient assumes a side-lying position and retracts the upper buttock with his hand to expose the anal area. **B,** The nurse sprays warm solution against the wound. Absorbent material is used to collect returning solution.

ing container about 2 feet above the level of the anal area, frees the tubing of air, lubricates the catheter generously with a water-soluble lubricant, and inserts it 1 to 1½ inches (Fig. 11-10, *A* and *B*). Further insertion or rapid injection of the fluid produces an enema effect, which is undesirable because the purpose of the irrigation is to cleanse the anal area. If the solution is administered correctly, it will return at the same rate at which it enters.

After 200 to 300 ml. of the solution has been used to irrigate the internal anal area, the nurse withdraws the catheter and uses the remaining solution to irrigate the external area (Fig. 11-10, *C*). For this part of the procedure, she holds the tip of the catheter 1 to 1½ inches away from the anal area. After the irrigation, the nurse gently pats the anal area dry with absorbent pledgets (Fig. 11-10, *D*).

Perineal care The physician may prescribe perineal cleansing following certain surgical and obstetric procedures. It is used at prescribed intervals and after defecation or urination. Until the patient can perform this procedure herself, the nurse must do it for her. This provides an opportunity to teach the technique and to stress the underlying principles used.

Regardless of the method used, the cleansing should always proceed from the vulva toward the anal area and from the midline outward. After each cleansing stroke, the used pledget is discarded. This prevents transfer of fecal contaminants to the urethra, vagina, and perineal wounds. The number of pledgets used should be guided by the purpose, which is to cleanse the area.

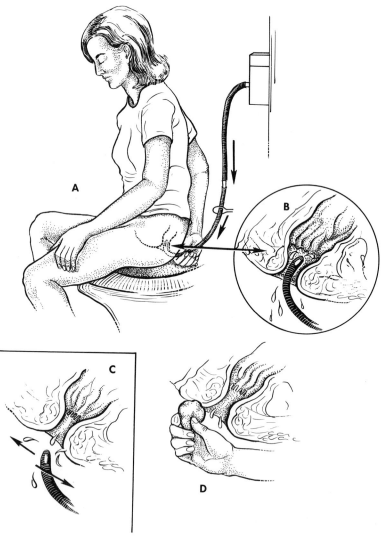

Fig. 11-10. Anal irrigation. **A,** The irrigating container is suspended about 2 feet above the anus. The patient, seated on a toilet, is permitted to insert the well-lubricated catheter. **B,** The catheter is inserted 1 to 1½ inches so that solution returns as rapidly as it enters. **C,** The remaining solution is directed toward the external anal area from a distance of 1 to 1½ inches. **D,** The area is patted dry with absorbent pledgets.

Sterile perineal care

Regardless of the exact technique used to cleanse the perineum, a sterile basin, pitcher, or graduated measure containing 300 to 500 ml. of solution, a forceps or gloves, and pledgets are needed. The nurse assists the patient in assuming the resired position, drapes her, and places her on a bedpan. She places several layers of newspaper or a waxed bag conveniently for receiving the soiled pledgets. Throughout the technique, she should ensure privacy. She may pour approximately 200 to 300 ml. of solution over the vulva (Fig. 11-11, *A*), using moistened pledgets held with forceps to further cleanse the area (Fig. 11-11, *B*). Then it is dried with pledgets, the bedpan is removed, the patient is

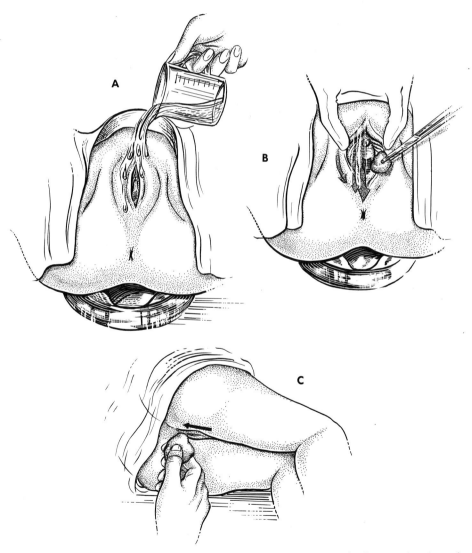

Fig. 11-11. Perineal care. **A,** The nurse places the patient on a bedpan and pours solution over the vulva. **B,** She uses sterile pledgets to cleanse, then dry the area. Arrows show direction of cleansing. **C,** After the bedpan is removed, the nurse dries the posterior area.

turned to one side, and the posterior area is dried (Fig. 11-11, *C*). The direction of cleansing and drying must always prevent contamination of the perineal area. Modifications of this procedure omit pouring of solution over the vulva. Cleansing may be done with moistened pledgets only. If sterile gloves are worn, the left hand may be used to separate the labia and the right to handle the pledgets.

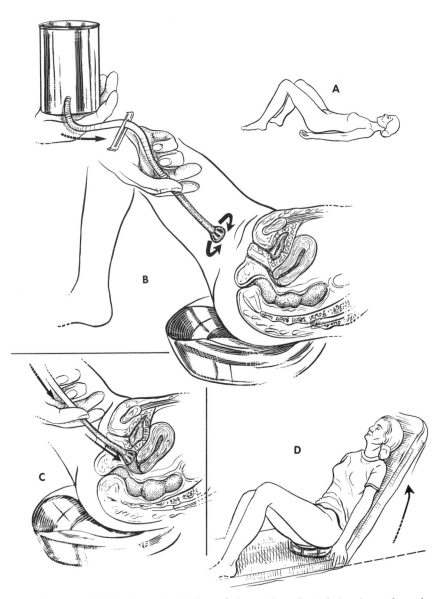

Fig. 11-12. Vaginal irrigation. **A,** Position of the patient. **B,** Solution is used to cleanse the vulva. **C,** Solution flows into the vagina through a vaginal irrigator that has been inserted to a depth of 1½ to 2 inches. **D,** Elevating the head of the bed hastens the rate at which solution is returned.

Clean perineal care The nurse may use disposable or clean washcloths to cleanse the perineal area. She follows the same principles that apply to sterile perineal care, using a clean, warm, wet cloth for each cleansing stroke. The principles of avoiding contamination should be emphasized when the nurse is teaching self-care.

Vaginal irrigation Vaginal irrigation differs from a douche in that the former introduces solution under low pressure, and the latter, under increased pressure. The nurse usually positions the patient as described for catheterization (Fig. 11-12, A) and places a bedpan beneath her. In some cases, the procedure may be carried out in the bathroom with the patient seated on the toilet.

The nurse may assemble necessary equipment on a tray. She should include an irrigating container, tubing, a clamp, and a douche tip. Temperature of the solution should not be greater than 105° F. (40.6° C.). Water or other nonirritating solutions may be prescribed. Amounts of solute needed to prepare 1 L. of commonly prescribed solutions are 2 tsp. of bicarbonate of soda, 2 tsp. of salt, or 1 tbsp. of vinegar.

Prior to the irrigation, the patient is asked to empty her bladder because a full bladder may cause discomfort and interfere with the irrigation itself. The nurse cleanses the vulva, either as described for perineal care or by allowing about 150 ml. of the prescribed solution to flow over the area (Fig. 11-12, B). She inserts the vaginal irrigator, commonly called a douche tip, into the vagina to a depth of 1½ to 2 inches (Fig. 11-12, C). If there are no contraindications, she may permit the patient to do this. The nurse holds the bottom of the irrigating container about 30 cm. (1 foot) above the vaginal orifice and permits the solution to flow into the vagina.

Following irrigation, the patient is allowed to assume a sitting position unless doing so is contraindicated (Fig. 11-12, D). This promotes the return flow of the solution.

Questions for discussion and exploration
1. What are the various purposes that irrigations may serve?
2. What information should the nurse have in order to accomplish the purpose of the irrigation ordered?
3. What may happen if high pressure is used to introduce irrigating solution into (a) a nasogastric tube, (b) a wound catheter, and (c) a urethral catheter?
4. Why is it important to start solution flowing close to the inner canthus of the eye and then move the irrigating solution slowly to the desirable distance from the eye to obtain some force?
5. Why is it uncomfortable to have solution directed at the cornea of the eye?
6. Why should solution not be directed toward the cornea of the eye following surgery on the eye? What will the patient probably do and what might the results of his action be?
7. Why should solution not be injected forcefully toward the eardrum? Of what might the patient complain if the solution is cold?
8. In carrying out a vaginal irrigation or douche, to cleanse and medicate

vaginal tissues, what should the nurse do if the returns obtained are bloody? On what information should her reasoning be based?

9. Why is the distance a catheter is inserted restricted for anal irrigation sometimes prescribed following hemorrhoidectomy? What happens if the catheter is inserted beyond the dentate margin and into the rectum, and why might this be a temptation for the patient?

10. What is the patient who is having oral irrigations likely to complain of if the irrigating container is placed too high above the oral cavity?

11. If an infected wound is being irrigated, how important is it to have the equipment, solution, and technique used sterile? What is your reasoning?

12. If, during a wound irrigation, the patient complains of severe pain as the solution is introduced, what nursing action is indicated?

Selected references   Herbut, H.: Clean perineal care, Amer. J. Nurs. **56**:1124, 1956.

Montague, J. F.: Better care for patients with rectal ailments, Amer. J. Nurs. **65**:83, 1965.

Saunders, W. H., Havener, W. H., Fair, C. J., and Hickey, J. T.: Nursing care in eye, ear, nose, and throat disorders, ed. 2, St. Louis, 1968, The C. V. Mosby Co.

Shafer, K. N., Sawyer, J. R., McCluskey, A. M., and Phipps, W. H.: Medical-surgical nursing, ed. 5, St. Louis, 1971, The C. V. Mosby Co.

Winter, C. C., and Roehm, M. M.: Sawyer's nursing care of patients with urologic diseases, ed. 2, St. Louis, 1968, The C. V. Mosby Co.

Chapter 12

Moisture and heat control

Local and systemic factors influence the need for increased heat, cold, moisture, or dryness, and the physiologic response to them is complex. If these agents are used in the presence of wounds, the transfer of microorganisms, the promotion of drainage, and the cellular response must be considered.

Factors known to alter tissue response are to be observed and evaluated in light of the expected effect. Any evidence of skin reactions, particularly those preceding the destruction of skin, is likely to be significant. It is known that impaired peripheral circulation, abnormal body weight, edema, thyroid dysfunction, general state of health, fatigue, muscular activity, extremes in age, and sensory perception alter tissue response. Individual tolerance to heat, cold, and moisture also varies. Although therapeutic applications are prescribed, the nurse is permitted to use reasonable measures to promote comfort unless definite contraindications are present.

The therapeutic order is likely to specify the area to be treated, the duration and frequency of treatment, and the general method of application. Temperature may be prescribed; otherwise, a safe temperature range is used.

Pressure should not be used to force such applications against a wound. Rather, the normal contour of the area to be treated, positioning, and auxiliary devices are used to keep the applications in place.

*Applications
of cold*

Cold may be applied for either a local or a systemic effect. Prolonged applications of cold may interfere with circulation, temperature, and function. Therefore, any signs of adverse reaction are important. Such signs include stiffness and bluish, purplish, mottled skin discoloration. Redness should never be disregarded, for it precedes freezing. Pallor, gray discoloration, or the appearance of blisters is ominous.

Alcohol sponge bath

Alcohol exerts a cooling effect by its rapid evaporation. For this method of lowering body temperature, a washcloth, four bath towels, a bath blanket, and a basin containing 25% to 50% alcohol are needed. Using a tepid solution of alcohol seems to reduce the reflex stimulation evidenced by shivering.

The nurse drapes the patient with a cotton bath blanket, folds the top linen to the foot of the bed, and places a towel beneath the extremity being sponged. If the bath is to last 25 to 30 minutes, the time believed necessary for physiologic adjustment, the nurse sponges each extremity and the entire back with the alcohol solution for 5 to 10 minutes. Only the extremity being sponged is exposed. If turning the patient is contraindicated, the nurse can depress the mattress with one hand while slipping the other hand beneath the patient to sponge the posterior area (Fig. 12-1).

To further increase the effectiveness of this treatment, the nurse may place cloths moistened with the solution or ice bags over areas containing large, superficial blood vessels. The areas most frequently so treated are the groin and the axilla. Application of an ice cap to the patient's head provides additional comfort. Sometimes one is allowed to apply a hot water bottle to the feet to promote comfort.

The nurse must observe the patient during and following this treatment. She takes the vital signs before the treatment is begun and 15 minutes after it is completed. Thereafter, she may take the vital signs at frequent intervals depending upon the trend and actual readings obtained. If the temperature is not lowered or continues to rise, she should notify the physician so that more vigorous treatment may be prescribed. She should also notify him if the pulse becomes rapid and weak, if respirations change, or if the lips or nail beds appear cyanotic. These changes may indicate impending heart failure.

Hypothermia

Several hypothermia machines are available. These are used to provide prolonged or profound cooling. Prolonged cooling is used in certain neurologic conditions, and profound cooling accompanies selected surgical procedures.

These machines circulate a liquid, specified by the manufacturer, from a reservoir through tubing contained within a

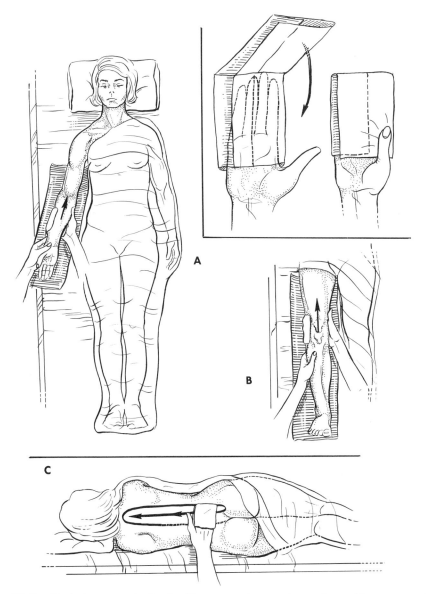

Fig. 12-1. Alcohol sponge bath. **A,** The nurse drapes the patient with a cotton bath blanket, folds the top linen to the foot of the bed, and places a towel beneath the part being sponged. She sponges each extremity and the entire back with alcohol solution for 5 to 10 minutes. The inset shows a method of wrapping the washcloth around the hand that makes it possible to work quickly and control the washcloth. **B,** Only the extremity being sponged is exposed. **C,** The nurse may sponge the posterior area after turning the patient to one side. If the patient is not to be turned, depression of the mattress permits the hand to contact the posterior area.

thin, mattress-like pad, commonly referred to as a hypothermia blanket. The tubing through which the cooling fluid circulates must not be allowed to become kinked because this will interrupt its flow. Directions supplied by the manufacturer should be consulted for details of operating the machine.

Orders concerning the rapidity of cooling, the desired body temperature, the area to be cooled, and the length of the treatment are obtained from the physician. In the clinical nursing situation, consideration should be given to both the patient and his family. The amount and kind of explanation given to the patient are influenced by his state of consciousness and his awareness of this therapy. Even though the patient appears unconscious, it is possible that he may have some sensory perception. Considerable support is likely to be needed by the family.

Individual response to this method of cooling necessitates careful observation of the patient. Shivering, a response that increases body temperature, thereby decreasing the effectiveness of the treatment, may occur. Shivering is seen less frequently when the level of consciousness is decreased. To combat this reaction, drug therapy may be ordered. Nursing responsibility for administration of the drugs necessarily varies with the prescribed drug, dose, and method of administration.

To protect the skin, the nurse places a sheet between the patient and the blanket (Fig. 12-2, *A*). It is common to place one hypothermia blanket beneath the patient, cover it with a sheet, place the patient on the sheet, then cover him with another sheet (Fig. 12-2, *B*). A drawsheet placed lengthwise serves this purpose. If the patient is to be enclosed in hypothermia blankets, the nurse may place a second one on top of the sheet covering the patient. The blankets may be fastened together with ties or a zipper. Pins must be avoided because these puncture the blanket. Use of additional covers is contraindicated because they produce warmth.

Monitoring the body temperature involves use of a rectal probe inserted approximately 2 inches and taped in place prior to arrangement of the top sheet (Fig. 12-2, *C*). The probe is attached to an electric thermometer that is part of the machine. Some units combine this with a thermostatic device that coordinates the temperature of the cooling agent with the desired temperature of the patient. If the thermostat is adjusted manually, the temperature of the coolant often needs to be 15° to 20° cooler than the desired body temperature. This will vary with the desired rate of lowering the body temperature.

Local application of cold

Hypothermia blankets. A small hypothermia blanket, ice bags, or moist, cold compresses may be used to apply cold to small areas. The nurse may be given specific instructions concerning the method of choice, or she may be permitted to use her own discretion. This is influenced largely by whether the application is used for comfort or as a part of planned therapy.

The hypothermia device is operated in accordance with the

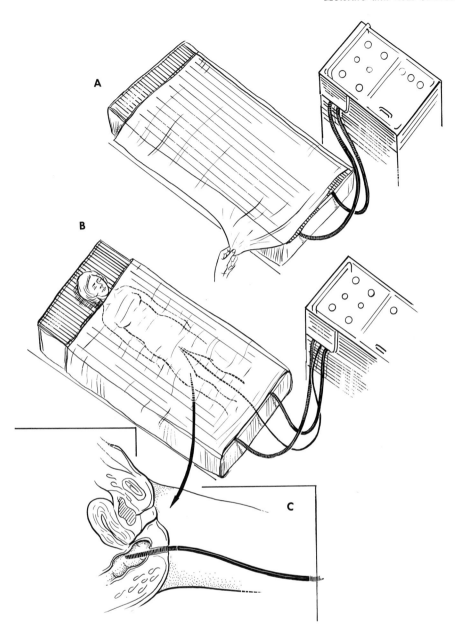

Fig. 12-2. Hypothermia. **A,** After the hypothermia blanket is placed on the bed, it is covered with a sheet. **B,** The patient lies on the covered hypothermia blanket and is covered with a top sheet. **C,** Cross section showing rectal probe used to monitor the body temperature.

manufacturer's directions and the prescribed temperature. As with the large blankets, a layer of cloth should be placed between the cooling blanket and the skin. The method of securing the blanket in place varies with the design and the area treated. If the blanket cannot be secured satisfactorily with the self-contained ties or fasteners, it can be enclosed in a cloth wrapper that can be secured. For example, the blanket applied to an

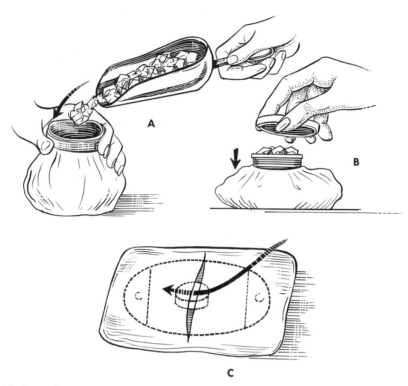

Fig. 12-3. Ice bags. **A,** An ice bag is filled with crushed or shaved ice. **B,** The bag is pressed against a flat surface to remove air and is sealed. **C,** The bag is enclosed with flannel.

extremity can be kept in place by wrapping it with a towel and tying the towel in place with roller bandage. Pins must not be placed in the blanket, and tape should not be applied to it.

Ice bags. Several types of ice bags, caps, and bottles are available commercially. They can also be created from plastic bags, which can be sealed with tape.

The nurse fills the container ⅓ to ½ full of crushed or shaved ice (Fig. 12-3, *A*). Before sealing the container, she removes the residual air, for air decreases thermal conductivity (Fig. 12-3, *B*). She does so by applying external pressure to the bag. Pressing it against a flat surface such as a tabletop is quite satisfactory. After the container is sealed, the nurse should cover it with flannel, which helps to absorb moisture that condenses on the outside of the bag (Fig. 12-3, *C*). The nurse should replace this cover with a dry one each time the bag is refilled. Refilling may be necessary at hourly intervals or oftener, depending upon the degree of environmental and local heat and the size of the container.

Moist, cold compresses. Moist, cold compresses provide another method of applying cold to a small area. These are fashioned by folding gauze, washcloths, towels, or other material to the size of the area treated. The nurse immerses the compress in ice water, frees it of excess moisture, and places it on the designated area. She changes the compresses according to the rate at which the body warms them, often every minute or two. The usual duration of this treatment is 15 to 20 minutes. Preparing the ice water with large pieces of ice reduces the rate of its melting and also reduces the probability of transferring pieces of ice to the skin. An ice bag may be applied over the compress to keep it cold for a longer period of time.

Applications of heat

The nurse may apply heat with hot water bottles, heating pads, moist compresses, baths, soaks, or lights.

Baths and soaks

Moist heat can be applied with baths or soaks. Unless otherwise specified, a temperature of 105° to 106° F. (41.1° C.) is desirable. It should not exceed 110° F. (43.3° C.). Because a higher temperature may produce thermal injury and tends to cause muscle contraction, a thermometer should be used for accurate determination of temperature. In addition, the nurse must see to it that the patient is not permitted to increase the temperature of the water, for his ability to perceive heat is not a reliable indicator of a safe temperature.

For this therapy, tubs designed for immersion of a particular part of the body are available. A regular bathtub may be used for sitz baths, or large containers may be used for immersion of an extremity.

The duration of treatment varies from a few minutes to half an hour. Unless specified, the usual time allowed for a tub bath is 10 to 30 minutes; for a sitz bath, 15 to 30 minutes; and for foot soaks, 15 to 20 minutes. Alternate application of heat and cold, called contrast baths, is done with the guidance of the physician or paramedical personnel. Higher temperatures are sometimes prescribed for these.

The comfort of the individual must be considered during this treatment. Rubber rings or pillows, covered with flannel, are used to relieve pressure on bony prominences and incision lines. These also help to preserve body alignment. Chilling and exposure are reduced with appropriate draping and control of drafts and environmental temperature.

Hot water bottle

Heat is applied with a hot water bottle in accordance with hospital policy and the physician's order. The temperature should not exceed 120° F. (49° C.), unless specifically ordered by the physician. Specialized knowledge is needed to determine when the application of a higher temperature is safe.

The temperature of the water is tested with a thermometer before it is placed in the hot water bottle (Fig. 12-4, *A*).

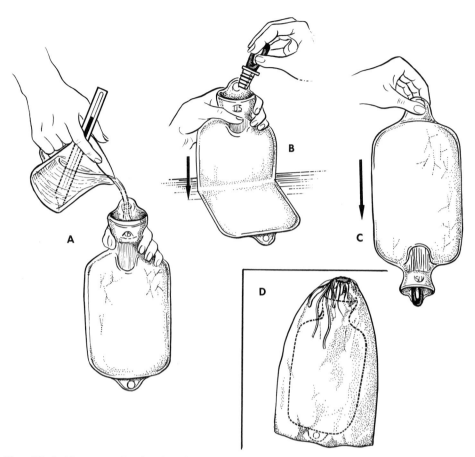

Fig. 12-4. Hot water bottle. **A,** After the temperature of the water has been tested, the bottle is filled about two-thirds full. **B,** Air is removed from the bottle, which is then sealed. **C,** The seal is tested for leakage. **D,** The bottle is enclosed in a cloth cover.

Residual air is removed from the bottle, which is then sealed, tested for leakage, and enclosed in a cloth cover (Fig. 12-4, *B* to *D*). Sometimes the hot water bottle is applied directly to the involved area; it may also be used to prolong the effectiveness of warm, moist dressings.

Lights   Light bulbs incorporated into frames may be used to apply dry heat (Fig. 12-5). The size, number, and kind of light bulbs and the distance between the source of light and the exposed tissue affect the amount of heat applied. Forty-watt or 60-watt light bulbs are used if the distance to the treated area is about 18 inches. The amount and type of covering applied over the cradle during treatment will influence heat loss due to convection.

Usually, heat is applied in this manner for 20 to 30 minutes. However, the first treatment commonly equals only half this time.

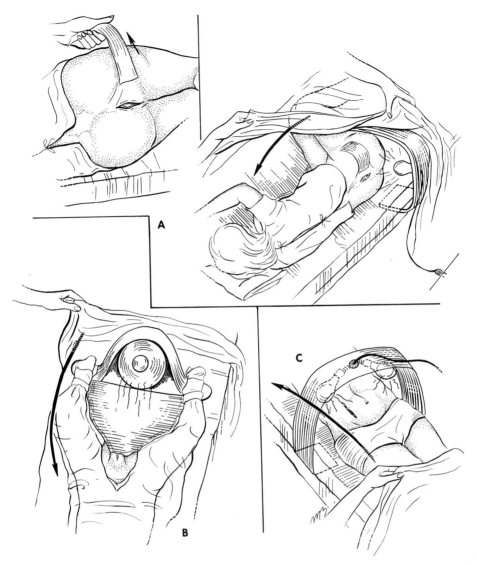

Fig. 12-5. Lights. **A,** Application of lights to a posterior wound. Inset shows a method of exposing the wound. Adhesive tape is used to retract the upper buttock during treatment. **B,** Method of applying perineal lights. **C,** Method of applying abdominal lights.

Hot packs   After selecting cloth material of an appropriate size for the area to be treated, the nurse may use one of several methods to prepare it with moisture and heat. The exact technique of application depends upon the method of preparation. Similarly, the frequency of changing the application also varies.

    Autoclave method. After moistening wool material with water, wringing it to free it of excess moisture, and folding it to a size slightly larger than the area to be treated, the nurse lays it in a metal container equipped with a cover and places it in the autoclave (Fig. 12-6, *A*). As soon as the pressure gauge

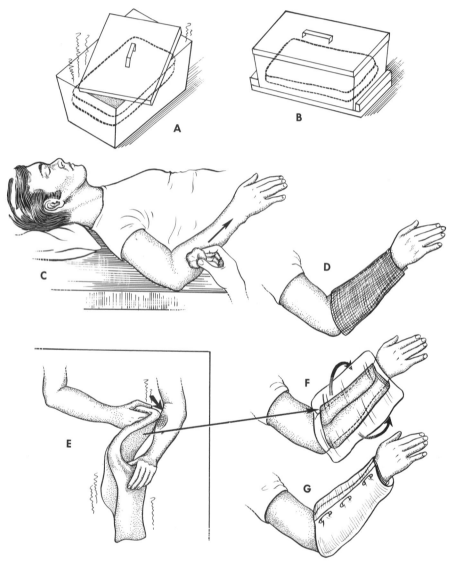

Fig. 12-6. Hot packs, autoclave method. **A,** Moist hot packs are placed in a metal container preparatory to heating. **B,** Method of transporting a metal container containing hot packs. **C,** Unless contraindicated, the nurse applies a thin coat of mineral oil to protect the skin. **D,** A layer or two of gauze placed over the area to be treated increases protection. **E,** The temperature of the hot pack is tested on the wrist or forearm or with a thermometer. **F,** After the hot pack is applied, it is covered with moistureproof material. **G,** Additional material covering the pack helps retain the heat.

registers 15 pounds, she removes the container. Otherwise, the wool fibers become very hard, changing the texture, odor, and heat retention of the material. The cover is placed on the container while it is carried to the nursing care center (Fig. 12-6, *B*). For this purpose, it is convenient to use a heavy board, constructed to prevent the container from slipping during transport.

Unless a wound is present or the hot packs are being applied to distend the veins for venipuncture, a thin coat of mineral oil is used to protect the skin (Fig. 12-6, *C*). A layer or two of gauze is placed over the area for the same purpose (Fig. 12-6, *D*). In the presence of a wound, a dry, sterile dressing is placed over the wound, and the surrounding skin is treated with oil and gauze. A sheet of plastic is placed over the wound dressing to keep it dry, thus preventing contamination.

The nurse removes the wool material, which is likely to be very hot, from the container and exposes it to air as necessary to dissipate the excess heat. Its temperature may be tested with a thermometer or on the wrist or forearm (Fig. 12-6, *E*). If the latter method is used, the nurse applies the hot pack slowly enough to permit the patient to decide whether he finds this temperature comfortable. If he thinks the hot pack is too warm, it should be removed immediately.

After the hot pack is applied, it is covered with moisture-proof material (Fig. 12-6, *F*). Additional material covering the pack helps retain the heat (Fig. 12-6, *G*). If continuous application is ordered, the nurse should change the packs every 2 hours or more often.

Hot water method. To apply moist heat by the hot water method, the nurse heats wool material in a hot water bath or folds Turkish towels, moistens them with hot water, and wrings them out (Fig. 12-7, *A* to *C*). The nurse should protect her hands from excess heat by using a stupe wringer or by the way she folds and wrings the material. The temperature of the material prepared by this method is less than when the autoclave method is used. She therefore may not need to treat the skin with mineral oil and gauze before she applies the hot pack. Hot packs prepared by this method will need to be changed frequently, often every 30 to 60 minutes unless additional external heat is applied.

Use of oil is definitely contraindicated if the purpose of the hot packs is to distend the veins prior to venipuncture. When used for this purpose, the hot pack should extend well beyond the chosen site for venipuncture. Thus, if a vein in the forearm is to be used, the hot pack should enclose the entire forearm, the hand, and the elbow (Fig. 12-7, *D* to *G*).

The nurse may preshape compresses to fit a specific area.

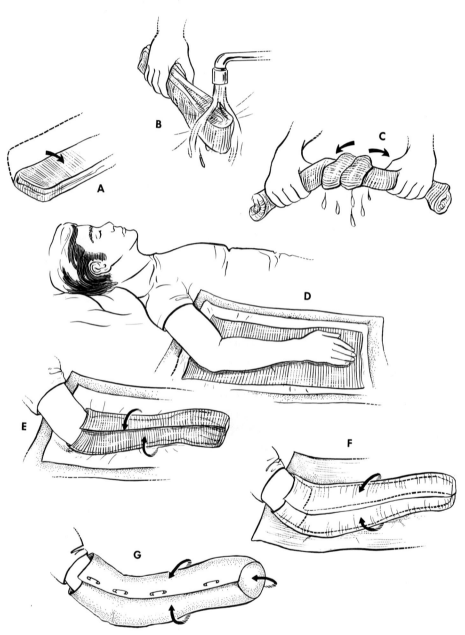

Fig. 12-7. Hot packs, hot water method. **A,** Method of folding a Turkish towel. **B,** Method of holding the towel during application of hot water. **C,** Method of wringing excess moisture from the towel. **D,** Area beneath the extremity protected with a Turkish towel and waterproof material. The hot pack is placed under the extremity. **E,** Hot pack wrapped around the extremity. **F,** Waterproof material wrapped around the hot pack. **G,** Dry Turkish towel used to stabilize the pack and to retain heat.

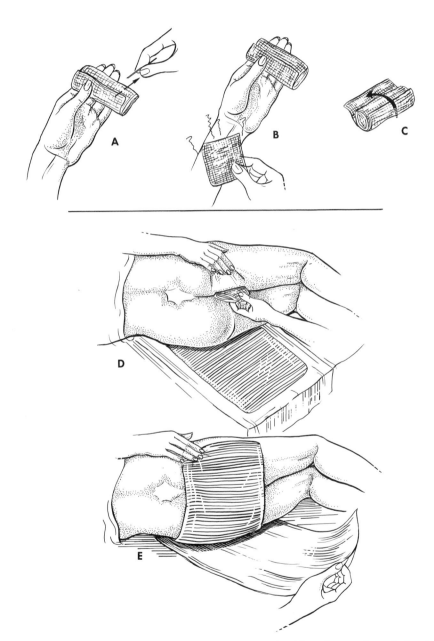

Fig. 12-8. Hot packs, preshaped for the anal area. **A,** After the preshaped dressing is heated, its fastener is removed. **B,** The outer dressing is removed to test its temperature. **C,** The cooled outer dressing is replaced around the heat-retaining core. **D,** The patient retracts his upper buttock during placement of the dressing. **E,** After a hyperthermia blanket or a special heating pad is in place, a large towel is used to maintain its position.

For example, she might shape hot packs applied to the anal area into a small roll. If the dressing is to be clean, rather than sterile, a 4-inch by 4-inch dressing can be rolled and then enclosed within another dressing. This permits the nurse to remove the outside dressing when she tests the temperature, while the inner dressing acts as a heat-retaining core. The outer dressing is cooled as necessary, then replaced about the core, and applied to the wound. After a hyperthermia blanket or a special heating pad is in place, a large towel is used to maintain its position (Fig. 12-8).

Warm, moist, sterile compresses

It is usual to apply these compresses four times a day. The schedule chosen should not interfere with the patient's rest. This, of course, requires knowledge of his rest and sleep patterns. After a specified length of time, often an hour, the compresses are removed and dry sterile dressings are applied. The exact method of preparing the compresses varies with the area to which they are to be applied and the available equipment.

Method 1. Prepared packs of cotton-filled 4-inch by 8-inch dressings are satisfactory for treating incisions. They are prepared by enclosing four dressings within a fifth dressing (Fig. 12-9, *A*). The number of packs needed varies with each incision. Thus, two to three packs might be needed to treat some abdominal incisions.

The nurse moistens the packs, wrings them as dry as possible, fluffs them, and arranges them in a dressing kettle (Fig. 12-9, *B* to *E*). She should place the folded edges of the packs so that they can be grasped securely with transfer forceps. The lid of the kettle should contain an opening for the forceps so that they are sterilized with the dressings. These are autoclaved for 15 minutes at 250° F.

The nurse tests the temperature of the compresses with a thermometer if the patient has diabetes or a vascular condition. In these cases, the temperature should never exceed 105° F. In all instances, the nurse should apply the dressing slowly, until it is known that the patient tolerates the temperature satisfactorily (Fig. 12-9, *F*). Applying the first pack so that it initially touches tissue distal to the incision permits temporary removal, if necessary, until it has cooled sufficiently. If this is done carefully, contamination can be avoided.

The nurse covers the moist compresses with dry, sterile dressings, moistureproof material, and additional reinforcement dressings (Fig. 12-9, *G* to *I*). The method of securing these dressings varies. An abdominal binder or tie tapes may be used when an abdominal incision is involved.

Method 2. A less desirable method involves sterilizing the

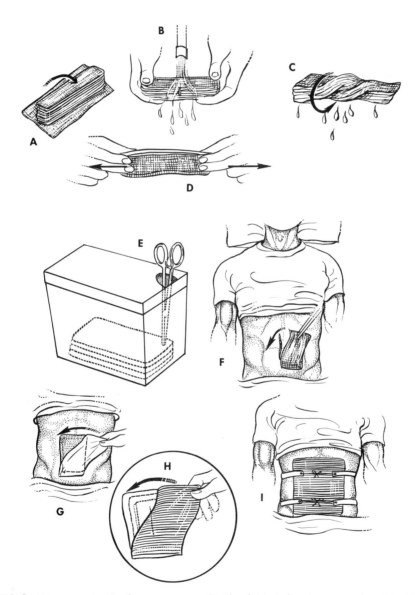

Fig. 12-9. Warm, moist sterile compresses. **A,** The folded dressings are placed inside the open dressing, thus forming a pack of dressings. **B,** The dressing pack is moistened. **C,** Excess moisture is removed. **D,** Method of fluffing the pack. **E,** Packs are placed in a kettle with dressing forceps for autoclaving. **F,** The dressing is applied slowly until it is certain that the patient tolerates its temperature. **G,** Additional dry sterile dressings cover the moist dressings. **H,** The dry dressings are covered with moistureproof material. **I,** Reinforcement dressings are applied and stabilized with Montgomery straps or an abdominal binder.

dressings by boiling or steaming them for 15 minutes. Maintenance of sterility by this method requires considerable effort and skill. The nurse uses sterile forceps to wring the moisture from the dressings and to fluff and apply them.

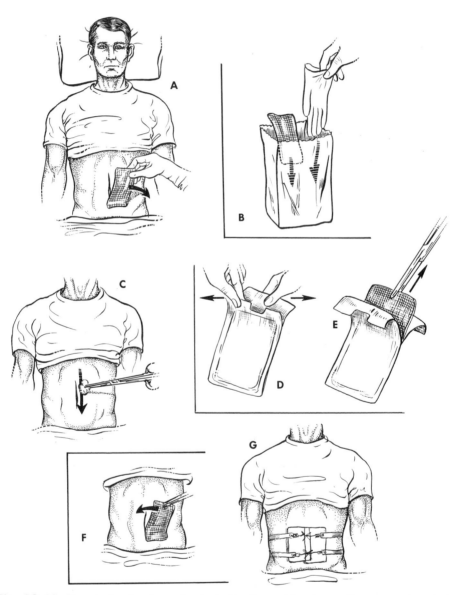

Fig. 12-10. Dry sterile dressings. **A,** A sterile disposable glove offers protection during removal of contaminated dressing. **B,** The soiled dressing and the glove are discarded. **C,** The wound is cleansed, if necessary, with sterile materials. **D,** Method of opening an individually packaged dressing. **E,** The dressing is removed from the wrapper with sterile forceps. **F,** A dressing being applied with sterile forceps. **G,** Completed dressing.

Hyperthermia pads

The nurse may apply external heat by using hyperthermia pads. These are available in various sizes. With the exception that the solution circulated within the pad is heated, these appear similar to hypothermia blankets. The nurse sets the temperature of the thermostat, often at 110° F., and allows the pad to heat for a specified time prior to application. The manufacturer's instructions should be consulted for details of operation.

The nurse applies the blanket to the specified area and secures it with ties incorporated into the design. It may be wrapped with a Turkish towel secured with strips of bandage. The purpose of the application will determine if the skin is to be enclosed in dry or moist material before applying the pad.

Dry sterile dressings

Dry sterile dressings serve to protect wounds from contamination and to absorb drainage. Selection of the type, thickness, size, and absorbency of dressings will be influenced by the nature of the wound, its anatomic location, and the amount and kind of drainage present.

The nurse should obtain the physician's approval before these dressings are changed. Often they may not be disturbed unless evidence of excess drainage or hemorrhage occurs. Even then, the nurse may be asked to reinforce, rather than change, the dressings. For this it may be permissible to replace the upper layers of a large dressing. The urgency of transmitting information concerning the quantity and kind of drainage present will differ with each situation.

Some physicians prefer to do the initial dressing change. Should this procedure be delegated to the nurse, she needs to know if drains are present and to avoid disturbing their placement, for they may adhere to the dressing.

It is imperative to maintain the sterility of the dressing by using sterile forceps or gloves (Fig. 12-10). It is also possible to maintain sterility through careful manipulation of the wrapper if dressings are packaged individually. Wearing a gown and mask to prevent contamination of the wound is recommended.

Questions for discussion and exploration

1. Presence of which conditions would indicate either heat or cold need to be applied with additional caution?
2. With what symptoms is the use of hot water bottles or other forms of local heat contraindicated?
3. What nursing observations indicate that the skin is reacting adversely to (a) heat? (b) cold?
4. For what conditions or symptoms would you expect hypothermia to be used?
5. What explanations should be given to the family and the patient when hypothermia is ordered?
6. When the patient is treated with hypothermia, he may begin to shiver. What is the cause, result, and treatment of shivering?

7. What must be done to prevent the skin from breaking down when hypothermia is used for a prolonged period of time?
8. Hypothermia blankets may lower the temperature of the patient within an hour or two. If the temperature of the patient drops profoundly within a 15-minute period, what would you check and why?
9. Why do some authorities recommend that the patient be placed directly in contact with the blanket instead of placing a sheet between the patient and the blanket? What modifications must be made in the care of the patient if the blanket is placed in direct contact with the patient?
10. What is meant by regional hypothermia? What are some examples of how hypothermia is applied regionally?
11. How might hypothermia be used to combat gastrointestinal bleeding?
12. Think through a plan for changing sterile dressings. The plan should include (a) nursing approach to the patient, (b) anticipation of supplies needed, (c) placement of supplies for your convenience but protecting them from contamination, (d) direction of removing dressing, (e) observations of drainage and wound, (f) how to learn if drains are present, (g) how to manage dressing that is adhering to drains or dressing or both, and (h) the advisability of gowning and masking.
13. Although you've just changed the dressings, an undesirable odor persists and is noticeable. What are some of the possible origins of the odor and what nursing action would be indicated?
14. If the tie tapes holding the dressing in place need to be changed, how can you remove the old ones with minimum trauma to the patient? Where should clean tie tapes be applied in relation to the sites from which the old ones were removed? How would you apply the tie tapes to prevent placing any of the tissues under pressure?

Selected references

Fernandez, J. P., and others: Rapid active rewarming in accidental hypothermia, J.A.M.A. **212**:153-156, 1970.

Hickey, M. C.: Hypothermia, Amer. J. Nurs. **65**:116-122, 1965.

Isler, C.: Hypothermia in action, RN **25**:36-47, 1962.

Larson, C. B., and Gould, M.: Orthopedic nursing, ed. 7, St. Louis, 1970, The C. V. Mosby Co.

Michenfelder, J., Terry, H., Daw, E., and Uehlein, A.: Induced hypothermia: physiologic effects, indications, and techniques, Surg. Clin. N. Amer. **45**:889-897, 1965.

Nugent, G. R.: Prolonged hypothermia, Amer. J. Nurs. **60**:967-969, 1960.

Saunders, W. H., Havener, W. H., Fair, C. J., and Hickey, J. T.: Nursing care in eye, ear, nose, and throat disorders, ed. 2, St. Louis, 1968, The C. V. Mosby Co.

Seldon, N. S.: Sterile warm wet compresses, Amer. J. Nurs. **59**:982-984, 1959.

Shafer, K. N., Sawyer, J. R., McCluskey, A. M., and Phipps, W. H.: Medical-surgical nursing, ed. 5, St. Louis, 1971, The C. V. Mosby Co.

Sheridan, B. A.: After hemorrhoidectomy; postoperative nursing care, Amer. J. Nurs. **63**:90-91, 1963.

Suddarth, D. S.: Individual dressing packs, Amer. J. Nurs. **60**:991-992, 1960.

Williams, M. E.: Chilled water mattress, Amer. J. Nurs. **70**:2377, 1970.

Glossary

Listed at the left are the symbols used in this glossary to indicate pronunciation. Listed at the right are common words using the sounds, which are indicated by boldface letters.

ă	h**a**t
ā	h**ay**
âr	p**are**
ä	f**a**ther
b	**b**id
ch	**ch**ild
d	**d**id, wille**d**
ĕ	w**e**t
ē	s**ee**
f	**f**ine, **ph**ase
g	**g**et
h	**h**it
hw	**wh**at
ĭ	s**i**t
ī	l**ie**, b**y**
îr	p**ier**
j	**j**ump, fu**dge**
k	**k**ick, **c**ot, pi**que**
l	**l**id
m	**m**ore
n	**n**ot
ng	si**ng**
ŏ	l**o**t, t**o**rrid
ō	w**oe**, s**oar**
ô	c**augh**t, l**aw**, f**or**
oi	n**oi**se
ŏŏ	l**oo**k
ōō	t**oo**t
ou	sn**ou**t
p	**p**ot
r	**r**ear
s	**s**ister
sh	**sh**op, da**sh**
t	**t**op, rap**p**ed

th	thick
th	that
ū	mute
ŭ	nut
ûr	urgent, stern, firm, heard, word
v	vane
w	wish
y	yoke
z	zenith, xylophone
zh	leisure, garage, visual
ə	around, item, circus, edible, gallop
ər	bitter

A *abdominal* (ăb-dŏm′ə-nəl) area of the body between the diaphragm and the pelvis

abduction (ăb-dŭk′shən) drawing away from the midline of the body

abrasion (ə-brā′zhən) injury produced by scraping away some skin or mucous membrane

activity (ăk-tĭv′ə-tē) motion; optimum activity refers to most favorable amount

adaptor (ə-dăp′tər) device used to join one part of equipment to another

adduction (ə-dŭk′shən) drawing toward the midline

adjacent (ə-jā′sənt) adjoining; next to

administer (ăd-mĭn′ĭs-tər) to give

aerosol (âr′ə-sôl) mist; fine spray

air conditioning (âr′kən-dĭsh′ən-ing) treatment of air that controls its temperature, movement, moisture, and dust content

airtight (âr′tīt′) impermeable to air

airway (âr′wā′) passageway for ventilation; may be natural or artificial

alcohol (ăl′kə-hôl′) colorless, flammable, volatile, liquid; used as an antiseptic as a vehicle for medicine; an intoxicating beverage

alignment (ə-līn′mənt) bringing into line for correct arrangement or position

allergen (ăl′ər-jən) anything that induces a state of allergy

allergic (ə-lûr′jĭk) hypersensitive

allergy (ăl′ər-jē) abnormal sensitivity to a substance

alveoli (ăl-vē′ə-lī′) air cells formed by the terminal dilatation of air passages in lungs

ambulation (ăm′byə-lā-shən) act of walking

ampule (ăm′pyo͞ol) sealed glass container of sterile drug; usually intended for injection

anatomic (ăn′ə-tŏm′ĭk) pertaining to the anatomy

anchor (ăng′kər) to fasten

anesthetic (ăn′ĭs-thĕt′ĭk) drug that causes loss of sensation; general anesthetic produces loss of consciousness, also

anomaly (ə-nŏm′ə-lē) deviation from normal anatomy

anorexia (ăn′ə-rĕk′sē-ə) loss of appetite

antacid (ănt-ăs′ĭd) counteracts acidity

antecubital (ăn′tĭ-kyo͞o′bĭ-təl) in front of the forearm

antihistamine (ăn′tĭ-hĭs′tə-mēn′) drug that acts against histamines

antiseptic (ăn′tə-sĕp′tĭk) drug or agent that arrests or prevents growth of microorganisms

appliance (ə-plī′əns) device designed for a particular use

apply (ə-plī′) to put on; to lay on

arrest (ə-rĕst′) to stop completely

arterial (är-tǐr′ē-əl) pertaining to the arteries; vessels through which the blood flows away from the heart

aspiration (ăs′pə-rā′shən) drawing into or out of, that is, drawing secretions into the lungs; suctioning secretions; withdrawal of secretions

astringent (ə-strǐn′jənt) medication that has the effect of limiting secretions by contracting and hardening tissues

atelectasis (ă-tə-lĕk′tə-sǔs) obstruction that prevents air from reaching a portion of the lung

auditory (ô′də-tôr′ē) pertaining to hearing

autoclave (ô′tō-klāv′) machine for sterilization under pressure

Aveeno (ə-vēē′nō) finely powdered oatmeal used for medicated baths

axilla (ăk-sǐl′ə) armpit

B   *baking soda* (bā′kǐng sō′də) bicarbonate of soda

balloon (bə-lōōn′) inflatable bag made of material impermeable to air or solution

Band-Aid (bănd′ād) trade name for small, commercially prepared, adhesive bandage with gauze dressing in the center

benzalkonium chloride (bĕn-zăl′kōn′ē-ŭm klôr′īd′) disinfectant; inactivated by presence of soap

bevel (bĕv′əl) slanted line but not at a right ˌangle; may refer to slanted portion at the end of a needle used for injection

bikini (bǐ-kē′nē) very brief swimsuit; refers to a cloth used to cover loin

bile (bīl) secretion of the liver; emulsifies fats during digestion

blister (blǐs′tər) saclike elevation of skin containing fluid

blot (blŏt) to touch gently; to dry with absorbent material by pressing gently

body mechanics (bŏd′ē mǐ-kăn′ǐks) concerned with the movements of the whole or parts of the body

bronchi (brŏng′kī) major branches leading from the trachea to the lungs

bronchitis (brŏng-kī′tǐs) inflammation of the trachea and bronchi

bronchogram (brŏng′kō-grăm) used for visualization and study of bronchi and bronchioli not accessible by bronchoscope; contrast medium injected and x-ray films taken

bronchographic (brŏng′ka-grăf′ĭk) pertains to examination of bronchi with x-ray and contrast medium

bubble suction (bŭb′əl sŭk′shən) *see* Suction

buccal (bŭk′əl) cheek; buccal cavity refers to area between the teeth and the cheek

burette (byōō-rĕt′) graduated device designed to measure fluid very accurately

buttocks (bŭt′əks) gluteal prominences

C   *calibration* (kăl′ə-brā′shən) marking that indicates a specific measurement of volume

canthus (kăn′thəs) corner of the eye; inner canthus refers to angle proximal to the nose; outer canthus refers to angle formed by eyelids at outside edge of the face

capillary (kăp′ə-lĕr′ē) very tiny blood vessel connecting artery and vein

cardiac massage (kär′dē-ăk mə-säzh′) rhythmically compressing and releasing the heart

cardiopulmonary (kär′dē-ō-pōōl′mə-nĕr′ē) pertaining to the heart and lungs

cardiotonic (kär′dē-ō-tŏn′ĭk) stimulating to the heart

cardiovascular (kär′dē-ō-văs′kyə-lər) pertaining to the heart and blood vessels

carminative (kär-mǐn′ə-tǐv) agent used to remove gases from the gastrointestinal tract

cast (kăst) moisturized materials that mold to body part and harden as drying occurs; used to immobilize parts in orthopedics

catheter (kăth′ə-tər) tube used to remove or instill fluids

catheterization (kăth′ə-tər-ī-zā′shən) insertion of a catheter

catheterize (kăth′ə-tə-rīz′) to insert a tube for removal or instillation of fluids; often used in reference to the urinary bladder

cellular response (sĕl′yə-lər rĭ-spŏns′) reaction of cells

cervix (sûr′vĭks) portion of uterus also known as the neck of the uterus

chemical (kĕm′ĭ-kəl) pertaining to the composition of substances

chest physical therapy (chĕst fĭz′ĭ-kəl thĕr′ə-pē) specialty that deals with medical prevention and treatment of diseases of the lungs

chill (chĭl) sensation of being very cold, accompanied by shivering

cilia (sĭl′ē-ə) tiny hairlike processes arising from the epithelial cells and possessing a waving or sweeping action

circular (sûr′kyə-lər) round; like a circle

circulation (sûr′kyə-lā′shən) movement in a recurrent fashion

clamp (klămp) to shut off; device used to press down and compress

clavicle (klăv′ĭ-kəl) collarbone

clean (klēn) free of soil

cleanse (klĕnz) to make clean

clinical response (klĭn′ĭ-kəl rĭ-spŏns′) reaction of the body to treatment

clitoris (klĭt′ə-rĭs) small organ of erectile tissue located behind the juncture of the labia minora

coagulation (kō-ăg′yə-lā′shən) change to a clot

colloid (kŏl′oid′) gelatinous; suspension of large particles in a solvent

colon (kō′lən) large intestine, specifically the portion from the cecum to the rectum

colostomy (kə-lŏs′tə-mē) surgically created artificial opening into the colon through the abdominal wall

compress (kəm-prĕs′) to press together; a dressing formed by several layers of material

compression (kəm-prĕsh′ən) act of pressing together

computation (kŏm′pyōō-tā′shən) method of determining an amount; mathematical

concentration (kŏn′sən-trā′shən) strength of a solution

conjunctiva (kŏn′jŭngt-tī′və) mucous membrane that lines eyelids and covers eyeball

conscious (kŏn′shəs) state of awareness

constrict (kən-strĭkt′) to squeeze, bind, tighten; to narrow the lumen as of vessels

contact (kŏn′tăkt′) to touch; exposure to an infectious disease

contaminant (kən-tăm′ə-nənt) anything that contaminates

contamination (kən-tăm′ə-nā′shən) impure state; may refer to act of rendering a sterile object unsterile

contiguous (kən-tĭg′yōō-əs) touching; neighboring

contour (kŏn′tōŏr) outline or boundary

contraindicated (kŏn′trə-ĭn′də-kāt′ĕd) treatment that is inappropriate due to adverse circumstances

costal (kŏs′təl) pertaining to the ribs

crepitation (krĕp′ə-tā′shən) crackling sound in tissues; grating sound of broken bones rubbing together

crevice (krĕv′ĭs) cleft, fissure, crack

crust (krŭst) hard covering, scab, eschar

cyanosis, cyanotic (sī′ə-nō′sĭs, sī′ə-nŏt′ĭk) bluish or grayish discoloration of skin due to insufficient oxygen

cycle (sī′kəl) a sequence that recurs at regular time intervals

D *Dakin's* (dā′kənz) a weak solution of sodium hypochlorite; used to cleanse wounds; a disinfectant

decompression (dē′kəm-prĕsh′ən) removal of pressure

decubiti (dĭ-kyōō′bĭ-tī) pressure sores

defecate (dĕf′ə-kāt′) evacuation of the bowels

deformity (dĭ-fôr′mĭ-tē) congenital or acquired disfigurement

dehiscence (dĭ-hĭs′ĕnz) breaking open a wound

deltoid (dĕl′toid′) triangular muscle originating at the shoulder *demarcation* (dē′mär-kā′shən) boundary; point of reference

denuded (dĭ-nōōd′ĕd) condition in which protective covering or layer such as the skin has been removed

dependent (dĭ-pĕn′dənt) hanging down; needing support

depilatory (dĭ-pĭl′ə-tôr′ē) agent used to remove hair

depression (dĭ-prĕsh′ən) area that is lower than the surface

dermatology (dûr′mə-tŏl′ə-jē) science of the skin and its diseases

deviation (dē′vē-ā′shən) departure from normal

diaphragm (dī′ə-frăm) anatomic structure that separates thorax from abdomen

diarrhea (dī′ə-rē′ə) frequent, liquid bowel movements

digital (dĭj′ə-təl) pertaining to the fingers

dilute (dĭ-lōōt′) to weaken as by adding water

disposable (dĭs-pō′zə-bəl) intended to be discarded after use

disruption (dĭs-rŭp′shən) separation or breaking apart

dissipate (dĭs′ə-pāt′) to scatter; to exhaust

distention (dĭs-tĕn′shən) to inflate; to stretch out

distill (dĭs-tĭl′) process of purifying water by vaporizing it and then condensing it

dorsal-recumbent (dôr′səl rĭ-kŭm′bənt) lying on one's back

douche (dōōsh) stream of solution directed against a part; often refers to cleansing vagina and vulva with a stream of solution

drain (drān) tube through which fluid escapes; to flow freely

drainage (drā′nĭj) fluids flowing from or being withdrawn from the body

dressing (drĕs′ĭng) protective covering for injured or diseased part

duodenum, duodenal (dōō′ə-dē′nəm, dōō′ə-dē′nəl) the part of the small intestine leading from the stomach to the jejunum

dysfunction (dĭs-fŭngk′shən) abnormal function or lack of function of an anatomic structure

dyspnea (dĭsp-nē′ə) labored or difficult breathing

E   *electrolyte* (ĭ-lĕk′trə-līt′) any substance that dissociates into ions when placed in solution; a solution that conducts electricity

elimination (ĭ-lĭm′ə-nā′shən) act of expelling; destruction

emollient (ĭ-mŏl′yənt) an agent that soothes and softens

enema (ĕn′ə-mə) solution injected into the rectum usually for the purpose of cleansing the rectum or the lower bowel or both

engorgement (ĕn-gôrj′mənt) distention or congestion

epigastric (ĕp′ĭ-găs′trĭk) over the abdomen; over the pit of the stomach

evaporation (ĭ-văp′ə-rā′shən) process of turning into vapor

exhale (ĕks-hāl′) to breathe out

extension (ĕk-stĕn′shən) anything that lengthens or stretches out

extremities (ĕk-strĕm′ə-tēs) the arms or legs

F   *fascia* (făsh′ē-ə) connective tissue that supports and separates muscles

fillers (fĭl′ərs) substances used to give bulk, absorbability, firmness, or other qualities to materials

filter (fĭl′tər) device that removes impurities; removal of impurities

flannel (flăn′əl) a soft fabric; often cotton but may be a blend of cotton and another fiber such as rayon

flare (flâr) to intensify; to spread; to increase in redness

flatus (flā′təs) an accumulation of gas in the digestive tract

flexion (flĕk′shən) bending as a joint of the body bends

fluctuation (flŭk′chōō-ā′shən) changing back and forth

fluoroscopic (flōōr′ə-skŏp′ĭc) type of examination using a screen to view shadows with the aid of x-rays

folliculitis (fə-lĭk′yə-līt′ĭs) inflammation of a follicle; hair follicle is an invagination of epidermis from which the hair develops

footboard (fōōt′bôrd′) upright device designed to support the feet

forceps (fôr′səps) instrument used for grasping and holding

Fowler's position (Fou'lər's) semisitting position

friable (frī'ə-bəl) easily broken or torn

G   *gag reflex* (găg rē'flĕks') act of retching that results from irritation of the fauces; may produce vomiting

gastrointestinal (găs'trō-ĭn-tĕs'tə-nəl) pertaining to the stomach and intestines

gastrostomy (găs-trŏs'tə-mē) surgically created opening that leads from the stomach through the abdominal wall; may be used for removal of secretions or for introducing tube for feeding

gauge (gāj) standard of measurement; used to indicate size of the diameter of a needle used for injection

gauze (gôz) a thin, loosely woven fabric

genitalia (jĕn'ə-tā'lē-ə) reproductive organs; usually refers to external sex organs

genitourinary tract (jĕn'ə-tō-yŏor'ə-nĕr'ē trăkt) reproductive and urinary systems

germicidal (jûr'mə-sīd'əl) agent that kills microorganisms

gloving (glŭv'ĭng) to put on gloves

gluteal area (glōō'tē-əl âr'ē-ə) the buttocks; specifically a portion of the upper outer quadrant

granulation (grăn'yə-lā'shən) small projections of tissue formed in healing process; usually observed when wound does not heal by first intention

gravitation (grăv'ə-tā'shən) tendency to move toward a particular point

gravity (grăv'ə-tē) possessing weight

green soap (grēn sōp) solution of soft soap in alcohol

groin (groin) depression or fold between the body and the thigh

gynecology (gī'nə-kŏl'ə-jē) study of the diseases of women

H   *hammock* (hăm'ək) specially designed cloth used to suspend the body in a lying position

harness (här'nĭs) a combination of straps; may be used to support the patient in a particular position

heat (hēt) degree of temperature; warmth

hematoma (hē'mə-tō'mə) tumor filled with blood

hemoptysis (hĭ-mŏp'tə-sĭs) expectoration of blood or bloody mucus from the level of the larynx or below

hemorrhage (hĕm'ə-rĭj) abnormal discharge of blood from the body; loss of large amount of blood

hepatitis (hĕp'ə-tī'tĭs) inflammation of the liver; may be caused by pathogens or toxins such as certain drugs to which the patient is sensitive

hernia (hûr'nē-ə) protrusion of an organ or its part through the wall of the cavity that normally contains it

humidifier (hyōō-mĭd'ə-fī'ər) device used to increase moisture content of inhaled gases

hydraulic (hī-drô'lĭk) operated by fluid pressure

hyperextend (hī'pər-ĭk'stənd) to stretch out as far as possible

hypotension (hī'pō-tĕn'shən) decrease in blood pressure to a level below the normal range

hypothermia (hī'pō-thûr'mĭ-ə) cooling; method of lowering the temperature of the body; may use a machine that circulates a coolant

I   *identification card* (ī-dĕn'tə-fĭ-kā'shən kärd) small cardboard on which is printed specific information; used to identify single dose of drug and the patient for whom it is intended

idiosyncrasy (ĭd'ē-ō-sĭng'krə-sē) characteristic or reaction peculiar to an individual

iliac crest (ĭl'ē-ək' krĕst) upper margin of the hipbone

immerse (ĭ-mûrs') to place under water or another solution

immobilization (ĭm-mō'bə-lī-zā'shən) fixation in an immovable position *impaction* (ĭm-păk'shən) pressing together tightly; fecal impaction refers to a hard mass of stool packed tightly and wedged; manual removal may be necessary

incision (ĭn-sĭzh'ən) cut made with a knife for surgical purposes

incontinent (ĭn-kŏn'tə-nənt) unable to retain urine or feces voluntarily

indwelling (ĭn-dwĕl'ĭng) to remain in place for an extended period of time

infection (ĭn-fĕk'shən) diseased state due to pathogenic organisms

infiltration (ĭn'fĭl-trā'shən) passing of liquid or gas substance into or through tissue

inflammation (ĭn'flə-mā'shən) a defensive reaction of the tissue to injury; characterized by redness, swelling, heat, and pain

inflation (ĭn-flā'shən) distention with a liquid or gas

inframammary (ĭn'frə-măm'ər-ē) below the breast

infusion (ĭn-fyōo'zhən) injection of a sterile solution into a vein or tissue

inguinal (ĭng'gwə-nəl) in the groin; pertaining to the groin

inhale (ĭn-hāl') to breathe in

injection (ĭn-jĕk'shən) introduction of a liquid into a vessel, cavity, or tissue; sterile equipment and solution are usually used

inline (ĭn'līn) incorporated into the main line of flow

insomnia (ĭn-sŏm'nē-ə) inability to sleep

inspire (ĭn-spīr') to breathe in

instillation (ĭn'stə-lā'shən) slow injection; putting in drop by drop

insufficiency (ĭn'sə-fĭsh'ən-sē) a deficiency; not enough for its purpose

interdigital (ĭn'tər-dĭj'ə-təl) between the fingers; sometimes used to pertain to the area between the toes

intermittent (ĭn'tər-mĭt'ənt) stopping periodically

intertriginous (ĭn'tər-trĭj'ə-nəs) folds of skin; areas in which two surfaces of the skin touch each other

intestinal (ĭn-tĕs'tən-əl) the part of the alimentary tract distal to the stomach

intramuscular (ĭn'trə-mŭs'kyə-lər) into or within a muscle

intravenous (ĭn'trə-vē'nəs) within a vein; often pertains to an injection or infusion into a vein

intravesical (ĭn'trə-vĕs'ĭ-kəl) within the bladder

intubate (ĭn'tōo-bāt') to insert a tube into the larynx

IPPB intermittent positive pressure breathing, inspiratory; often refers to machines that assist or control ventilation

irreversible (ĭr'ĭ-vûr'sə-bəl) cannot be changed back to its former state

irrigate (ĭr'ĭ-gāt') to wash out with a flow of solution

irritation (ĭr'ə-tā'shən) anything that stimulates an adverse reaction

isolation (ī'sə-lā'shən) separation from others; used to prevent transmission of organisms from one person to another

K   *knee-chest* (nē'chĕst') position in which patient rests his weight on his knees and chest; head is supported by his forearms

L   *labia* (lā'bē-ə) folds of tissue surrounding the orifice of the vulva

larynx (lăr'ĭngks) voice box

Lassar's paste (Lăs'ărz pāst) thick preparation of zinc oxide

lateral (lăt'ər-əl) on the side; may refer to side-lying position

leverage (lĕv'ər-ĭj) mechanical advantage

Levin tube (Lĕv'ən tōob) straight tube used to decompress the stomach or to introduce food into it

lint (lĭnt) bits of thread

liter (lē'tər) a unit of measure

lithotomy (lĭ-thŏt'ə-mē) also called dorsosacral; position in which patient lies on back with thighs flexed toward abdomen and legs abducted but at a right angle to the thighs

lotion (lō'shən) liquid preparation containing medicine patted onto the skin

lozenge (lŏz'ĭnj) small, flat, discoid preparation containing medicine intended to be held in the mouth until it dissolves

lubricate (lōo'brĭ-kāt') to make slippery

lumbar (lŭm′bər) part of the body on either side of the spinal column; between the ribs and the hip

M **maceration** (măs′ər-ā′shən) process that softens tissue

macroscopic (măk′rə-skŏp′ĭk) visible with the naked eye

malignancy (mə-lĭg′nən-sē) tendency to spread and produce death

manipulate (mə-nĭp′yə-lāt′) to handle with a degree of skill

mastication (măs′tə-kā′shən) act of chewing

meatus (mē-ā′təs) opening

mechanical (mĭ-kăn′ĭ-kəl) pertaining to machinery

medication (mĕd′ə-kā′shən) drug used to prevent or treat illness; application of a drug

medication card (mĕd′ə-kā′shən kärd) *see* Identification card

meniscus (mə-nĭs′kəs) curvature on upper surface of fluid; caused by fluid clinging to the sides of the container

microbe (mī′krōb′) organism too small to be seen with the naked eye

microorganism (mī′krō-ôr′gən-ĭz′əm) tiny plant or animal that cannot be seen without magnification

micturition (mĭk′chə-rĭsh′ən) voiding of urine; urination

midanterior (mĭd′ăn-tĭr′ē-ər) midpoint and front

midstream (mĭd′strēm′) middle of the flow; neither at the beginning nor at the end

milk (mĭlk) pertains to milking a chest tube; to alternately apply and release pressure on the tube by squeezing it with the hand

milliliter (mĭl′lə-lē′tər) unit of metric measure; equivalent to a cubic centimeter

moisture (mois′chər) water

mottled (mŏt′tləd) patterned with irregular discolorations or blotches

mucosa (myōō-kō′sə) mucous membrane

musculoskeletal (mŭs′kyə-lō-skĕl′ə-təl) pertaining to the muscles and skeleton

myocardium (mī′ō-kär′dē-əm) muscle of the heart

N **narcotic** (när-kŏt′ĭk) drug with addicting properties that also depresses the central nervous system

nasogastric (nā′zō-găs′trĭk) pertaining to the nose and stomach

nebulization (nĕb′yə-lĭ-zā′shən) act of breaking a liquid into a fine spray; vaporization

negative pressure (nĕg′ə-tĭv prĕsh′ər) mechanical withdrawal of force

nephrectomy (nə-frĕk′tə-mē) removal of a kidney

neurosurgery (nōōr′ō-sûr′jər-ē) surgery on the nervous system

nostril (nŏs′trəl) external opening of the nose

nutrition (nōō-trĭsh′ən) food; process of converting food into tissue

O **obstruction** (əb-strŭk′shən) blockage of a passageway; prevents normal functioning

occlusive (ə-klōō′sĭv) tending to shut in moisture or heat, often applied to dressings used for this purpose

ointment (oint′mənt) semisolid preparation of medicine in a fatty base; applied externally by stroking

oral (ôr′əl) pertaining to the mouth

orifice (ôr′ə-fĭs) opening; an entrance or outlet

orogastric (ôr′ō-găs′trĭk) pertaining to the mouth and stomach

orthopedic (ôr′thə-pē′dĭk) locomotor structures of the body, their diseases and deformities

overdosage (ō′vər-dōs′ĭj) excessive amount or dose of medicine

oxygen (ŏk′sĭ-jən) colorless, odorless gas necessary for life; supports combustion but does not burn

P **palate** (păl′ĭt) roof of the mouth

pallor (păl′ər) unnatural paleness

paralyzed (păr'ə-līz'd) unable to move because of loss of motor and sensory function

patency (pāt'n-sē) state of being open; not obstructed

pathogen (păth'ə-jən) organism capable of producing disease

pathophysiologic (păth'ə-fĭz'ē-ə-lŏj'ĭk) study of disease state as it is related to normal functioning of the body

pelvic (pĕl'vĭk) pertaining to the area of the body formed by the innominate bones, the pubis, the sacrum, the coccyx, and the ligaments uniting them

percussion (pər-kŭsh'ən) tapping or striking a part of the body to diagnose or treat

perineum (pĕr'ə-nē'əm) area between the vulva or the scrotum and the anus; sometimes includes the vulva

peripheral (pə-rĭf'ər-əl) near the outside

pharynx (făr'ĭngks) anatomic area between the oronasal passages and the esophagus

physical therapist (fĭz'ĭ-kəl thĕr'ə-pĭst) person trained to treat with physical and mechanical means

physiologic (fĭz'ē-ə-lŏj'ĭk) related to normal body functioning

pivot (pĭv'ət) to turn or rotate

pledget (plĕj'ət) a small mass of cotton or rayon fibers

pleural cavity (plŏŏr'əl kăv'ə-tē) space between the two layers of membrane that enclose the lungs

ply (plī) thickness

pneumothorax (nŏŏ'mō-thôr'ăks') air in the pleural cavity; causes collapse of the lung

popliteal (pŏp'lĭ-tē'əl) behind the knee

positioning (pə-zĭsh'ən-ĭng) manner of arranging the body

posterior (pŏ-stîr'ē-ər) caudal end of the body, dorsal side or back

postural drainage (pŏs'chər-əl drā'nĭj) positioning of patient that promotes drainage of secretions from the lungs and bronchi

precaution (prĭ-kô'shən) to guard against

precipitation (prĭ-sĭp'ə-tā'shən) separation of solid from liquid by allowing or causing it to settle out

pregnancy (prĕg'nən-sē) period of time during which a developing fetus is present within the uterus

pressure, direct (prĕsh'ər, dĭ-rĕkt') compression or force exerted on a part

probe (prōb) instrument inserted into a body cavity

profound (prə-found') extreme or intense, as profound cooling

prostatic fluid (prō-stăt'ĭk) secretion produced by the prostate gland.

prosthesis (prŏs-thē'sĭs) an artificial part used to replace a missing part or to correct a defect

pruritus (prŏŏ-rī'təs) itching

psoriasis (sə-rī'ə-sĭs) a chronic skin disease identified by characteristic lesions

pulmonary (pŏŏl'mə-nĕr'ē) pertaining to the lungs

pylorus (pī-lôr'əs) opening from the stomach into the duodenum

R *radiopaque* (rā'dē-ō-pāk') property of not being penetrated by x-ray; visible with x-ray

radius (rā'dē-əs) outer bone of the lower arm

range of motion (rānj ŭv mō'shən) extent to which the body part can be moved

rectal (rĕk'təl) pertaining to the lower part of the rectum; between the sigmoid flexure and the anus

recumbent (rĭ-kŭm'bənt) lying down; *see also* Dorsal-recumbent

reducing sock (rĭ-dŏŏs'ing sŏk) device made of stockinette and used to cover stump following amputation

regurgitation (rē-gûr'jə-tā'shən) return of stomach contents to the mouth; may refer to backflow of blood

resection (rĭ-sĕk'shən) excision of part of a body structure *reservoir* (rĕz'ər-vwär') collecting or storage container for fluids

residual (rĭ-zĭj'ōō-əl) quantity remaining or left over

respiration (rĕs'pə-rā'shən) act of breathing

respirator (rĕs'pə-rā'tər) machine, such as the IPPB machine, used for artificial breathing or used to assist respiration

restrain, restraint (rĭ-strān', rĭ-strănt') to hinder or restrict action; ·device or method used to prevent patient from injuring himself

resuscitation (rĭ-sŭs'ə-tā'shən) bringing back to life

resuscitator (rĭ-sŭs'ə-tā'ter) person who resuscitates or machine used

retract (rĭ-trăkt') to draw back or curl away

reverse isolation (rĭ-vûrs' ī'sə-lā'shən) special precautions or methods used to protect patient whose resistance to microorganisms is low; *see also* Isolation

rinsing (rĭns'ing) washing lightly with water or another liquid

S   *salivary* (săl'ə-vĕr'ē) glands that discharge secretions into the mouth

scale (skāl) thin, flat, hard, flakelike materials on the skin that resemble the scales on a fish

scalp (skălp) integument of head containing hair

scapula (skăp'yə-lə) shoulder blade

scrub (skrŭb) to cleanse the hands as thoroughly as possible; surgical scrub includes the forearms

sebaceous (sĭ-bā'shəs) pertaining to fat; pertains to glands in the skin that secrete oil

secretion (sĭ-krē'shən) product produced by glands; a fluid

sedative (sĕd'ə-tĭv) a drug that calms; the effect of lowering activity

sediment (sĕd'ə-mənt) residual matter that settles out of a liquid

sensitivity (sĕn'sə-tĭv'ə-tē) state of being affected readily by outside influences

septum (sĕp'təm) partition between two body cavities

shampoo (shăm-poo') washing the hair; may include gentle massage of the scalp

shivering (shĭv'ər-əng) to shake from cold; a physiologic reaction that tends to increase body temperature

shock (shŏk) state of collapse resulting from circulatory failure; known to be precipitated by many causes; recognized by many signs and symptoms

shoulder blade (shōl'dər blād) scapula

sidearm (sīd'ärm) extension of, but to one side of, an apparatus

sigh (sī) periodic deep inspiration

silicone (sĭl'ĭ-kōn') chemical that provides lubrication; gel is a semisolid form

Sims' position (Sĭms' pə-zĭsh'ən) patient lying on side with upper leg, flexed forward and toward abdomen

single dose (sĭng'gəl dōs) amount of medicine to be administered at one time; used to refer to units prepared and packaged by manufacturer or by a pharmacist

siphon (sī'fən) to remove liquids with the aid of a tube and atmospheric pressure

sitz bath (sĭts băth) bath that patient sits in for designated period of time; water usually covers the hips

skate (skāt) device attached to foot for purpose of exercising leg

sling (slĭng) device used to support an injured extremity; used on some mechanical lifts to aid in transferring patient

solution (sə-lōō'shən) homogenous mixture of gas, liquid, or solid in one of the former; parts cannot be separated by ordinary means

Soyaloid (soi'ə-loyd') commercial product prepared from soybeans and used in the treatment of selected skin diseases

spasm (spăz'əm) a muscular contraction that is sudden and involuntary

specimen (spĕs'ə-mən) a part intended to be representative of the whole, such as a specimen of urine

sphincter (sfĭngk'tər) band of muscle that encircles a body orifice; its relaxation and constriction are voluntary or involuntary depending on its function

sphygmomanometer (sfĭg′mō-mə-nŏm′ə-tər) device used to measure arterial blood pressure

splint (splĭnt) any of a number of devices used to immobilize a body part

sponge (spŭnj) absorbent material used to remove fluids

spontaneous (spŏn-tā′nē-əs) unaided

sterile (stĕr′əl) free of living organisms; unfertile

sterilization (stĕr′ə-lə-zā′shən) act of making sterile

stertorous (stûr′tər-ŭs) breathing characterized by snoring sounds

stethoscope (stĕth′ə-skōp′) instrument used to hear sounds within the body

stimulus (stĭm′yə-ləs) anything that causes part or all of organism to react with activity

stockinet, stockinette (stŏk′ə-nĕt′) machine-knitted fabric; used to line orthopedic casts

stoma (stō′mə) opening, either artificial or a small natural opening

stopcock (stŏp′kŏk′) a special valve used to control flow of fluid from a reservoir

strip (strĭp) referring to chest tubes: to remove contents from the tube with a simultaneous stroking and compressing motion

stump (stŭmp) part of an extremity or organ remaining following amputation

stylet (stī′lĭt) a slender piece of rigid material inserted through a catheter, needle, or cannula to make it rigid or to block its opening; may be solid or hollow

subcutaneous (sŭb′kyōō-tā′nē-əs) lying directly under the skin

sublingual (sŭb′lĭng′gwəl) beneath the tongue

suction (sŭk′shən) removal of gases or liquids by reducing the atmospheric pressure

suffocation (sŭf′ə-kā′shən) asphyxiation; effective ventilation is decreased appreciably or stopped; results in death if untreated

sump drain (sŭmp drān) tube used to remove accumulated secretions from deep body cavities; usually attached to suction machine for this purpose

superficial (soo′pər-fĭsh′əl) near the top; without depth

surgery (sûr′jə-rē) medical specialty that treats and diagnoses with operative procedures; area in which operative procedures are done

swallow (swä′lō) to move food from mouth to stomach without the aid of tubes or other devices

symphysis pubis (sĭm′fə-sĭs pyōō′bĭs) anterior point at which pubic bones join

syringe (sə-rĭnj′) instrument used to instill or inject solutions into cavities, vessels, or tissues; sometimes attached to a needle for injection

systemic (sĭ-stĕm′ĭk) pertaining to the whole body or one of its organs

T *temperature* (tĕm′pər-ə-chōōr′) degree of warmth or coldness

temporary (tĕm′pə-rĕr′ē) for a period of time; not permanent

tepid (tĕp′ĭd) lukewarm

termination (tûr′mə-nā′shən) bringing to an end or close, as termination of an infusion

therapeutic (thĕr′ə-pyōō′tĭk) treatment of an illness; possessing healing properties

therapy (thĕr′ə-pē) treatment of an illness

thermal (thûr′məl) pertaining to heat

thermostatic (thûr′mə-stăt′ĭk) regulation of temperature automatically

thigh (thī) part of leg between the knee and the hip joint

thrombophlebitis (thrŏm′bō-flĭ-bī′tĭs) clot accompanied by inflammation of the affected vein

thyroid (thī′roid) a ductless gland lying on either side of the upper part of the trachea and the lower part of the larynx

tidal drainage (tīd′l drān′ĭj) automatic irrigation of the urinary bladder characterized by periodic rising and falling of the level of fluid in a tube

tidal volume (tĭd'l vŏl'yo͝om) amount of air moved into and out of the respiratory system

topical (tŏp'ĭ-kəl) the surface of the body; a definite area

tourniquet (to͝or'nĭ-kĭt) any device used to decrease bleeding by compressing blood vessels; encircles extremity and applies pressure

trachea (trā'kē-ə) the windpipe;. a tube-shaped anatomic structure leading from the larynx to the bronchi

tranquilizing (trăn'kwə-līz'ĭng) making calm; often refers to a group of drugs used to treat emotionally disturbed persons

transfusion (trăns-fyo͞o'zhən) injection of another person's blood; used less commonly to mean infusion of liquids other than blood

transmission (trăns-mĭsh'ən) act of transferring; applies to transfer of organisms from one person to another

transurethral (trăns'yo͞o-rē'thrəl) through the urethra; as a transurethral resection of the prostate gland

trauma (trou'mə) injury to the body

Trendelenburg (Trĕn-dĕl'ən-bûrg) dorsal-recumbent position with the head lower than the trunk of the body and the trunk lower than the legs; sometimes called the shock position

trial (trī'əl) a test, such as trying a medication; an experiment

trochanter roll (trō-kăn'tər rōl) roll of material placed against the hip to maintain its position and to prevent its outward rotation

trough (trôf) long, narrow receptacle used to channel direction of flow of fluids

trunk (trŭngk) torso of body, all of the body except the head, neck, and extremities

T *tube* (tē' to͞ob) connector shaped like the letter T; also refers to drains similar to the letter T

tube (to͞ob) long, hollow cylinder used to provide a passageway for liquids and gases

Turkish towel (Tûr'kĭsh tou'əl) thick cotton towel made with loops of fiber; very absorbent due to its long nap

twist (twĭst) to rotate, wind together, intertwine

U   *ulcerated* (ŭl'sə-rāt'əd) affected with an open lesion or lesions on the skin or on the mucous membrane; manifested by disintegration of tissues

ulna (ŭl'nə) long bone on inner aspect of forearm

ultraviolet (ŭl'trə-vī'ə-lĭt) invisible light rays; abbreviated U. V.

umbilicus (ŭm'bĭl'ĭ-kəs) navel; depression in midpoint of abdomen that indicates the place at which the umbilical cord was attached

unconscious (ŭn'kŏn'shəs) state in which one is not aware of himself

undine (ŭn-dēn') small device used to irrigate the eye

unilateral (yo͞o'nĭ-lăt'ər-əl) affecting one side only

unsterile (ŭn'stĕr'əl) not known to be free of organisms or other contaminants

urination (yo͝or'ə-nā'shən) act of discharging urine

urology (yo͞o-rŏl'ə-jē) science that deals with the urinary and genitourinary tracts

V   *vacuum* (văk'yo͞o-əm) space devoid of gases and other matter

vagina (və-jī'nə) musculomembranous, tubelike structure or passageway between the uterus and the vulva

vaporizer (vā'pə-rī'zər) device that converts water to steam or a mist

vastus lateralis (văs'təs lăt'ər-əl-ĭs) muscle in the thigh; extends the knee

venipuncture (vĕn'ə-pŭngk'chər) piercing of a vein with a needle, usually for the purpose of injecting fluid or medicine or to obtain a sample of blood

venous (vē'nəs) pertaining to the vein

venous outflow (vē'nəs out'flō) flowing out of the veins, away from the heart through the veins

venous pattern (vē'nəs păt'ərn) design or layout formed by the veins *venous pressure* (vē′nəs prĕsh′ər) pressure within the veins

venous return (vē′nəs rĭ-tûrn′) flowing back to the heart through the veins

ventilate (vĕnt′l-āt) to transport air to and from the alveolar surfaces

ventilation (vĕn′tə-lā′shən) act of ventilating

ventilator (vĕnt′l-ā′tər) machine or person who ventilates

ventrogluteal (vĕn′trō-glōō′tē-əl) anterior portion of the gluteal muscle

vertebra (vûr′tə-brə) bony segment of the spinal column; pl., *-brae* or *-bras*

vial (vī′əl) sealed glass container for medicine

vibration (vī-brā′shən) shaking movement; to oscillate

viscosity (vĭs-kŏs′ə-tē) quality demonstrated by the resistance of a fluid to flow

viscous (vĭs′kəs) tending to adhere to a surface; to flow slowly or with resistance

vital signs (vī′təl sīns) usually refers to temperature, pulse, and respiration; commonly includes blood pressure also

vulva (vŭl′və) external female genitalia

vulvectomy (vŭl-vĕk′tă-mē) removal of external vulva surgically; radical vulvectomy includes removal of lymph nodes in groin

W *water-sealed drainage* (wô′tər sēl′d drā′-nĭj) drainage system in which the tube leading from the body to the drainage receptacle is under water; water seals the drainage tube and prevents gases from ascending through it

X *xiphoid process* (zĭf′oid′ prŏs′ĕs′) distal end of the sternum

Z *zephiran chloride* (zĕf′ĭ-rən klôr′īd′) same as benzalkonium chloride

z *track* (zē′ trăk) method of applying tension that displaces the subcutaneous tissue during insertion of a needle; refers to Z formed in overlying tissue when tension is applied; used to inject irritating drugs, especially those containing heavy metals; useful when drugs are to be injected into the gluteal area

Index